Understanding Developmental Disorders of Auditory Processing, Language and Literacy Across Languages

International Perspectives

A Volume in
Research on Sociocultural Influences on Motivation and Learning

Series Editor:
Dennis Michael McInerney, *The Hong Kong Institute of Education*

Research on Sociocultural Influences on Motivation and Learning

Dennis Michael McInerney, Series Editor

Volume 1: *Research on Sociocultural Influences on Motivation and Learning* (2001)
edited by Dennis M. McInerney and Shawn Van Etten

Volume 2: *Research on Sociocultural Influences on Motivation and Learning* (2002)
edited by Dennis M. McInerney and Shawn Van Etten

Volume 3: *Sociocultural Influences and Teacher Education Programs* (2003)
edited by Dennis M. McInerney and Shawn Van Etten

Volume 4: *Big Theories Revisited* (2004)
edited by Dennis M. McInerney and Shawn Van Etten

Volume 5: *Focus on Curriculum* (2005)
edited by Dennis M. McInerney and Shawn Van Etten

Volume 6: *Effective Schools* (2006)
edited by Dennis M. McInerney, Martin Dowson, and Shawn Van Etten

Volume 7: *Standards in Education* (2007)
edited by Dennis M. McInerney, Shawn Van Etten, and Martin Dowson

Volume 8: *Teaching and Learning: International Best Practice* (2008)
edited by Dennis M. McInerney and Gregory Arief Daranegara Liem

Volume 9: *Student Perspectives on Assessment: What Students Can Tell Us About Assessment for Learning* (2009)
edited by Dennis M. McInerney, Gavin T. L. Brown, and Gregory Arief D. Liem

Volume 10: *Sociocultural Theories of Learning and Motivation: Looking Back, Looking Forward* (2011)
edited by Dennis M. McInerney, Richard A. Walker, and Gregory Arief D. Liem

Volume 11: *Understanding Developmental Disorders of Auditory Processing, Language and Literacy Across Languages: International Perspectives* (2014)
edited by Kevin Kien Hoa Chung, Kevin Chi Pun Yuen, and Dennis Michael McInerney

Understanding Developmental Disorders of Auditory Processing, Language and Literacy Across Languages

International Perspectives

edited by

Kevin Kien Hoa Chung

Kevin Chi Pun Yuen

and

Dennis Michael McInerney

The Hong Kong Institute of Education

IAP

INFORMATION AGE PUBLISHING, INC.

Charlotte, NC • www.infoagepub.com

Library of Congress Cataloging-in-Publication Data

A CIP record for this book is available from the Library of Congress
http://www.loc.gov

ISBN: 978-1-62396-664-5 (Paperback)
978-1-62396-665-2 (Hardcover)
978-1-62396-666-9 (ebook)

Printed and bound by CPI Group (UK) Ltd, Croydon, CR0 4YY

CONTENTS

PREFACE

The Global Conference on Disorders in Auditory Processing, Literacy, Language and Related Sciences 2012 (APLL2012) was successfully hosted by the Department of Special Education and Counselling of the Hong Kong Institute of Education, January 4-7, 2012. APLL2012 attracted close to 300 registrations from Hong Kong, China, Singapore, Taiwan, the United States, the UK, Australia, India, Japan, Indonesia, and the Philippines.

APLL 2012 originated from conversations held among the organizing committee members of the conference that it is imperative to have more cross-disciplinary discussions on issues relating to auditory processing disorders, reading and writing disorders, language disorders, and other related disorders. From historical and professional practice perspectives, these disorders seem distinct from one another, but more recent research suggests that they in fact overlap in many ways, including clinical presentations, suspected underlying causes, diagnostic criteria, and re/habilitation strategies. By bringing together respective leaders in the fields, APLL2012 opened new windows to promote cross-disciplinary discussions and collaborations on ways that professionals can better service individuals with these closely related disorders and develop collaborative research in the future.

Presentations were delivered by an unprecedented number of world renowned keynote and invited speakers who are prominent scholars, scientists, and leading practitioners in their respective fields. We would like to show our great appreciation to these eminent speakers who formed the cadre of APLL2012.

Understanding Developmental Disorders of Auditory Processing, Language and Literacy Across Languages: International Perspectives, pp. vii–ix

Keynote Speakers (in alphabetical order)

Prof. Teri James Bellis, The University of South Dakota
Dr. Piers Dawes, The University of Manchester, UK

Prof. Usha Goswami, University of Cambridge, UK

Prof. Kenneth Hugdahl, University of Bergen, Norway

Prof. Nina Kraus, Northwestern University

Dr. Carol Miller, University of Pennsylvania

Prof. David Moore, Institute of Hearing Research, Medical Research Council, Nottingham, UK

Prof. Kenneth Pugh, University of Connecticut, Yale University, Haskins Laboratories, and The Yale Reading Center

Prof. Stuart Rosen, University College London, UK

Prof. Frank Vellutino, University at Albany, State University of New York

Invited Speakers (in alphabetical order)

Prof. Hin Tat Cheung, The Hong Kong Institute of Education
Dr. Fuk Chuen Ho, The Hong Kong Institute of Education

Dr. Catherine Lam Chi Chin, JP, Department of Health,
The Government of the Hong Kong Special Administrative Region

Dr. Dan Lin, The Government of the Hong Kong Special
Administrative Region Hong Kong Institute of Education

Dr. Jenny Loo, National University of Singapore

Prof. Catherine McBride-Chang, The Chinese University of
Hong Kong

Prof. Bradley McPherson, The University of Hong Kong

Dr. I-Fan Su, The University of Hong Kong

Dr. Shelley Xiuli Tong, The University of Hong Kong

Dr. Lena Wong, The University of Hong Kong

Their presentations were at the forefront of theorizing and research on the areas of auditory processing disorders, literacy disorders, language disorders, and other related disorders across different languages and cultures. Due to the huge success of APLL2012, to promote continuous discussions of the conference theme, the conference organizing committee decided to invite scholars, scientists, and practitioners to contribute their work to the 11th volume in the *Research on Sociocultural Influences on Motivation and Learning* research monograph series. This volume is focused on issues in typical and disordered developments in auditory processing, literacy, and language across different cultural and linguistic contexts in Asia, Europe, and North America. The contributors of this volume offer insightful theoretical and practical ideas to shape future directions in research, assessment, intervention, and education. This is an intriguing and inspiring volume for students, researchers, and practitioners in the fields of speech-language pathology, audiology, developmental psychology, educational psychology, neuropsychology, and other related disciplines.

We are very grateful to all the contributors and editorial board members for their unfailing support for making this publication project possible. We are also very thankful to the Department of Special Education and Counselling, the Hong Kong Institute of Education for the generous financial support for this project.

On behalf of all the contributors, we invite your reflections and comments to generate future dialogues on the fascinating research areas in disorders in auditory processing, literacy, language, and related sciences.

—Kevin K. H. Chung, Kevin C. P. Yuen, and Dennis M. McInerney,
The Hong Kong Institute of Education

ACKNOWLEDGMENTS

We wish to acknowledge the excellent contributions of all the authors. They have brought us one step forward to understand the normal and disordered developments in auditory processing, literacy, language, and related sciences. We sincerely thank the reviewers for their generous support of this project: Dr. Doris Bamiou, Dr. Chow Wing Yin Bonnie, Dr. Benjamin J. Lovett, Dr. Bradley McPherson, Dr. Wong Kwok Shing Richard, Dr. Wong Mei-Yin Anita and Dr. Patcy P. S. Yeung, and several anonymous reviewers. We are indebted to Mr. Edmond Lau, Ms. Vicki Fan Pui Hang, Ms. Silvia Kwok Sze Wai, and Ms. Julian Yip Wai Shan for their seamless and efficient administration on this project. It has been a wonderful experience to work with all the authors, reviewers, and administrative staff on this important and gratifying project.

—Kevin K. H. Chung, Kevin C. P. Yuen, and Dennis M. McInerney

Understanding Developmental Disorders of Auditory Processing, Language and Literacy Across Languages: International Perspectives, pp. xi–xi

CHAPTER 1

AUDITORY PROCESSING DISORDER IN CHILDREN AND ITS RELATION TO LANGUAGE AND LITERACY DISORDERS

David R. Moore

What is an auditory processing disorder? The children under assessment at APD clinics in the U.K. have usually been through two stages of referral (detailed as follows), but their presenting symptoms appear to be similar to those seen in other APD clinics across the world. Audiologists often interpret the children's primary complaint as one of difficulty hearing in noisy environments, but the actual statements made by parents or other caregivers paint a slightly different and broader picture. Consider the following statements:[1]

1. "If there is any noise (TV, others talking) she is unaware that she is being spoken to . . . "
2. "He often has a blank stare in response to questions or instructions ... It is unclear whether he forgot or didn't hear or understand ... "

Understanding Developmental Disorders of Auditory Processing, Language and Literacy Across Languages: International Perspectives, pp. 1–18

3. "She ... has trouble with attention and directions, even within the family."
4. "He has difficulty understanding information and directions at school."

While the first statement may suggest a speech-in-noise problem, it may also indicate either inattentiveness or conversely an excessive level of attentive focus. The second statement could describe a child with listening, language, attention, or memory problems. The important points from these and the other examples are (a) that listening problems usually co-occur with other developmental issues (Sharma, Purdy, & Kelly, 2009) that may be of a primarily cognitive[2] rather than a sensory nature, and (b) that audiologists and other medical and related professionals tend to arrive at diagnoses based on their particular fields of expertise. In fact, the selection pathway toward a diagnosis of APD begins before the APD clinic. Among other possibilities, children may receive primary referrals from (a) their schools due to listening difficulties, (b) their family doctors due to initial complaints from parents or (c) speech/language therapists due to their apparently normal productive language (Hind et al., 2011). In each of these instances, the initial suspicion may be that the child has experienced hearing loss, so the audiology referral is intended to explore this possibility. Some children turn out not to have an audiometric hearing loss but are still referred by audiologists who are aware of APD. We (Ferguson, Hall, Riley, & Moore, 2011) and others (Dawes & Bishop, 2010; Sharma et al., 2009) have shown that children diagnosed with or suspected of APD may be nearly indistinguishable symptomatically from those diagnosed with language disorders.

Sound Processing in the Auditory System

One way to understand the problem(s) that a child with listening difficulties experiences is to consider the processing and perception of sounds within the auditory system. I recently expanded on the neuroscience of this issue elsewhere (Moore, 2012a). Here, I discuss some recently discovered and newly reappraised aspects of the auditory system function directly related to APD. We know that the biophysical aspects of hearing in several ways resemble the behavioral audiogram. However, we also know that because the cochlea is highly nonlinear, it is difficult to predict high-level outputs based on what is observed at low sound levels. This could contribute, for example, to the imperfect relationship between the audiogram and hearing assessments based on speech-in-noise intelligibility (Füllgrabe, 2013). We also know that moderate levels of sound exposure can lead to a neurodegeneration of the cochlear nerve that is not reflected in the audiogram, but is observed functionally when higher-level sounds are presented (Kujawa & Liberman, 2009). These findings suggest that APD could be influenced by either normal or abnormal cochlear function.

We know that experience-based neuroplasticity can alter brain function, for example, in response to abnormal binaural input caused by otitis media with effusion in children (Hogan & Moore, 2003). In the auditory cortex, recent studies have shown that levels of noise exposure formerly thought to be "safe" (pp. 65–70 dB SPL) and that do not produce any known peripheral damage can lead to reductions (Pienkowski & Eggermont, 2012; Zhou & Merzenich, 2012) or other changes (Zheng, 2012) in neuron activity and parallel behavioral abnormalities in laboratory animals. These findings have provided possible routes and mechanisms for APD generated by auditory experience, including passive noise exposure. In addition, there is a vast superstructure of cortical processing pathways exerting transmodal and cognitive modulatory influence on the auditory system (Rauschecker & Scott, 2009) in addition to a descending, efferent system extending from the cortex to the ear, the function of which is also influenced by auditory experience (e.g., auditory learning in the absence of sensorineural hearing loss (Bajo, Nodal, Moore, & King, 2010; de Boer & Thornton, 2008; Irving, Moore, Liberman, & Summer, 2011).

How Has the Audiology Profession Dealt With APD?

This question may be addressed by considering a recent article in *Journal of Speech, Language and Hearing Research*. Wilson and colleagues (2011) made an important observation among children aged 7–14 attending an audiology clinic. The results of three commonly used screening tests did not correlate well with the children's performance on four diagnostic tests for APD. It was concluded that the screens, of which two were questionnaires, were therefore inappropriate for diagnosis referral. However, an alternative conclusion could be that the currently used diagnostic tests may be inappropriate follow-ups to the screens. I make this point not as a mere exercise in logic, but due to the very real concern that the current and most commonly used diagnostic tests for APD are out of touch with "clinical presentation," the reason why people seek help for their listening difficulties.

We must consult history to understand the origins of current APD diagnostic tests. The American Speech-Language-Hearing Association (ASHA) defined APD as

> difficulties in the perceptual processing of auditory information in the central nervous system (CNS), as demonstrated by poor performance in one or

> more of the following skills: sound localization and lateralization; auditory discrimination; auditory pattern recognition; temporal aspects of audition, including temporal integration, temporal discrimination (e.g., temporal gap detection), temporal ordering, and temporal masking; auditory performance in competing acoustic signals (including dichotic listening); and auditory performance with degraded acoustic signals. (ASHA, 2005a)

This definition grew out of an earlier task force convened by ASHA (1996) and consisting of both basic and clinical auditory scientists, in which the participants attempted to list every auditory function that involved central auditory processing. Because the purpose of this meeting was to arrive at a consensus on an APD definition, it seemed reasonable to imagine that any or all of these functions may go awry in people who had otherwise normal hearing (i.e., pure tone sensitivity) but nevertheless complained of listening difficulties.

Those familiar with the diagnostic tests used by Wilson et al. (2011), including low-pass filtered speech, competing sentences, two-pair dichotic digits, and frequency pattern tests, should recognize that several of the functions included in the ASHA definition (e.g., dichotic listening) were actually based on tests already in use to diagnose APD at the time of the meeting. Others (e.g., sound localization) have been common and enduring themes in psychoacoustics and auditory neuroscience. I suggest that there is no good evidence to link any of the functions listed in the definition to the clinical presentation of APD. On the contrary, studies that have specifically sought such a link (Dawes & Bishop, 2010; Moore, Ferguson, Edmondson-Jones, Ratib, & Riley, 2010; Watson & Kidd, 2009) have failed to find one. Instead, we (Moore et al., 2010) found that the significant if modest correlations between performance on several psychoacoustic tests and questionnaires related to APD, such as the Children's Auditory Processing Performance Scales (CHAPPS; Smoski, Brunt, & Tannahill, 1992) used as a screening test by Wilson et al. (2011), were primarily attributable to the cognitive rather than sensory demands of the psychoacoustic tests. This idea is discussed further below.

It appears that a fundamental error in the current professional conception of APD might have occurred because normal peripheral sensitivity was initially equated with normal peripheral function and then with abnormal function during the early stages of auditory processing by the brain. APD must be reformulated based on the listening problems people actually report when they present at audiology clinics. These problems appear to be primarily cognitive in origin.

CLINICAL DIAGNOSIS AND MANAGEMENT

Clinical management of APD will not progress until we better understand the listening problems we are dealing with and the best strategy for dealing with them. Anecdotal clinical reports and broadly based research studies have shed some light on the nature of the listening problems experienced by children. As mentioned previously, these reports and studies have suggested that cognitive difficulties (language, attention, and memory) are primarily responsible, that the difficulties are shared with other learning problems of childhood, and that they may interact with coding problems in the ear and classically defined central auditory system (CAS). However, I know of no clear evidence showing this to be the case. The optimal management strategy is clearly dependent on further understanding the nature of the problems, and several promising recent developments have offered interim solutions that are compatible with current concepts and address ever-present clinical needs.

Diagnosis

Although a complete consideration and specification of the range of listening problems in children is beyond the scope of this largely conceptual and strategic chapter, such a review is badly needed. A frequent report on developmental APD that has also been shared with other learning problems (see the following) is that it is very heterogeneous. Nevertheless, some common threads can be discerned, for example, from the quotations of parents, shown previously. Like adults, children have limited cognitive resources and can generally attend to only one thing at a time. If the focus of their attention is speech, auditory signals must be grouped together into phonologically meaningful objects. Auditory objects of any kind must be stored in working memory, either for immediate action or for further rehearsal and storage in their long-term memory (Rönnberg, Rudner, Foo, & Lunner, 2008). Finally, the contents of memory must be read out into action, mediated by motor systems or subjected to further mental manipulation. Note here that the processing of auditory signals by the ear and CAS are but the first stages in a chain that must be completed before the outcome can be meaningful to the individual or apparent to others, including parents and professionals.

Our research into the listening and hearing problems of children has tended to focus on attention as a potential bottleneck in the chain. Isolating the relevant aspects of attention and measuring them are undertakings fraught with potential problems because the literature has described many forms of attention (e.g., Zhang, Barry, Moore, & Amitay, 2012). Every distinct task seems to have its own form of attention demand. One solution to this problem is to determine the most relevant measure of attention for the task of interest, for example, the intelligibility of speech in an acoustically challenging environment. We have suggested that measuring response variability during a task's performance both captures relevant behavior and provides a parallel index to perceptual performance (e.g., the number of words correctly identified) in real time. For this reason, we have called the variability a measure of "intrinsic attention" (Moore et al., 2010). We may alternatively hypothesize that attention to relevant auditory targets (e.g., speech) consists of attention modules that are relevant to various other tasks (e.g., visual spatial attention). In common with a long tradition in cognitive psychology, modular attention may be measured using reaction time (RT) to the presentation of a simple sound stimulus that itself does not present a discriminative challenge. When paired with a cue stimulus and a simple decision requirement, RT tasks can quickly measure several modular aspects of attention. We have proposed that such measures could be useful in clinics, including in APD assessment (Zhang et al., 2012). A full APD diagnostic assessment of the future may thus consist of a series of auditory and speech perception tests, during which both (threshold) performance and (intrinsic) attention are measured, and some additional stand-alone tests of auditory attention and working memory.

Management

In principle, clinical management can be effective without knowledge of the underlying nature of the problem being managed. It may be desirable to treat APD symptom(s) selectively (Dillon, Cameron, Glyde, Wilson, & Tomlin, 2012). However, while we await a better understanding of those symptoms, children are turning up at audiology clinics in need of help. A recent comprehensive review of APD management (BSA, 2011) recommended two broad and intersecting types of management strategy: environmental control and auditory training. Controlling the environment via the use of good-listening strategies, reverberation reduction, and other measures to improve signal-to-noise (S/N) levels is an obvious approach to universally improving listening, but may not be readily achieved. For children, noisy classroom (Dockrell & Shield, 2006) and home (Roberts et al., 2004) environments have both been implicated in impaired listening as having long-lasting and far-reaching consequences, especially when inadequately interspersed with periods of high S/N levels. It is a general principle of neural plasticity that a brain system will develop and continue to function normally if even a relatively small amount of normal experience is available, and this seems to be the case for the development of both hearing and language (Halliday and Moore, 2010; Hogan & Moore, 2003). Encouraging even modest amounts of time without the masking noise of a disruptive pupil or a loud television may therefore have disproportionate benefits for a child with listening difficulties. The increasing availability of inexpensive wireless communication systems (generically known as "FM systems") that dramatically improve S/N through speaker-worn microphone(s) and hearing-aid-like receivers also offers a simple and effective means for capturing the attention of a child with listening difficulties. In a recent study, Hornickel, Zecker, Bradlow, and Kraus (2012) showed improved communicative abilities and associated brainstem function in children with dyslexia who wore wireless communication devices during a school year. Similar improvements could be predicted in children with APD.

Improved listening as a result of using an S/N-enhancing device is hardly surprising. However, the finding that listening remains enhanced when the device is removed after a period of use (Hornickel et al., 2012) is evidence of auditory learning. The sensorimotor systems of the brain in both children and adults have generally resulted in measureable improvement after a training period (Moore, 2012b). However, the gains have tended to be modest and potentially functionally insignificant (Halliday, Taylor, Millward, & Moore, 2012) unless the training stimulus and task are similar or identical to the skill being learned (Wright & Zhang, 2009). Improving the "generalization" or "transfer" of the training to a broader range of more functionally useful goals has become the primary goal of many involved in sensorimotor learning research. This may be achieved through a large amount of training. For example, visual training, which is an alternative to conventional eye patching, could have a significant effect on amblyopia ("brain blindness") through computer-based visual acuity training, but only if many thousands of trials ("kilotrials") are practiced over many weeks (Levi & Li, 2009). Although children often like to play computer games, this practice intensity is something that most children would find impossible, especially if they are inattentive. One alternative is to practice a task that is more suited to the individual's interests. Musical training is widely available and has been shown to have a positive effect on APD symptoms (e.g., improved auditory attention and speech-in-noise intelligibility) (Parbery-Clark, Strait, Anderson, Hittner, & Kraus, 2011; Strait, Parbery-Clark, Hittner, & Kraus, 2012). Although it remains unclear how much musical training is needed to see an improvement that is functionally significant, as with computer-based training, there is a positive relationship between improvement and the amount of practice. The same group showed very recently that training in a second language could likewise improve listening skills and executive function (Kraus, 2012; Krizman, Marian, Shook, Skoe, & Kraus, 2012).

Recent research has explored the relationship between sensorimotor learning and cognition. That such a relationship exists has been shown in several sensory learning studies in which manipulations of attention (Amitay, Irwin, & Moore, 2006; Xiao et al., 2008), motivation (Amitay, Halliday, Taylor, Sohoglu, & Moore, 2010) or memory (Zhang, Moore, Guirard, Molloy, & Amitay, 2013) have led to learning changes that might not have been predicted based on the stimuli or tasks. In applied studies of adult "brain training," one approach has involved the use of auditory training to affect memory enhancement (Mahncke et al., 2006). In one study, working memory and auditory training were shown to work reciprocally, with each skill improving the other (Zhang et al., 2013). This research has led to the hypothesis that sensorimotor learning is based entirely on cognitive factors, indicating that learning involves an improvement in the "level of engagement" of the learner with the task and stimuli rather than some sort of bottom-up fine-tuning of primary sensory coding. From an auditory rehabilitation perspective, a major interest of this work is its potential to address the biggest training challenge, that is, the need for long periods of practice. If training that focuses on top-down cognitive processes were effective, it could greatly widen the opportunity to try more innovative and motivating forms of training. For example, using handheld devices such as the Nintendo DS in conjunction with the "Dr. Kawashima's Brain Training" software suite may improve hearing and listening.[3]

LANGUAGE AND LITERACY DISORDERS—AN AUDITORY AND NEUROSCIENCE PERSPECTIVE

Language and Literacy Disorders

The suggestion that auditory "processing" difficulties may underlie or contribute to language (LI) and literacy (RD) difficulties is nearly as old as the recognition that each of these difficulties exists (Miller, 2011; Rosen, 2003). Much has been written on the nature of LI (Bishop, 1997; Leonard, 1998) and RD (Snowling, 2000), including other chapters in this volume, and I provide only the briefest of overviews here before focusing on how hearing applies. There have been two main contrasting views. The first is that language problems are "domain specific," and that the problem sources are specific to linguistic processing and particularly to phonological awareness. The assumption is that the sensory input generated by speech sounds and words and conveyed to the cerebral cortex is normal in children with language problems. The second view is that sensory processing problems underpin LI and RD. In an extreme form such as the temporal processing hypothesis (Stein & Talcott, 1999; Tallal, 2004), according to which language and reading impairments are caused specifically by slow or imprecise neural coding in the CAS, impaired sensory processing is *the* reason for LI and RD (and APD; Tallal, 2012). More recently, the notion that there are two main forms of RD (i.e., those with and without specifically phonological problems, but incorporating attention and working memory impairments such as slow attention shifting [SAS]) has been gaining traction (Guirard & Ramus, 2012; Lallier, Thierry, & Tainturier, 2013) and opened the possibility of a hybrid version of the two traditional views. Note that these developments parallel the development of opinions on the nature of APD in several ways.

Auditory Basis of LI and RD

Several questions relevant to the role of hearing in LI and RD are introduced in the preceding discussion of APD. The normality of the peripheral auditory system comes into question, as it is universally assumed outside auditory science on the basis of pure tone audiometry. The recognition that the suprathreshold perception is not always well predicted by and therefore not simply related to pure tone sensitivity has long been recognized in hearing science. However, the knowledge of the reasons for this disparity is in its infancy and has not yet had any effect on the childhood learning literature that I am aware of. The new interest in nonphonological, neurological, and genetic explanations of LI and RD has made it essential to recognize that suprathreshold auditory processing deficits may play a role, and to initiate suitable experiments to test this hypothesis.

A second question relates to the contribution of different sources of neural activity to hearing. We cannot assume that performance on any psychoacoustic or electrophysiological test (Moore et al., 2013) necessarily reflects activity in a particular brain pathway. For example, as explained elsewhere (Moore, 2012a), auditory perception necessarily involves *both* sensory and cognitive contributions. Thus, performance on any of the basic auditory functions specified by ASHA (2005a, 2005b) as contributors to APD and on auditory tasks such as the Tallal Auditory Repetition Test (Tallal & Piercy, 1973), which is used to generate sensory explanations for LI and RD, also involves cognitive contributions that may often include language skills (e.g., labeling stimuli). Physiological measures said to be "objective" or "preattentive" (e.g., the "mismatch negativity" [MMN]) have similarly been necessarily influenced by descending inputs, either directly and on a cyclical basis or indirectly via longer-term brain plasticity. For example, there has recently been great interest in the findings of Nina Kraus's lab that complex sensorimotor/cognitive tasks, specifically musical and foreign language training (Krizman et al., 2012; Skoe & Kraus, 2012), influence the timing of neural signals in the auditory brainstem. However, training exerts influence on and may result primarily from the cortical and descending modulation of afferent (ascending) activity in the CAS (Bajo et al., 2010; de Boer & Thornton, 2008; Irving et al., 2011). Evidence has also shown that descending pathways substantially influence processing in the auditory cortex (Rauschecker & Scott, 2009) and, according to some studies and to a lesser extent, in the brainstem (Lukas, 1980) in real time. Statements such as the following should thus be considered with skepticism:

> In the present study, we use a neurophysiological paradigm that circumvents these limitations by relying exclusively on bottom-up cortical responses to passively heard auditory stimuli, thus tapping into the first steps of auditory cortical integration without calling upon any explicit task. (Lehongre, Ramus, Villiermet, Schwartz, & Giraud, 2011, p. 1080)

> … both studies found the genetic effects to affect the late (300–700 ms) MMN component, but not the early one (100–200 ms). This presumably reflects intact auditory discrimination ability, but alterations at later stages of auditory/phonological processing. (Giraud & Ramus, 2012, p. 2)

In sum, the reviewed studies showed that auditory perception and its underlying neural processing are much more complex and difficult to interpret than studies of LI and RD have universally assumed. However, disorders expressed in the CAS are still disorders in the CAS, whatever their origin. It may therefore be reasonable to attribute some aspects of impaired language to impaired auditory processing, if that is understood to be what the CAS delivers to cortical linguistic processing areas.

A third question relates to the nature of auditory temporal processing. Despite strong evidence that some children with RD (about one third to one half) have problems performing a range of auditory temporal perception tasks, the same children also tend to experience more problems with auditory spectral perception and other aspects of hearing (Amitay, Amitay, Ben-Yehudah, Banai, & Ahissar, 2002; White et al., 2006). Moreover, the remaining children (about one half to two thirds) appear to be perceptually normal. Nevertheless, the idea that a specific temporal processing problem underpins LI and RD has been remarkably resilient (e.g., Tallal, 2012). Recent evidence has also suggested that different types of temporal disorder may be responsible. In a classic review, Rosen (1992) proposed three temporal processing speeds in audition. The speeds, ascribed modern/speech-based labels are envelope/syllable processing (0.5–20 Hz), periodic/phonemic processing (20–200 Hz), and temporal fine structure (200–6,000 Hz). Temporal processing problems accompanying normal audiograms have mainly been associated with the two slower speeds, especially envelope processing. Intrinsic brain rhythms across many brain systems have been found to operate at these speeds. These rhythms have generally been associated with multimodal cognitive processing, raising the possibility that the neural implications of language problems such as SAS represent a form of temporal processing deficit (e.g., Lehongre et al., 2011), although they are clearly of a different variety and function to those originally proposed by Tallal and colleagues.

A fourth question that brings us full circle relates to the latest developments in the neurogenetics of RD. Giraud and Ramus (2012) and Pinel et al. (2012) drew a link between the location (in the inferior frontal cortex and temporo-parietal junction) of auditory-cognitive-related processing areas that have been co-localized in experiments, showing (a) the location of aberrant expression (SNPs) in certain genes (e.g., KIAA0319) associated with LI, RD, and other developmental learning problems; (b) the location of structural alterations (microlesions, white matter abnormalities, grey matter ectopias); and (c) diminished auditory steady state responses (to 30 Hz noise; Lehongre et al., 2011). While these neurogenetic issues have intriguingly been observed in adults with the dominant phonological-deficit-based variety of RD, their location (in the posterior fiber tracts that lie within the superior longitudinal fasciculus and the corpus callosum, and those linking the left medial temporal gyrus with angular and supramarginal gyri) corresponds to a proposed role of corpus callosum in APD (Musiek & Weihing, 2011) based on older studies showing a reduced right ear advantage in dichotic listening (Berlin et al., 1973; Hugdahl & Andersson, 1986; Kimura, 1961). Note that the RD literature has considered the phonological form of RD *not* to be associated with impaired sensory processing.

Multimodal Processing—A Central Generator?

In considering all of the evidence related to the nature of APD and its association with other learning problems, it has been proposed that APD symptoms may be those of a broader neurodevelopmental disorder (BSA, 2011; Moore & Hunter, 2013). Similar thoughts have been associated with a wide range of other developmental learning problems (Bishop, 2009; Karmiloff-Smith, 1998) due to their extensive overlap (comorbidity). This suggestion has two important implications, one being that at least some common mechanisms may underlie many of these problems, the other that common diagnosis and management protocols may be handled by a single, appropriately trained professional. Experts in LI and RD have been quick to point out that they have spent many years demonstrating defining differences between the disorders, while also acknowledging a continuity (Catts, Adlof, Hogan, & Weismer, 2005; Snowling & Hulme, 2012). Although differences in certain defining skills (e.g., reading) have been acknowledged, these differences may reflect relatively small asymmetries in a "circle of common difficulties" that affect productive and receptive language, reading, listening, task engagement, social awareness, and behavior control. Common mechanisms may include genes (Giraud & Ramus, 2012), patterns of protein expression, neural pathways (e.g., the arcuate fasciculus; see Dick & Tremblay, 2012), and environmental influences. Implicit in this conceptualization is that common underpinning cognitive mechanisms (attention, working memory) are multimodal and handle a variety of sensorimotor processes under the influence of interacting inputs (e.g., auditory, visual).

In terms of the second implication, some proponents of a reevaluation of APD have suggested that unimodal dysfunction should be a defining quality of the disorder (McFarland & Cacace, 2009). This suggestion appears to be motivated by the worthy desire to separate a distinctly "auditory" deficit from other forms of learning problems that may contain an auditory component (e.g., LI and RD). However, I believe that this and other "axioms" of APD (e.g., that it has nothing to do with cognitive processes or that it should be diagnosed purely on the basis of nonspeech processing) falsely constrain the range of plausible explanations for the clinical presentation of APD. They also appear to be partly motivated by a perceived primary role of the audiology profession in the diagnosis and management of APD. While a multidisciplinary assessment of sensorimotor learning problems is often advocated and may be necessary in differentiating the elements of the "circle," it does not seem beyond the abilities of most relevant professionals such as audiologists to receive training in some carefully researched multimodal assessment and intervention techniques.

CONCLUDING REMARKS

The invitation to prepare this chapter provided me with the opportunity to summarize my current views as an auditory scientist on APDs and the possible role of hearing in LI and RD. Because the research in the latter two areas has been much more mature than that on APD, the most recent developments in genetics, imaging, electrophysiology, and psychology should be reviewed to further our understanding of APDs. It seems clear that, with a general recognition of the similarity of these disorders, APD research has been moving toward examination of the nature of the listening difficulties that may contribute to the disorders. One specific opportunity that has not yet been discussed is the growing concern over the increasing levels of autism spectrum disorder (ASD) and their relation to APD (Dawes & Bishop, 2010). Children with apparent listening difficulties may be slipping through the current diagnostic net because their high-functioning ASD symptoms are relatively difficult to detect (Karmiloff-Smith et al., 2012). The measurement of listening difficulties in this group may be one of the more sensitive objective methods for detecting a broader problem. In general, a greater focus on holistic development and the way in which the expression of different behavior changes with age, that is, a "neuroconstructivist" perspective (Karmiloff-Smith, 1998; Karmiloff-Smith et al., 2012) would seem to provide a particularly appropriate framework for the further study of neurodevelopmental disorders, including APD, LI, and RD.

Despite my reservations over multidisciplinary clinical assessment, I feel that multidisciplinary research, whether conducted by individuals or teams, is absolutely necessary to take these fields forward. APD has been and remains difficult to characterize because the audiology profession has largely acted alone in dealing with a disorder whose behavioral aspects are much better understood by others. I am hopeful that uniting professionals across traditional fields, as the Hong Kong conference did and this book attempts to do, will mark a significant step toward achieving a greater shared understanding.

NOTES

1. These are actual quotations from parents of children being assessed for APD at the Pediatric Audiology Clinic at Cincinnati Children's Hospital, kindly provided by Dr. Lisa Hunter.
2. I use the term "cognitive" throughout this chapter in reference to the interpretation of sensory signals.
3. The author declares no interest in any currently commercially available learning method or device.

ACKNOWLEDGMENTS

The preparation of this chapter is a result of many years of generous funding provided by the intramural program of the Medical Research Council to myself, my research team, and the MRC Institute of Hearing Research in Nottingham, UK. I would particularly like to thank Mel Ferguson, Johanna Barry, Justin Cowan, Alison Riley, Dorothy Bishop, and Stuart Rosen for their contributions to my thinking about APD and to the research reported here.

REFERENCES

Amitay, S., Ben-Yehudah, G., Banai, K., & Ahissar, M. (2002). Disabled readers suffer from visual and auditory impairments but not from a specific magnocellular deficit. *Brain, 125*(10), 2272–2285.

Amitay, S., Halliday, L., Taylor, J., Sohoglu, E., & Moore, D. R. (2010). Motivation and intelligence drive auditory perceptual learning. *PloS One, 5*(3), e9816.

Amitay, S., Irwin, A., & Moore, D. R. (2006). Discrimination learning induced by training with identical stimuli. *Nature Neuroscience, 9*(11), 1446–1448.

American Speech-Language-Hearing Association (ASHA). (1996). Central auditory processing: Current status of research and implications for clinical practice. *American Journal of Audiology, 5*(2), 41–54.

American Speech-Language-Hearing Association (ASHA). (2005a). *(Central) auditory processing disorders*. Retrieved from http://www.asha.org/members/deskref-journals/deskref/default

American Speech-Language-Hearing Association (ASHA). (2005b). *(Central) auditory processing disorders: The role of the audiologist (Position statement)*. Retrieved from http://www.asha.org/members/deskref-journals/deskref/default

Bajo, V. M., Nodal, F. R., Moore, D. R., & King, A. J. (2010). The descending corticocollicular pathway mediates learning-induced auditory plasticity. *Nature Neuroscience, 13*(2), 253–260.

Berlin, C. I., Hughes, L. F., Lowe-Bell, S. S., & Berlin, H. L. (1973). Dichotic right ear advantage in children 5 to 13. *Cortex, 9(*4), 394-402.

Bishop, D. V. M. (1997). *Uncommon understanding: Development and disorders of language comprehension in children*. Hove, UK: Psychology.

Bishop, D. V. (2009). Genes, cognition, and communication: Insights from neurodevelopmental disorders. *Annals of the New York Academy of Sciences, 1156*, 1–18.

British Society of Audiology (BSA). (2011). An overview of current management of auditory processing disorder (APD). *British Society of Audiology*. Retrieved from http://www.thebsa.org.uk/images/stories/docs/BSA_APD_Management_1Aug11_FINAL_amended17Oct11.pdf

Catts, H. W., Adlof, S. M., Hogan, T. P., & Weismer, S. E. (2005). Are specific language impairment and dyslexia distinct disorders? *Journal of Speech, Language and Hearing Research, 48*(6), 1378–1396.

Dawes, P., & Bishop, D. V. (2010). Psychometric profile of children with auditory processing disorder and children with dyslexia. *Archives of Disease in Childhood, 95*(6), 432–436.

de Boer, J., & Thornton, A. R. (2008). Neural correlates of perceptual learning in the auditory brainstem: Efferent activity predicts and reflects improvement at a speech-in-noise discrimination task. *Journal of Neuroscience, 28*(19), 4929–4937.

Dick, A. S., & Tremblay, P. (2012). Beyond the arcuate fasciculus: Consensus and controversy in the connectional anatomy of language. *Brain, 135*(12), 3529-3550.

Dillon, H., Cameron, S., Glyde, H., Wilson, W., & Tomlin, D. (2012). An opinion on the assessment of people who may have an auditory processing disorder. *Journal of the American Academy of Audiology, 23*(2), 97–105.

Dockrell, J., & Shield, B. (2006). Acoustical barriers in classrooms: The impact of noise on performance in the classroom. *British Educational Research Journal, 32*(3), 509–525.

Ferguson, M. A., Hall, R. L., Riley, A., & Moore, D. R. (2011). Communication, listening, speech and cognition in children with auditory processing disorder (APD) or specific language impairment (SLI). *Journal of Speech, Language and Hearing Research, 54*(2), 211–227.

Füllgrabe, C. (2013). Age-dependent changes in temporal-fine-structure processing in the absence of peripheral hearing loss. *American Journal of Audiology, 22,* 313-315. doi:10.1044/1059-0889(2013/12-0070)

Giraud, A.-L., & Ramus, F. (2012). Neurogenetics and auditory processing in developmental dyslexia. *Current Opinion in Neurobiology*. Retrieved from http://dx.doi.org/10.1016/ j.conb.2012.09.003

Halliday, L. F., & Moore, D. R. (2010). Auditory basis of language and learning disorders. In C. J. Plack (Ed.), *OUP handbook of auditory science: Hearing* (pp. 349–374). Oxford, UK: Oxford University Press.

Halliday, L. F., Taylor, J. L., Millward, K. E., & Moore, D. R. (2012). Lack of generalization of auditory learning in typically developing children. *Journal of Speech, Language and Hearing Research, 55*(1), 168–181.

Hind, S. E., Haines-Bazrafshan, R., Benton, C. L., Brassington, W., Towle, B., & Moore, D. R. (2011). Prevalence of clinical referrals having hearing thresholds within normal limits. *International Journal of Audiology, 50*(10), 708–716.

Hogan, S. C., & Moore, D. R. (2003). Impaired binaural hearing in children produced by a threshold level of middle ear disease. *Journal Association for Research in Otolaryngology, 4*(2), 123–129.

Hornickel, J., Zecker, S. G., Bradlow, A. R., & Kraus, N. (2012). Assistive listening devices drive neuroplasticity in children with dyslexia. *Proceedings of the National Academy of Sciences USA, 109*(41), 16731–16736.

Hugdahl, K., & Andersson, L. (1986). The "forced-attention paradigm" in dichotic listening to CV-syllables: A comparison between adults and children. *Cortex, 22*(3), 417–432.

Irving, S., Moore, D. R., Liberman, M. C., & Sumner, C. J. (2011). Olivocochlear efferent control in sound localization and experience-dependent learning. *Journal of Neuroscience, 31*, 2943–2501.

Karmiloff-Smith, A. (1998). Development itself is the key to understanding developmental disorders. *Trends in Cognitive Sciences, 2*(10), 389–398. doi:S1364-6613(98)01230-3 [pii]

Karmiloff-Smith, A., D'Souza, D., Dekker, T.M., Van Herwegen, J., Xu, F., Rodic, M. & Ansari, D. (2012). Genetic and environmental vulnerabilities in children with neurodevelopmental disorders. *Proceedings of the National Academy of Sciences of the United States of America, 109*(Suppl 2), 17261-17265.

Kimura, D. (1961). Cerebral dominance and the perception of verbal stimuli. *Canadian Journal of Psychology, 15*(3), 166–171.

Kraus, N. (2012). Biological impact of music and software-based auditory training. *Journal of Communication Disorders, 45*(6), 403–410.

Krizman, J., Marian, V., Shook, A., Skoe, E., & Kraus, N. (2012). Subcortical encoding of sound is enhanced in bilinguals and relates to executive function advantages. *Proceedings of the National Academy of Sciences USA, 109*(20), 7877–7881.

Kujawa, S. G., & Liberman, M. C. (2009). Adding insult to injury: Cochlear nerve degeneration after "temporary" noise-induced hearing loss. *Journal of Neuroscience, 29*(45), 14077–14085.

Lallier, M., Thierry, G., & Tainturier, M. J. (2013). On the importance of considering individual profiles when investigating the role of auditory sequential deficits in developmental dyslexia. *Cognition, 126*(1), 121–127.

Lehongre, K., Ramus, F., Villiermet, N., Schwartz, D., & Giraud, A. L. (2011). Altered low-gamma sampling in auditory cortex accounts for the three main facets of dyslexia. *Neuron, 72*(6), 1080–1090.

Leonard, L. B. (1998). *Children with specific language impairment*. Cambridge, MA: MIT Press.

Levi, D. M., & Li, R. W. (2009). Perceptual learning as a potential treatment for amblyopia: A mini-review. *Vision Research, 49*(21), 2535–2549.

Lukas, J. H. (1980). Human auditory attention: The olivocochlear bundle may function as a peripheral filter. *Psychophysiology, 17*(5), 444–452.

Mahncke, H. W., Connor, B. B., Appelman, J., Ahsanuddin, O. N., Hardy, J. L., Wood, R. A., ... Merzenich, M. M. (2006). Memory enhancement in healthy older adults using a brain plasticity-based training program: A randomized, controlled study. *Proceedings of the National Academy of Sciences USA, 103*(33), 12523–12528.

McFarland, D. J., & Cacace, A. T. (2009). Modality specificity and auditory processing disorders. In A. T. Cacace & D. J. McFarland (Eds.), *Controversies in central auditory processing disorder* (pp. 93–107). San Diego, CA: Plural.

Miller, C. A. (2011). Auditory processing theories of language disorders: Past, present, and future. *Language, Speech, and Hearing Services in Schools, 42*(3), 309–319.

Moore, D. R. (2012a). Listening difficulties in children: Bottom-up and top-down contributions. *Journal of Communication Disorders, 45*(6), 411–418.

Moore, D. R. (2012b). Stroke recovery and sensory plasticity: Common mechanisms? *Developmental Psychobiology, 54*(3), 326–331.

Moore, D. R., Ferguson, M. A., Edmondson-Jones, A. M., Ratib, S., & Riley, A. (2010). The nature of auditory processing disorder in children. *Pediatrics, 126*(2), e382–e390.

Moore, D. R., & Hunter, L. L. (2013). Auditory processing disorder (APD) in children: A marker of neurodevelopmental syndrome. *Hearing, Balance and Communication, 11*, 160-167.

Moore, D. R., Rosen, S., Bamiou, D.-E., Campbell, N. G., & Sirimanna, T. (2013) Evolving concepts of developmental auditory processing disorder (APD): A British Society of Audiology APD Special Interest Group "white paper." *International Journal of Audiology, 52*(1), 3-13.

Musiek, F. E., & Weihing, J. (2011) Perspectives on dichotic listening and the corpus callosum. *Brain and Cognition, 76*(2), 225-232.

Parbery-Clark, A., Strait, D. L., Anderson, S., Hittner, E., & Kraus, N. (2011). Musical experience and the aging auditory system: Implications for cognitive abilities and hearing speech in noise. *PLoS ONE, 6*(5), e18082.

Pienkowski, M., & Eggermont, J. J. (2012). Reversible long-term changes in auditory processing in mature auditory cortex in the absence of hearing loss induced by passive, moderate-level sound exposure. *Ear and Hearing, 33*(3), 305–314.

Pinel, P., Fauchereau, F., Moreno, A., Barbot, A., Lathrop, M., Zelenika, D., ... Dehaene, S. (2012). Genetic variants of FOXP2 and KIAA0319/TTRAP/THEM2 locus are associated with altered brain activation in distinct language-related regions. *Journal of Neuroscience, 32*(3), 817–825.

Rauschecker, J. P., & Scott, S. K. (2009). Maps and streams in the auditory cortex: Nonhuman primates illuminate human speech processing. *Nature Neuroscience, 12*(6), 718–724.

Roberts, J., Hunter, L., Gravel, J., Rosenfeld, R., Berman, S., Haggard, M., ... Wallace I. (2004). Otitis media, hearing loss, and language learning: Controversies and current research. *Journal of Developmental and Behavioral Pediatrics, 25*(2), 110–122.

Rönnberg, J., Rudner, M., Foo, C., & Lunner, T. (2008). Cognition counts: A working memory system for ease of language understanding (ELU). *International Journal of Audiology, 47*(2), S99–S105.

Rosen, S. (1992). Temporal information in speech: Acoustic, auditory and linguistic aspects. *Philosophical Transactions of the Royal Society of London. Series B, Biological Sciences, 336*(1278), 367–373.

Rosen, S. (2003). Auditory processing in dyslexia and specific language impairment: Is there a deficit? What is its nature? Does it explain anything? *Journal of Phonetics, 31*, 509–527.

Sharma, M., Purdy, S. C., & Kelly, A. S. (2009). Comorbidity of auditory processing, language, and reading disorders. *Journal of Speech, Language, and Hearing Research, 52*(3), 706–722.

Skoe, E., & Kraus, N. (2012). A little goes a long way: How the adult brain is shaped by musical training in childhood. *Journal of Neuroscience, 32*(34), 11507–11510.

Smoski, W. J., Brunt, M. A., & Tannahill, J. C. (1992). Listening characteristics of children with central auditory processing disorders. *Language, Speech, and Hearing Services in Schools, 23*(2), 145–152.

Snowling, M. J. (2000). *Dyslexia*. Oxford, UK: Blackwell.

Snowling, M. J., & Hulme, C. (2012). Interventions for children's language and literacy difficulties. *International Journal of Language and Communication Disorders, 47*(1), 27–34.

Stein, J. F., & Talcott, J. B. (1999). The magnocellular theory of dyslexia. *Dyslexia, 5*(2), 59–78.

Strait, D. L., Parbery-Clark, A., Hittner, E., & Kraus, N. (2012). Musical training during early childhood enhances the neural encoding of speech in noise. *Brain and Language, 123*(3), 191–201.

Tallal, P. (2004). Improving language and literacy is a matter of time. *Nature Reviews: Neuroscience*, *5*(9), 721–728. doi:10.1038/nrn1499nrn1499 [pii]

Tallal, P. (2012). Improving neural response to sound improves reading. *Proceedings of the National Academy of Sciences USA*, *109*(41), 16406–16407. doi:10.1073/pnas.1214122109 1214122109 [pii]

Tallal, P., & Piercy, M. (1973). Defects of non-verbal auditory perception in children with developmental aphasia. *Nature*, *241*, 468–469.

Watson, C. S., & Kidd, G. R. (2009). Associations between auditory abilities, reading, and other language skills, in children and adults. In C. A. McFarland (Ed.), *Current controversies in central auditory processing disorder (CAPD)*. San Diego, CA: Plural.

White, S., Milne, E., Rosen, S., Hansen, P., Swettenham, J., Frith, U., & Ramus, F. (2006). The role of sensorimotor impairments in dyslexia: A multiple case study of dyslexic children. *Developmental Science*, *9*(3), 237–255.

Wilson, W. J., Jackson, A., Pender, A., Rose, C., Wilson, J., Heine, C., & Khan, A. (2011). The CHAPS, SIFTER, and TAPS-R as predictors of (C)AP skills and (C)APD. *Journal of Speech, Language and Hearing Research*, *54*(1), 278–291.

Wright, B. A., & Zhang, Y. (2009). A review of the generalization of auditory learning. *Philosophical Transactions of the Royal Society of London. Series B, Biological Sciences*, *364*(1515), 301–311.

Xiao, L. Q., Zhang, J. Y., Wang, R., Klein, S. A., Levi, D. M., & Yu, C. (2008). Complete transfer of perceptual learning across retinal locations enabled by double training. *Current Biology*, *18*(24), 1922–1926.

Zhang, Y.-X., Barry, J., Moore, D. R., & Amitay, S. (2012). A new test of attention in listening (TAIL) predicts basic auditory performance. *PLoS ONE*, *7*(12), e53502.

Zhang, Y.-X., Moore, D. R., Guirard, J., Molloy, K., & Amitay, S. (2013). Bridging perceptual and cognitive learning: Mutual transfer between tone frequency discrimination and working memory. Annual meeting presentation. *British Society of Cognitive Neuroscience*.

Zheng, W. (2012). Auditory map reorganization and pitch discrimination in adult rats chronically exposed to low-level ambient noise. *Frontiers in Systems Neuroscience*, *6*, 65.

Zhou, X., & Merzenich, M. M. (2012). Environmental noise exposure degrades normal listening processes. *Nature Communications*, *3*, 843.

CHAPTER 2

A FRAMEWORK FOR EVALUATING THE ROLE OF AUDITORY PROCESSING IN LANGUAGE-LEARNING DISORDERS

Carol Miller

There is a long and lively history of hypotheses proposing that auditory processing deficits cause language-learning disorders (LLDs). In 1973, auditory processing hypotheses had enough traction in the field to prompt a trenchant critique by Rees. Thirty years later, Rosen (2003) reviewed the auditory processing hypotheses of oral and written language disorders and concluded that the presence of auditory deficits does not provide a satisfactory causal explanation for LLDs. Another decade has since passed, and auditory processing hypotheses have continued to receive considerable clinical and research attention despite the cautionary conclusions of Rees, Rosen, and others (e.g., Kamhi, 2011; Moore, Ferguson, Edmondson-Jones, Ratib, & Riley, 2010; Watson & Kidd, 2009). Among the reasons for the continued interest are promising neuroscience discoveries related to the auditory system (see Banai & Kraus, 2007, 2009 for reviews) and

Understanding Developmental Disorders of Auditory Processing, Language and Literacy Across Languages: International Perspectives, pp. 19–40

evolving definitions of auditory processing (Giraud & Poeppel, 2012; Goswami, 2011; Song, Skoe, Banai, & Kraus, 2011). It seems that our understanding of the role of auditory processing in typical and atypical language development is progressing. At the same time, the more we learn about the complexity of the auditory system, the more we realize how much we have yet to learn.

I believe that there is another reason for both the enduring popularity of auditory processing hypotheses among clinicians and the motivation of researchers to devote resources to investigating them. It is my perception that many students and clinicians, and perhaps some researchers, feel that auditory processing hypotheses are superior to other hypotheses about the causes of LLDs. Perhaps this is because intuitively, it seems that auditory processing hypotheses are somehow more "fundamental" than other types of hypotheses and that auditory processing is basic and concrete in a way that, say, phonological processing is not. However, what makes one hypothesis better than another is not the level of explanation it assumes but its ability to make testable predictions that are supported by empirical data and explained in a precise, coherent manner. In this chapter, I aim to show that there are many ways to think about LLDs and their causes, each of which potentially has validity, explanatory value and psychological reality. That is not to say that all these ways of thinking produce equally useful hypotheses about the causes of LLDs. However, each hypothesis should be evaluated on the basis of what it can explain, what evidence is available to support it, and whether it leads to effective interventions. Auditory processing hypotheses are not special; they can and should be evaluated by the same criteria as other hypotheses.

LLDs are defined in terms of language difficulties. The "pieces" of deficient language vary across disorders and individuals, but every LLD is described in terms of language constructs,—whether very broad, such as "oral language," or more narrow, such as "phonological processing." Any hypothesis about the cause of an LLD attempts to link observable language deficits to other mental constructs that are less directly observable. For example, what we observe in dyslexia is slow, error-ridden reading of individual words. One explanation for this observed behavior claims that the reader has a flawed phonological system. (There have been several different accounts of the nature of the flaw.) However, we cannot directly observe anyone's phonological system; we can only make inferences about it based on observable behavior. In this chapter, I categorize the hypotheses according to the types of unobservable construct they appeal to in explaining the observable deficits of LLDs.

HYPOTHESIS CATEGORIES

Some hypotheses explain language deficits in terms of linguistic constructs. The extended optional infinitive (EOI) hypothesis is an example of a linguistic account of oral language disorders (Rice & Wexler, 1996; Rice, Wexler, & Cleave, 1995). Observed deficits in subject-verb agreement are explained in terms of the components of phrase structure grammar. Certain relationships among phrasal types are not obligatory in the immature grammar. A language disorder occurs when an immature grammar persists for a period much longer than usual during development. For written language disorders, the phonological deficit hypothesis is a linguistic-level explanation. There have been various proposals regarding the specific nature of the phonological deficit (Kamhi & Catts, 2012).

Some hypotheses explain language difficulties in terms of nonlinguistic constructs. One category comprises hypotheses that attribute LLDs to deficits in domain-general cognitive functions. Among the cognitive functions that have been proposed as deficient in both oral and written LLDs are working memory, attention, processing speed, and (more broadly) limited processing capacity (Windsor & Kohnert, 2009).

A third group of hypotheses that explain language difficulties in terms of nonlinguistic constructs comprises those that invoke perceptual processing deficits. These differ from the cognitive functions described previously in that the deficits are thought to be limited to a single sensory system, such as the auditory or visual system. In contrast, functions such as working memory can operate upon input from any sensory system and indeed may be crucial in integrating data from different systems. Some of the hypotheses posit that visual processing deficits underlie written language disorders. However, auditory processing deficits have been proposed as causal factors in both oral and written LLDs.

These different explanations of LLD causes need not be mutually exclusive. For example, both phonological and processing speed deficits may contribute to written LLDs, as in the double deficit hypothesis (Wolf, Bowers, & Biddle, 2000). In this chapter, however, I focus on example hypotheses at each level to illustrate how the hypotheses can be evaluated using the same criteria.

LANGUAGE-LEARNING DISORDERS

I use the term "language-learning disorders" or LLDs to indicate developmental disorders that are primarily characterized by deficits in spoken or written language. These deficits do not occur due to sensory impairments, cognitive impairments, social-behavioral disorders, or frank neurological disease or damage and are not the result of inadequate opportunities to learn. Specific language impairment (SLI) (Leonard, 1998; Windsor & Kohnert, 2004) is an LLD of spoken language. In the domain of written language, dyslexia is an LLD that refers to a specific deficit in word recognition (Lyon, Shaywitz, & Shaywitz, 2003). Kamhi and Catts (2012) described a model based on the Simple View of reading (Hoover & Gough, 1990) that includes both word recognition and listening comprehension; poor readers may be deficient in either or both skills. While I include all of these reading difficulty subtypes under the LLD umbrella, auditory processing hypotheses typically focus on dyslexia (poor word recognition in the presence of adequate listening comprehension), which is also a focus in the discussion that follows. Auditory processing disorder (APD) is a diagnosis based on the presence of listening difficulties and deficits in one or more specific auditory skills where peripheral hearing is normal (ASHA, 2005). Children with APD usually demonstrate oral and/or written language difficulties that are very similar to those observed in children with SLI and/or dyslexia (Ferguson, Hall, Riley, & Moore, 2011; Miller & Wagstaff, 2011; Sharma, Purdy, & Kelly, 2009). If LLDs are defined by primary deficits in language, then should APD be considered an LLD? I return to this question later in the chapter.

Although I use the term “LLD” to describe more than one disorder, I do not claim that every LLD has the same etiology or that they all can be considered a single clinical entity. However, because auditory processing hypotheses have been proposed for each of the LLDs discussed here (in the case of APD, auditory processing deficits *define* the disorder), I therefore feel justified in discussing them together.

Let us consider a representative hypothesis from each of the three categories described earlier: those that explain LLDs using linguistic constructs, nonlinguistic cognitive constructs, and perceptual processing constructs. The descriptions of each hypothesis and the summaries of the evidence bearing on them are necessarily brief and gloss over many nuances. However, the purpose is not to choose a “winner” but to demonstrate that every hypothesis is subject to the same process of interrogation.

LINGUISTIC ACCOUNTS OF LLDs

A Linguistic Account of SLI

A well-known hypothesis that invokes linguistic constructs is the EOI hypothesis (Rice & Wexler, 1996; Rice, Wexler, & Cleave, 1995) of SLI. This hypothesis, which is based on a generativist theoretical approach to language, posits that every child passes through a developmental stage in which he/she uses a grammar that differs from the grammar of mature language users (although perhaps not in every language). In the child's grammar, tense and agreement features are not obligatory in matrix clauses. This aspect of the immature grammar results in occasional omissions of tense and/or agreement morphology from the sentences the child produces.

a. *The girl walk_ to school every day.
b. The girl walks to school every day.
c. *Yesterday the puppy bark_ at me.
d. Yesterday the puppy barked at me.
e. *The girls walks to school every day.

For example, the child may produce (a) or (c), wherein the morphologically marked form is replaced with an infinitival form, that is, the "optional infinitive" rather than the corresponding mature forms in (b) and (d). However, children rarely produce overt errors such as the sentence in (e). The low incidence of such errors indicates that the tense and agreement system is intact in the grammar, but not used consistently. Typically developing children emerge from the optional infinitive stage by the age of 3, using tense and agreement consistently (Wexler, 2003). Children with SLI remain in the optional infinitive stage for an extended period. Thus, according to the EOI hypothesis, SLI is caused by a deficit in the child's grammatical system.

Evidence

Some of the clearest evidence pertaining to the EOI hypothesis came from two longitudinal studies (reported in Rice, Tomblin, Hoffman, Richman & Marquis, 2004 and Rice, Wexler, & Hershberger, 1998, among other publications) that examined the production of grammatical morphology in children with and without language impairment over several years. Both studies included the morphemes third person singular *–s* (3S) and regular and irregular past tense. In addition, Rice et al. (1998) included copula and auxiliary *be* and auxiliary *do*. The children with SLI in both studies consistently lagged behind children of the same age in producing these forms that marked finiteness in English, but not in producing control morphemes that did not mark finiteness. In the study by Rice et al. (1998), by the age of 8, the children with SLI had not yet reached the near-perfect levels of performance shown by typically developing children at ages 5 or 6. Similar results in the study by Rice et al. (2004), which used an epidemiologically ascertained sample, showed that children with SLI did not exceed a 95% correctness level on finiteness markers until at least grade 3 (approximately 8 years of age). Rice, Wexler, and Redmond (1999) obtained grammaticality judgments from the same participants as those in the study by Rice et al. (1998) and found that the children tended to accept sentences with missing finiteness markers similar to those they produced. The children with SLI performed at accuracy levels below those of typically developing children 2 years younger.

A Linguistic Account of Dyslexia

The most commonly accepted causal hypothesis on dyslexia is that it results from a deficit in phonological processing (e.g., Ramus, 2003; Shaywitz, Gruen, Mody, & Shaywitz, 2009; Shaywitz & Shaywitz, 2005; Snowling & Hulme, 2012a; Vellutino, Fletcher, Snowling, & Scanlon, 2004). Although the precise nature of the phonological deficit remains a matter of investigation and debate, most reading researchers have agreed that reading well requires one to isolate phonological units in spoken language and the written code and match them to one another. Phonological awareness skills such as rhyming, blending sounds, and combining sounds are indicators of phonological processing ability and good predictors of reading outcomes (e.g., Catts, Fey, Zhang, & Tomblin, 2001; Share & Stanovich, 1995; Wagner & Torgeson, 1987). Deficits in phonological processing, indicated by poor performance on phonological awareness and phonological memory tasks, make the decoding of words slow and inaccurate.

Evidence

For each of the hypotheses reviewed in this chapter, summarizing the pertinent evidence in a few paragraphs presents a challenge, one that is particularly acute for the phonological deficit hypothesis of dyslexia. The large amount of relevant literature has addressed a number of issues on the precise nature of various phonological skills and how they are related to aspects of reading development. I summarize the findings of a few recent reviews to give a broad view of the current status of the phonological deficit hypothesis. One large meta-analysis of studies comparing children with dyslexia with age- or reading-level-matched control subjects suggested that "there is a specific and substantial association between concurrent measures of phonemic awareness and children's word reading skills" (Melby-Lervåg, Lyster, & Hulme, 2012, p. 340). The results were similar for English and other orthographies. Melby-Lervåg et al. (2012) further argued that there is reason to suppose that phonemic awareness plays a causal role in reading development.

Vellutino et al. (2004) summarized evidence for a causal role of phonological processing in dyslexia. They noted that both adults and children who were poor readers also had poor phonological processing, that phonologically based interventions were effective in remediating dyslexia, and that phonological processing was implicated in dyslexia for readers of several different orthographies. However, the specific phonological skills that predicted language outcomes varied depending on the transparency of the orthography (i.e., the directness of the relation between sound and spelling).

In a recent review of neuroimaging findings, Diehl, Frost, Mencl, and Pugh (2011) argued that there is strong evidence for a left-hemisphere reading circuit consisting of

> a. an anterior system primarily in the posterior portion of the inferior frontal gyrus,
> b. a posterior dorsal system in temporo-parietal cortex [including Wernicke's area and the angular gyrus], and
> c. a posterior ventral system in occipito-temporal cortex and adjacent areas. (p. 218)

While the location and function of these areas are important, so are the interconnections between the areas. For example, a functional connectivity analysis (i.e., correlations of activity among brain areas) by Pugh et al. (2000) suggested that dyslexic adults had a decreased connectivity in the left-hemisphere reading circuit, but only for tasks that required complex phonological processing. On those same tasks, the dyslexic readers showed more right-hemisphere connectivity compared with unimpaired controls.

What Linguistic Accounts Explain

One advantage that linguistic hypotheses have over those that invoke general or specific cognitive and perceptual processes is that the chain of logic linking the hypothesized constructs to the observed behavior is relatively short. For spoken language, the crucial deficit is proposed to reside in the grammatical system that generates spoken sentences. A disadvantage of the EOI hypothesis and some other linguistic hypotheses is that they rely on the accuracy of the linguistic theory on which they are predicated. In this case, the theory assumes that every human is born with an innate universal grammar that constrains language learning. If this assumption is incorrect, the EOI hypothesis is untenable. Another disadvantage of the EOI hypothesis in comparison with other hypotheses that invoke nonlinguistic constructs is that its explanatory scope is limited to syntax. The Computational Grammatical Complexity account (van der Lely, 2005), another linguistic hypothesis of SLI, also attempts to explain deficits in morphology and phonology. However, no linguistic account, by its nature, attempts to explain the causes of the full cognitive profile of SLI, and some researchers in the field have viewed this as a serious limitation.

Like the EOI hypothesis, the phonological deficit hypothesis requires few logical steps between the hypothesized deficit and observed behavior. These hypotheses also share the limitation of explaining a fairly narrow range of behavior in SLI and dyslexia, disorders that have broader phenotypes (see Leonard, 1998 for SLI and Vellutino et al., 2004 for dyslexia). Unlike the EOI hypothesis, the phonological deficit hypothesis does not rely too heavily on a specific linguistic theory. Challenges to the phonological deficit hypothesis are more likely to be based on claims that the phonology construct can be deconstructed into sensory processes. I return to this notion in the section on perceptual processing accounts.

Linguistic Accounts and Intervention

The EOI hypothesis can be clinically applied more readily to diagnosis than to intervention. Rice and colleagues suggested that omitting tense and agreement constitutes a clinical marker for SLI (e.g., Rice & Wexler, 1996). The Test of Early Grammatical Impairment (Rice & Wexler, 2001) is a published test that probes for tense and agreement morphology to identify children with SLI. Because the EOI hypothesis emphasizes maturation as a developmental mechanism that drives growth in the use of tense and agreement morphology, it may inform intervention timing (Rice, 2004) and the selection of clinical goals, but it does not suggest therapeutic techniques.

In contrast, the phonological deficit account suggests a clear direction for intervention: if phonological processing can be improved, better reading should follow. As Snowling and Hulme (2012b) noted, evidence for a causal theory may be obtained from intervention studies. If interventions based on the phonological deficit hypothesis are effective, the hypothesis is supported. Recent reviews (Duff & Clarke, 2011; Shaywitz, Morris, & Shaywitz, 2008; Snowling & Hulme, 2012a) of research in the United Kingdom and the United States have indicated that the most effective interventions include explicit training in phonological awareness and letter-sound correspondences along with reading practice. Indeed, it is considered educational best practice to teach beginning readers phonological awareness skills, and to provide explicit instruction in grapheme-phoneme correspondence rules (National Institute of Child Health and Human Development, 2000; Rose, 2009).

NONLINGUISTIC COGNITIVE ACCOUNTS OF LLDs

A Processing Speed Account of SLI

Speed of information processing is a nonlinguistic cognitive construct that has been proposed as an explanation for SLI (Kail, 1994; Miller, Kail, Leonard, & Tomblin, 2001; Miller et al., 2006); that is, slow processing speed may lead to the language deficits observed in SLI. Comprehension of running speech may be affected by speed limitations if the child is unable to fully process a word or morpheme before the following material interferes. According to the surface hypothesis (Leonard, 1998), because a child must sometimes abandon processing of linguistic forms to keep up with incoming speech, it takes him/her longer to build up complete, accurate linguistic representations than it does for typically developing peers. Poor quality representations cause further comprehension problems and adversely affect sentence production. Production may also be negatively affected by speed limitations, because the child faces time pressure to produce a spoken message. Grammatical morphemes may be omitted due to a lack of the necessary time to access and generate them (Bishop, 1994).

Evidence

Several studies have demonstrated that many children with SLI have slow processing speeds compared with peers of the same age. A few illustrative examples are described here. Miller et al. (2001, 2006) administered a battery of response time tasks to a single sample of children during 3rd grade and 8th grade. The majority of the children with SLI were slower than their typically developing peers across the tasks. Kohnert and Windsor (2004) found that children with SLI were slower than their typically developing peers on several nonlinguistic tasks. Montgomery (2005) administered online sentence processing tasks to children with and without SLI. The children with SLI were slower overall than their typically developing peers and benefited when sentences were presented at a slower rate, although their peers did not.

These and other studies have suggested that slow processing is characteristic of the majority of children with SLI. The evidence to connect slow processing with language performance has been more mixed. In a study by Montgomery and Windsor (2007), response time on a nonlinguistic task predicted real-time sentence processing but did not predict language test performance independently of phonological memory. Lahey, Edwards, and Munson (2001) found that response times on several tasks did not predict language test scores. In contrast, Leonard et al. (2007) found that processing speed predicted language test scores. Using data from a large longitudinal study (Miller et al., 2001, 2006, reported data from the same study), the authors evaluated the ability of processing speed and working memory measures to predict language performance in 14-year-olds with and without SLI. Both predictors accounted for significant variance in language performance, although working memory was a stronger predictor than processing speed.

A Processing Speed Account of Dyslexia

Processing speed has also been proposed as a causal factor in dyslexia (Breznitz & Misra, 2003; Horowitz-Kraus & Breznitz, 2011; Wolf et al., 2000). One measure that is widely used to assess individuals with dyslexia is naming speed, that is, how quickly an individual can speak the names of a series of letters, numbers, colors, or common objects. Although slow naming speed is a good predictor of dyslexia (e.g., Denckla & Rudel, 1976; Wolf et al., 2000), its relation to reading is not fully understood. Wolf et al. (2000) advanced some hypotheses about the role of processing speed in reading, such as the hypothesis that a general slowed processing speed could interfere with many component processes in reading (e.g., visual and motor processing, construction of orthographic representations, phonological retrieval) and with the coordination of these processes (see also Breznitz & Misra, 2003), resulting in poor reading fluency that is perhaps moderated by slow naming speed.

Evidence

Evidence in support of the processing speed hypothesis of dyslexia includes the work of Kail and Hall (1994), who found that general processing speed contributed significantly to naming speed in a sample of typically developing children. Catts, Gillispie, Leonard, Kail, and Miller (2002) found that poor readers were slower than normal readers on a variety of response time (RT) tasks. They further found that RT accounted for unique variance in word recognition and that rapid object naming did not, suggesting that naming speed may reflect general processing speed. However, Norton and Wolf (2012) cited evidence from studies using multivariate modeling to suggest that naming speed does not reduce to general processing speed. Several studies have shown that naming speed is a good predictor of reading outcomes. This is true of nonalphabetic orthographies in addition to both more and less transparent alphabetic orthographies (Norton & Wolf, 2012).

Breznitz and colleagues undertook a comprehensive investigation of processing speed in child and young-adult normal and dyslexic readers (reviewed in Breznitz & Berman, 2003). The researchers varied the participants' reading rates and measured both their behavior (reaction time) and electrophysiological responses (event-related potentials (ERPs)). The results suggested that for all groups, speed of processing varied according to whether the task was simple or complex, visual or auditory, and linguistic or nonlinguistic. Speed of processing was most strongly associated with discrimination of auditory phonemes in children with dyslexia, and in adults with dyslexia, it was most strongly associated with word-level phonological processing. When the reading rate of the adult dyslexics was accelerated, the ERP data suggested that they became speedier at an earlier stage of perceptual and attentional processing and at a later stage of working memory updating. For typical readers, the reading rate acceleration affected their processing speed only at the later stage.

What Processing Speed Accounts Explain

The speed of processing accounts of SLI and dyslexia must explain more logical steps between the observed deficits and the presumed cause compared with linguistic accounts. Exactly which processes are slowed, and how do they contribute to speaking, listening, and reading? The answers rely on the theoretical models of these activities to some extent. Although there has been consensus on the broad outlines of such models for the most part, the details do matter. At this point, the most elaborated processing speed model for either spoken or written language has come from Breznitz and colleagues (Breznitz, 2006; Breznitz & Berman, 2003). In particular, Breznitz's group offered evidence from experimental manipulations of processing speed, described further in the following section on intervention. More such experimental work is required to complement the bulk of the evidence, which has come from correlation-regression and structural equation modeling approaches.

Processing Speed Accounts and Intervention

If processing speed is not merely associated with LLDs but also plays a causal role, then intervention that increases processing speed should decrease LLD deficits. Is it possible to increase processing speed? Developmentally, general processing speed increases through childhood, plateaus in young adulthood, and then decreases with age (Cerella & Hale, 1994). This developmental pattern may reflect biological changes (e.g., myelination). Naming speed deficits tend to remain stable throughout development, and even if naming speed could be changed through intervention, that alone may not be enough to meaningfully improve reading fluency (Norton & Wolf, 2012). Little of the SLI research has considered whether processing speed could be changed through intervention. However, Breznitz and colleagues (e.g., Breznitz, 1997; Breznitz & Berman, 2003) have shown that when dyslexic readers voluntarily increase their reading rate, their decoding accuracy and comprehension improve, and the latencies of the relevant ERP components correspondingly decrease.

PERCEPTUAL PROCESSING ACCOUNTS OF LLDs

An Auditory Processing Account of SLI and Dyslexia

Hypotheses that propose a causal role for auditory processing deficits are found in both the SLI and dyslexia literatures, and often are proposed for LLDs in general. The rapid auditory processing (RAP) account of Tallal and colleagues (Fitch & Tallal, 2003; Merzenich et al., 1996; Tallal, 1988, 2004; Tallal & Piercy, 1973; Tallal et al., 1996) is one well-known hypothesis that proposes that auditory processing deficits cause both SLI and dyslexia. It claims that many individuals with LLDs experience a deficit in discriminating acoustic differences (e.g., frequency differences) that occur very rapidly, as in speech. According to Tallal (2004), children with LLDs

> are specifically impaired in both their ability to discriminate between and to produce speech sounds that are characterized by brief, rapidly successive acoustic changes, such as the brief formant transitions (40 msec) preceding the steady-state portion of the vowel, which are the sole differentiating feature between syllables such as /ba/ and /da/. (p. 722)

This auditory processing impairment makes it difficult for children with LLDs to isolate phonemic units, which negatively affects phonological representation and processing (Fitch & Tallal, 2003).

Some more recent auditory processing accounts of LLDs have focused on cortical oscillations at slower rates, consistent with syllable-sized acoustic units, as well as rates that correspond to phoneme-sized acoustic units. An example of an oscillation account may be found in Goswami (2011). She proposed a temporal sampling framework (TSF) in which individuals with dyslexia (and perhaps other LLDs; see also Goswami & Szűcs, 2011) experience specific deficits in processing lower-frequency speech components (1.5–10 Hz) that lead to poor phonological representations. Both the RAP and TSF accounts supplement the phonological deficit hypothesis of dyslexia, while also broadening it to include SLI. The linguistic deficit is part of these hypotheses, but is given an explanation at the perceptual level.

Kraus and colleagues (e.g., Banai, Nicol, Zecker, & Kraus, 2005; Johnson, Nicol, Zecker & Kraus, 2007) have proposed that children with

LLDs experience deficits in the auditory brainstem response (ABR) to speech sounds. In typical listeners, the speech signal is encoded fairly directly in distinct components of the ABR that correspond to syllable onsets and steady-state vowels (Johnson et al., 2008). The ABR is less well synchronized to the speech signal in many children with LLDs (Johnson et al., 2007), particularly in the presence of background noise (Cunningham, Nicol, Zecker, Bradlow, & Kraus, 2001).

Evidence

There has been a great deal of conflicting evidence on auditory processing in LLDs. Some studies have found evidence of auditory processing difficulties in individuals with LLDs and some have not, and even when LLD groups have differed from control groups, some participants with LLDs have performed within normal limits (McArthur & Bishop, 2001; Rosen, 2003). Some of the evidence in support of the RAP has come from longitudinal studies of infants at risk of LLD due to a positive family history of such a disorder (Benasich, Thomas, Choudhury, & Leppänen, 2002). Infants with a positive family history required a longer interval between two tones to discriminate them. Furthermore, the discrimination threshold was the best predictor of language outcome at age 3 compared with other variables. Another type of evidence often cited as support for the RAP is the success of Fast ForWord, a computer-based intervention designed to improve RAP (Tallal, 2004). In this intervention, a series of computer games uses acoustically altered speech and individualized modification of the speed at which the stimuli are presented. However, one meta-analysis of Fast ForWord studies (Strong, Torgerson, Torgerson, & Hulme, 2011) found no evidence that the intervention improved the language or reading skills of children with LLDs. Two systematic reviews that considered computerized auditory training interventions more generally (including Fast ForWord) also found little or no evidence of improved language and/or reading outcomes for children with LLDs (Fey et al., 2011; Loo, Bamiou, Campbell, & Luxon, 2010).

Goswami (2011) reviewed behavioral and electrophysiological data pertaining to dyslexia that were consistent with the TSF. Some examples of relevant evidence for the TSF have come from studies of rise-time perception, that is, the discrimination of different rates of the change in amplitude in an acoustic signal. Corriveau, Pasquini, and Goswami (2007) found that children with SLI had difficulty discriminating rise-time differences. However, Fraser, Goswami, and Conti-Ramsden (2010) found rise-time discrimination problems in children with dyslexia, with or without co-morbid SLI, whereas children with only SLI did not perform significantly worse than their typically developing peers. Beattie and Manis (2013) also studied dyslexic children with and without language impairments and found that each of the two groups performed more poorly than the control group, but on different rise-time tasks. Based on regression analyses, Fraser et al. (2010) concluded that auditory processing influenced reading by way of phonological awareness. Beattie and Manis (2013) found that auditory processing was not significantly correlated with any reading or language measures in the LLD groups but was correlated with one reading measure in the control group.

There has been a substantial body of evidence showing ABR deficits in children with LLDs, not only from Kraus and colleagues, who have typically used synthesized speech syllables as stimuli, but also from researchers who have used tones and clicks (Basu, Krishnan, & Weber-Fox, 2010; Marler & Champlin, 2005). Evidence for a relation between ABR deficits and reading skills comes from an intervention study (Hornickel, Zecker, Bradlow, & Kraus, 2012) in which children with dyslexia were provided with assistive listening devices for one academic year and compared to a control group of children with dyslexia who did not use such devices. The results suggested that in about half of the children using assistive listening devices, ABR responses to speech became more consistent, and the degree of consistency predicted improvements in phonological awareness.

What Auditory Processing Accounts Explain

Accounts of LLDs that are founded on perceptual mechanisms, such as the RAP, TSF, and ABR hypotheses described previously, have more of an explanatory distance to travel than do accounts that explain LLDs in terms of linguistic or cognitive constructs. Proponents of the RAP (Tallal, 2004), TSF (Goswami, 2011), and ABR (Banai & Kraus, 2007) hypotheses have offered suggestions related to the neural mechanisms that may underlie the hypothesized auditory processing deficits. Proposals about neural mechanisms for the RAP, such as white-matter disruptions, neuronal migration abnormalities, or reduced thalamic volumes (Fitch & Tallal, 2003), are perhaps the most speculative. Goswami (2011) based the TSF on well-documented cortical oscillation frequencies, and the properties of ABRs in response to speech are becoming increasingly well understood (Chandrasekaran & Kraus, 2010b). However, in each case, establishing a causal chain between the proposed neural mechanism and the observed language deficits has thus far been based on associations rather than established cause-and-effect relationships.

What about APD? The three auditory processing hypotheses discussed here have focused on dyslexia and/or SLI. I earlier asked whether APD should also be considered an LLD. In APD, listening problems are considered to compose the primary deficit, and spoken and written language problems are considered secondary. However, APD is behaviorally indistinguishable from SLI and dyslexia (Ferguson et al., 2011; Miller & Wagstaff, 2011; Sharma et al., 2009). Given the hypotheses that propose that auditory processing deficits underlie SLI and dyslexia, it may be most parsimonious to consider APD as an LLD in which the auditory processing deficits are more readily observable than in "traditional" LLDs. The causal chain from auditory processing deficits to language deficits, when and if it is established, may be the same for APD, SLI, and dyslexia. However, it is possible that distinguishable auditory processing deficits may underlie each of these disorders such that different causal chains may be established, although each terminates in similar observable language difficulties.

Auditory Processing Accounts and Intervention

The auditory processing hypotheses related to LLDs suggest intervention techniques, and the RAP has already led to the development of the Fast ForWord computer-based intervention program (Tallal, 2004). As noted previously, the intervention has existed long enough for several studies to be conducted, and reviews have concluded that Fast ForWord is no more effective than other methods in remediating spoken and written language difficulties (Fey et al., 2011; Loo et al., 2010; Strong et al., 2011). The TSF and ABR hypotheses are relatively new, and few interventions based on these accounts have been developed and tested. As noted previously, promising results were obtained with an intervention using assistive listening devices, presumably because the devices increased the signal-to-noise ratio (Hornickel et al., 2012). Both Goswami (2011) and Kraus (Chandrasekaran & Kraus, 2010a) suggested musical training as a direction for intervention.

EVALUATING AUDITORY PROCESSING HYPOTHESES IN CONTEXT

This chapter describes only a small sample of the many hypotheses related to LLD causes. Some of the hypotheses compete directly and some are complementary. For example, auditory processing hypotheses may support phonological deficit hypotheses by explaining the source of the phonological deficit. In any case, research that directly compares one hypothesis to another has been rare. To facilitate comparisons, I attempt to outline a framework that makes it easier to understand how different LLD accounts are related to one another, regardless of whether they are competing or complementary. Within this framework, it should be clear that auditory processing hypotheses are neither special nor privileged. They can be evaluated in the same way as hypotheses that invoke other types of perceptual processes, nonlinguistic cognitive constructs, or linguistic constructs. Auditory processing hypotheses do differ from other types of hypotheses in one way: they endeavor to follow a lengthy causal chain from perception to observed language behaviors. This ambition is laudable, as we ultimately aspire to understand the entire pathway from hearing and seeing to speaking and reading. However, due to the current limitations on how much we know about the central nervous system, there remain sizable gaps in the causal chain. Hypotheses that start from constructs closer to observed behavior may be more successful in suggesting directions for effective interventions. To consider one clear example, interventions based on the phonological deficit hypothesis of dyslexia have had a strong record of success in improving reading performance. Interventions based on auditory processing hypotheses that claim to explain why phonological deficits exist have been much less successful. As auditory processing hypotheses become more refined and the gaps in our understanding of the central nervous system are filled in, this situation will probably change. In the meantime, I recommend that clinicians and educators choose evidence-based interventions for LLDs, taking into consideration the hypotheses on which the interventions are founded, the empirical support for those hypotheses, and the applicability of the hypotheses to individual children. Although there is no shortcut to the best theory or intervention, the evidence base for informed clinical decision making is growing.

REFERENCES

American Speech-Language-Hearing Association (ASHA). (2005). *(Central) Auditory Processing Disorders* [Technical report]. Retrieved from http://www.asha.org/docs/html/TR2005-00043.html

Banai, K., & Kraus, N. (2007). Neurobiology of (central) auditory processing disorder and language-based learning disability. In F. E. Musiek & G. D. Chermak (Eds.), *Handbook of (central) auditory processing disorder Volume I: Auditory neuroscience and diagnosis* (pp. 89–116). San Diego, CA: Plural.

Banai, K., & Kraus, N. (2009). The dynamic brainstem: Implications for auditory processing disorder. In A. T. Cacace & D. J. McFarland (Eds.), *Controversies in central auditory processing disorder* (pp. 269–289). San Diego, CA: Plural.

Banai, K., Nicol, T., Zecker, S. G., & Kraus, N. (2005). Brainstem timing: Implications for cortical processing and literacy. *Journal of Neuroscience, 25*(43), 9850–9857.

Basu, M., Krishnan, A., & Weber-Fox, C. (2010). Brainstem correlates of temporal auditory processing in children with specific language impairment. *Developmental Science, 13*, 77–91.

Beattie, R. L., & Manis, F. R. (2013). Rise time perception in children with reading and combined reading and language difficulties. *Journal of Learning Disabilities, 46,* 200–209. doi:10.1177/0022219412449421

Benasich, A. A., Thomas, J. J., Choudhury, N., & Leppänen, P. H. T. (2002). The importance of rapid auditory processing abilities to early language development: Evidence from converging methodologies. *Developmental Psychobiology, 40,* 278–292.

Bishop, D. V. M. (1994). Grammatical errors in specific language impairment: Competence or performance limitation? *Applied Psycholinguistics, 15,* 507–550.

Breznitz, Z. (1997). Effects of accelerated reading rate on memory for text among dyslexic readers. *Journal of Educational Psychology, 89,* 289–297.

Breznitz, Z. (2006). *Fluency in reading: Synchronization of processes.* Mahwah, NJ: Lawrence Erlbaum.

Breznitz, Z., & Berman, L. (2003). The underlying factors of word reading rate. *Educational Psychology Review, 15,* 247–265.

Breznitz, Z., & Misra, M. (2003). Speed of processing of the visual-orthographic and auditory-phonological systems in adult dyslexics: The contribution of "asynchrony" to word recognition deficits. *Brain and Language, 85,* 486–502.

Catts, H. W., Fey, M. E., Zhang, X., & Tomblin, J. B. (2001). Estimating the risk of future reading difficulties in kindergarten children: A research-based model and its clinical implementation. *Language, Speech, and Hearing Services in Schools, 32,* 38–50.

Catts, H. W., Gillispie, M., Leonard, L. B., Kail, R. V., & Miller, C. A. (2002). The role of speed of processing, rapid naming, and phonological awareness in reading achievement. *Journal of Learning Disabilities, 35,* 509–524.

Cerella, J., & Hale, S. (1994). The rise and fall in information-processing rates over the life span. *Acta Psychologica, 86,* 109–197.

Chandrasekaran, B., & Kraus, N. (2010a). Music, noise exclusion, and learning. *Music Perception, 27*(4), 297–306.

Chandrasekaran, B., & Kraus, N. (2010b). The scalp-recorded brainstem response to speech: Neural origins and plasticity. *Psychophysiology, 47,* 236–246.

Corriveau, K., Pasquini, E., & Goswami, U. (2007). Basic auditory processing skills and specific language impairment: A new look at an old hypothesis. *Journal of Speech, Language, and Hearing Research, 50,* 647–666.

Cunningham, J., Nicol, T., Zecker, S. G., Bradlow, A., & Kraus, N. (2001). Neurobiologic responses to speech in noise in children with learning problems: Deficits and strategies for improvement. *Clinical Neurophysiology, 112,* 758–767.

Denckla, M. B., & Rudel, R. G. (1976). Naming of object-drawings by dyslexic and other learning disabled children. *Brain and Language, 3,* 1–15.

Diehl, J. J., Frost, S. J., Mencl, W. E., & Pugh, K. R. (2011). Neuroimaging and the phonological deficit hypothesis. In S. A. Brady, D. Braze, & C. A. Fowler (Eds.), *Explaining individual differences in reading: Theory and evidence* (pp. 217–237). New York, NY: Psychology.

Duff, F. J., & Clarke, P. J. (2011). Practitioner review: Reading disorders: What are the effective interventions and how should they be implemented and evaluated? *Journal of Child Psychology and Psychiatry, 52,* 3–12.

Ferguson, M. A., Hall, R. L., Riley, A., & Moore, D. R. (2011). Communication, listening, cognitive and speech perception skills in children with auditory processing disorder (APD) or specific language impairment (SLI). *Journal of Speech, Language, and Hearing Research, 54*, 211–227.

Fey, M., Richard, G. J., Geffner, D., Kamhi, A. G., Medwetsky, L., Paul, D., ... Schooling, T. (2011). Auditory processing disorders and auditory/language interventions: An evidence-based systematic review. *Language, Speech, and Hearing Services in Schools, 42*, 246–264.

Fitch, R. H., & Tallal, P. (2003). Neural mechanisms of language-based learning impairments: Insights from human populations and animal models. *Behavioral and Cognitive Neuroscience Reviews, 2*, 155–178.

Fraser, J., Goswami, U., & Conti-Ramsden, G. (2010). Dyslexia and specific language impairment: The role of phonology and auditory processing. *Scientific Studies of Reading, 14*(1), 8–29.

Giraud, A., & Poeppel, D. (2012). Cortical oscillations and speech processing: Emerging computational principles and operations. *Nature Neuroscience, 15*, 511–517.

Goswami, U. (2011). A temporal sampling framework for developmental dyslexia. *Trends in Cognitive Sciences, 15*, 3–10. doi:10.1016/j.tics.2010.10.001

Goswami, U., & Szûcs, D. (2011). Educational neuroscience: Developmental mechanisms: Towards a conceptual framework. *Neuroimage, 57*, 651–658. doi:10.1016/j.neuroimage.2010.08.072

Hoover, W. A., & Gough, P. B. (1990). The simple view of reading. *Reading and Writing: An Interdisciplinary Journal, 2*, 127–160.

Hornickel, J., Zecker, S. G., Bradlow, A. R., & Kraus, N. (2012). Assistive listening devices drive neuroplasticity in children with dyslexia. *Proceedings of the National Academy of Sciences, 109*, 16731–16736. doi:10.1073/pnas.1206628109

Horowitz-Kraus, T., & Breznitz, Z. (2011). Reaction time and accuracy in erroneous vs correct responses among dyslexic and regular readers: From letters to sentences. *Dyslexia, 17*, 72–84.

Johnson, K. L., Nicol, T., Zecker, S. G., Bradlow, A. R., Skoe, E., & Kraus, N. (2008). Brainstem encoding of voiced consonant-vowel stop syllables. *Clinical Neurophysiology, 119*, 2623–2635.

Johnson, K. L., Nicol, T., Zecker, S. G., & Kraus, N. (2007). Auditory brainstem correlates of perceptual timing deficits. *Journal of Cognitive Neuroscience, 19*(3), 376–385.

Kail, R. (1994). A method for studying the generalized slowing hypothesis in children with specific language impairment. *Journal of Speech and Hearing Research, 37*, 418–421.

Kail, R., & Hall, L. K. (1994). Processing speed, naming speed, and reading. *Developmental Psychology, 30*, 949–954.

Kamhi, A. G. (2011). What SLPs need to know about APD. *Language, Speech, and Hearing Services in Schools, 42*, 265–272. doi:10.1044/0161-1461(2010/10-0004)

Kamhi, A. G., & Catts, H. W. (2012). *Language and reading disabilities* (3rd ed.). Boston, MA: Pearson.

Kohnert, K., & Windsor, J. (2004). The search for common ground: Part II. Nonlinguistic performance by linguistically diverse learners. *Journal of Speech, Language, and Hearing Research*, *47*, 891–903.

Lahey, M., Edwards, J., & Munson, E. (2001). Is processing speed related to severity of language impairment? *Journal of Speech, Language, and Hearing Research*, *44*, 1354–1361.

Leonard, L. B. (1998). *Children with specific language impairment.* Cambridge, MA: MIT Press.

Leonard, L. B., Ellis Weismer, S., Miller, C. A., Francis, D., Tomblin, J. B., & Kail, R. V. (2007). Speed of processing, working memory, and language impairment in children. *Journal of Speech, Language, and Hearing Research*, *50*, 408–428.

Loo, J. H. Y., Bamiou, D.-E., Campbell, N., & Luxon, L. M. (2010). Computer-based auditory training (CBAT): Benefits for children with language- and reading-related learning difficulties. *Developmental Medicine & Child Neurology*, *52*, 708–717.

Lyon, G. R., Shaywitz, S. E., & Shaywitz, B. A. (2003). A definition of dyslexia. *Annals of Dyslexia*, *53*, 1–14.

Marler, J. A., & Champlin, C. A. (2005). Sensory processing of backward-masking signals in children with language-learning impairment as assessed with the auditory brainstem response. *Journal of Speech, Language, and Hearing Research*, *48*, 189–203.

McArthur, G. M., & Bishop, D. V. M. (2001). Auditory perceptual processing in people with reading and oral language impairments: Current issues and recommendations. *Dyslexia*, *7*, 150–170.

Melby-Lervåg, M., Lyster, S.-A. H., & Hulme, C. (2012). Phonological skills and their role in learning to read: A meta-analytic review. *Psychological Bulletin*, *138*, 322–352.

Merzenich, M., Jenkins, W., Johnston, P., Schreiner, C., Miller, S., & Tallal, P. (1996). Temporal processing deficits of language-learning impaired children ameliorated by training. *Science*, *271*(5245), 77–81.

Miller, C. A., Kail, R., Leonard, L. B., & Tomblin, J. B. (2001). Speed of processing in children with specific language impairment. *Journal of Speech, Language, and Hearing Research*, *44*, 416–433.

Miller, C., Leonard, L., Kail, R., Zhang, X., Tomblin, B., & Francis, D. (2006). Response time in 14-year-olds with language impairment. *Journal of Speech, Language, and Hearing Research*, *49*, 712–728.

Miller, C. A., & Wagstaff, D. A. (2011). Behavioral profiles associated with auditory processing disorder and specific language impairment. *Journal of Communication Disorders*, *44*, 745–763.

Montgomery, J. (2005). Effects of input rate and age on the real-time language processing of children with specific language impairment. *International Journal of Language and Communication Disorders*, *40*, 171–188.

Montgomery, J., & Windsor, J. (2007). Examining the language performances of children with and without language impairment: Contributions of phonological short-term memory and speed of processing. *Journal of Speech, Language, and Hearing Research*, *50*, 778–797.

Moore, D. R., Ferguson, M. A., Edmondson-Jones, A. M., Ratib, S., & Riley, A. (2010). Nature of auditory processing disorder in children. *Pediatrics, 126*, e382–e390. doi:10.1542/peds.2009–2826

National Institute of Child Health and Human Development. (2000). *Report of the National Reading Panel. Teaching children to read: An evidence-based assessment of the scientific research literature on reading and its implications for reading instruction* (NIH Publication No. 00-4769). Washington, DC: U.S. Government Printing Office.

Norton, E. S., & Wolf, M. (2012). Rapid automatized naming (RAN) and reading fluency: Implications for understanding and treatment of reading disabilities. *Annual Review of Psychology, 63*, 427–452.

Pugh, K. R., Mencl, W. E., Shaywitz, B. A., Shaywitz, S. E., Fulbright, R. K., Constable, R. T., ... Gore, J. C. (2000). The angular gyrus in developmental dyslexia: Task-specific differences in functional connectivity within posterior cortex. *Psychological Science, 11*, 51–56.

Ramus, F. (2003). Developmental dyslexia: Specific phonological deficit or general sensorimotor dysfunction? *Current Opinion in Neurobiology, 13*, 212–218. doi:10.1016/S0959-4388(03)00035-7

Rees, N. S. (1973). Auditory processing factors in language disorders: The view from Procrustes' bed. *Journal of Speech and Hearing Disorders, 38*, 304–315.

Rice, M. (2004). Growth models of developmental language disorders. In M. Rice & S. Warren (Eds.), *Developmental language disorders: From phenotypes to etiologies* (pp. 207–240). Mahwah, NJ: Erlbaum.

Rice, M. L., Tomblin, J. B., Hoffman, L., Richman, W. A., & Marquis, J. (2004). Grammatical tense deficits in children with SLI and nonspecific language impairment: Relationships with nonverbal IQ over time. *Journal of Speech and Hearing Research, 47*, 816–834.

Rice, M. L., & Wexler, K. (1996). Toward tense as a clinical marker of specific language impairment in English-speaking children. *Journal of Speech and Hearing Research, 39*, 1239–1257.

Rice, M. L., & Wexler, K. (2001). *Rice/Wexler test of early grammatical impairment.* San Antonio, TX: Psychological Corporation.

Rice, M. L., Wexler, K., & Cleave, P. L. (1995). Specific language impairment as a period of extended optional infinitive. *Journal of Speech, Language, and Hearing Research, 38*, 850–863.

Rice, M. L., Wexler, K., & Hershberger, S. (1998). Tense over time: The longitudinal course of tense acquisition in children with specific language impairment. *Journal of Speech, Language, and Hearing Research, 41*, 1412–1431.

Rice, M. L., Wexler, K., & Redmond, S. M. (1999). Grammaticality judgments of an extended optional infinitive grammar: Evidence from English-speaking children with specific language impairment. *Journal of Speech, Language, and Hearing Research, 42*, 943–961.

Rose, J. (2009). *Identifying and teaching children and young people with dyslexia and literacy difficulties.* Report to the Secretary of State for Children, Schools and Families.

Rosen, S. (2003). Auditory processing in dyslexia and specific language impairment: Is there a deficit? What is its nature? Does it explain anything? *Journal of Phonetics, 31*, 509–527.

Share, D. L., & Stanovich, K. E. (1995). Cognitive processes in early reading development: Accommodating individual differences into a model of acquisition. *Issues in Education, 1*(1), 1–57.

Sharma, M., Purdy, S. C., & Kelly, A. S. (2009). Comorbidity of auditory processing, language, and reading disorders. *Journal of Speech, Language, and Hearing Research, 52*, 706–722.

Shaywitz, S. E., Gruen, J. R., Mody, M., & Shaywitz, B. A. (2009). Dyslexia. In R. G. Schwartz (Ed.), *The handbook of child language disorders* (pp. 115–139). New York, NY: Psychology.

Shaywitz, S. E., Morris, R., & Shaywitz, B. A. (2008). The education of dyslexic children from childhood to young adulthood. *Annual Review of Psychology, 59*, 451–475.

Shaywitz, S. E., & Shaywitz, B. A. (2005). Dyslexia (specific reading disability). *Biological Psychiatry, 57*, 1301–1309.

Snowling, M. J., & Hulme, C. (2012a). Annual research review: The nature and classification of reading disorders—A commentary on proposals for DSM-5. *Journal of Child Psychology and Psychiatry, 53*, 593–607.

Snowling, M. J., & Hulme, C. (2012b). Intervention for children's language and literacy difficulties. *International Journal of Language and Communication Disorders, 47*, 27–34.

Song, J. H., Skoe, E., Banai, K., & Kraus, N. (2011). Perception of speech in noise: Neural correlates. *Journal of Cognitive Neuroscience, 23*(9), 2268–2279.

Strong, G. K., Torgerson, C. J., Torgerson, D., & Hulme, C. (2011). A systematic meta-analytic review of evidence for the effectiveness of the "Fast ForWord" language intervention program. *Journal of Child Psychology and Psychiatry, 52*, 224–235.

Tallal, P. (1988). Developmental language disorders. In J. F. Kavanagh & T. J. Truss, Jr. (Eds.), *Learning disabilities: Proceedings of the national conference* (pp. 181–272). Parkton, MD: York.

Tallal, P. (2004). Improving language and literacy is a matter of time. *Nature Reviews Neuroscience, 5*, 721–728.

Tallal, P., & Piercy, M. (1973). Developmental aphasia: Impaired rate of non-verbal processing as a function of sensory modality. *Neuropsychologia, 11*, 389–398.

Tallal, P., Miller, S., Bedi, G., Byma, G., Wang, X., Nagarajan, S., ... Merzenich, M. M. (1996). Language comprehension in language-learning impaired children improved with acoustically modified speech. *Science, 271*(5245), 81–84.

van der Lely, H. K. J. (2005). Domain-specific cognitive systems: Insight from grammatical-SLI. *Trends in Cognitive Sciences, 9*(2), 53–59.

Vellutino, F. R., Fletcher, J. M., Snowling, M. J., & Scanlon, D. M. (2004). Specific reading disability (dyslexia): What have we learned in the past four decades? *Journal of Child Psychology and Psychiatry, 45*, 2–40.

Wagner, R. K., & Torgesen, J. K. (1987). The nature of phonological processing and its causal role in the acquisition of reading skills. *Psychological Bulletin, 101*, 192–212.

Watson, C. S., & Kidd, G. R. (2009). Associations between auditory abilities, reading, and other language skills, in children and adults. In A. T. Cacace & D. J. McFarland (Eds.), *Controversies in central auditory processing disorder* (pp. 217–242). San Diego, CA: Plural.

Wexler, K. (2003). Lenneberg's dream: Learning, normal language development, and specific language impairment. In Y. Levy & J. Schaeffer (Eds.), *Language competence across populations: Toward a definition of specific language impairment* (pp. 11–61). Mahwah, NJ: Erlbaum.

Windsor, J., & Kohnert, K. (2004). The search for common ground: Part I. Lexical performance by linguistically diverse learners. *Journal of Speech, Language, and Hearing Research*, *47*, 877–890.

Windsor, J., & Kohnert, K. (2009). Processing speed, attention, and perception in child language disorders. In R. G. Schwartz (Ed.), *The handbook of child language disorders* (pp. 445–461). New York, NY: Psychology.

Wolf, M., Bowers, P. G., & Biddle, K. (2000). Naming-speed processes, timing, and reading: A conceptual review. *Journal of Learning Disabilities*, *33*, 387–407.

CHAPTER 3

AUDITORY PROCESSING AND COGNITION

Kenneth Hugdahl

The asymmetrical functioning of the two cerebral hemispheres (Hugdahl & Westerhausen, 2010) is closely linked to research on speech and language, and in particular to issues in relation to language and auditory processing deficits in children (Moncrieff, 2010; Musiek, Reeves, & Baran, 1985; Obrzut & Mahoney, 2011). In this chapter, I consider the relevance of an experimental procedure, dichotic listening (DL), to unravel the secrets of the two hemispheres of the brain for speech processing and also when deficits of hemispheric asymmetry occur due to developmental or other problems. The chapter focuses on recent modifications of the standard DL procedure and introduces both bottom-up and top-down cognitive processing strategies for modulating the ear advantage in reports of simple consonant-vowel (CV) syllable sounds.

I begin by introducing the concepts of structural and functional brain asymmetry and how the different functions of the hemispheres may have evolutionary benefits. I then give a brief overview of the DL task and of administration and data scoring procedures and consider validation studies such as functional neuroimaging and brain lesion studies. The rest of the chapter examines the application of DL to different normal and clinical states and conditions, including reading and language processing studies

Understanding Developmental Disorders of Auditory Processing, Language and Literacy Across Languages: International Perspectives, pp. 41–65

and to auditory processing deficits. DL involves pairwise presentations of CV syllables wherein the subject orally reports the syllable that he/she perceived in each trial. By instructing the subject to focus attention on either the right or left ear stimulus and to only report from that ear, it is possible to add a cognitive dimension to the task and thus study how higher cognition may modulate or shape low-level perceptual processes.

FUNCTIONAL VERSUS STRUCTURAL BRAIN ASYMMETRY

From an evolutionary standpoint, humans have a unique ability to decode the phonetic information in an acoustic signal and to merge units of perception to meaningful words, sentences, and discourse. This process occurs automatically whenever the brain encounters an acoustic input composed of phonetic information (phonemes, syllables, words, sentences). Furthermore, speech perception primarily engages neurons in the left temporal lobe (Hugdahl et al., 1999; Sininger & Bhatara, 2012; Zatorre, Evans, Meyer, & Gjedde, 1992) and is thus one of the most profound examples of hemispheric asymmetry or functional laterality, that is, the specialization of functions to one of the cerebral hemispheres (see Hugdahl & Westerhausen, 2009 for a discussion of the foundations of hemispheric asymmetry for language). However, a "paradoxical" problem in studies of functional laterality of language in the visual domain is that there is little or no evidence of a corresponding structural asymmetry in the visual cortex. Thus, from a gross anatomy viewpoint, the two cerebral hemispheres are essentially symmetrical in shape in the visual areas. This is different in the auditory domain wherein functional asymmetry has a structural correlate. The Heschl's gyrus (HG) and the adjacent planum temporale (PT) areas in the upper posterior part of the auditory speech perception areas in the temporal lobe, including the superior temporal gyrus and sulcus, have larger grey matter volume on the left side compared with the right side (Dorsaint-Pierre et al., 2006) (see Figure 3.1).

Heschl's Gyrus and the Planum Temporale

Studies have shown that the left PT area is about 30%–35% larger on the left side, and that such an asymmetry pattern is seen in about 60%–65% of individuals (Geschwind & Levitsky, 1968). The volume asymmetry correlates with more widely spaced cellular columns on the left side, which could point toward greater connectivity per neuron and more heavily myelinated axons connecting the neurons, which could point toward an increased action potential traveling speed on the left side. Both instances

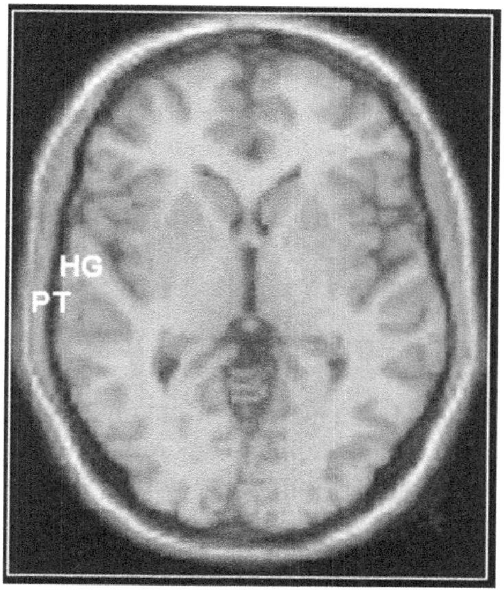

Figure 3.1. Axial (horizontal) structural MR image from a single individual in the temporal lobe plane, showing the asymmetry of the Heschl's gyrus (HG) and planum temporale (PT) with left > right grey matter volumes.

would result in superior processing in the left PT compared with the right PT, with an increased speed of decoding the phonetic structure of the acoustic signal, which parallels the transfer of the phonetic units from the ear to the brain. The HG and PT leftward asymmetry fits with another structural asymmetry in the brain: the so-called Yakelovian torque (Toga & Thompson, 2003; Yakovlev & Rakic, 1966). This involves the twisting of the brain along the longitudinal axis, with the right frontal and left occipital poles protruding beyond the corresponding left and right sides, which is necessary for the expansion of the left peri-Sylvian region and right occipito-parietal regions. It could be argued that an expanded PT area on the left side would "push" the brain parenchyma backward from the PT, resulting in a protrusion of the left posterior occipital lobe in comparison with the right lobe, as seen in the Yakelovian torque.

Evolutionary Significance

Functional asymmetry of speech perception is thus supported by an asymmetry in the gross anatomy and favors a rapid processing of the phonetic structure of the speech signal. It should be noted that Gannon et al.

(1998; see also Gannon, 2010) reported on a leftward asymmetry of the chimpanzee PT area that was similar to the asymmetry found in the human brain. One can only speculate as to the evolutionary significance of such a coincidence, as chimpanzees never developed speech understanding (or speech production). It could be that speech and language were evolutionarily "prepared" in the primate brain but sacrificed during evolutionary history due to other more salient developments such as quadrupedia and a shorter vocal tract.

THE DICHOTIC LISTENING PARADIGM

In addition to studies of brain anatomy and animal investigations, studies of brain-lesioned subjects (e.g., aphasia or similar conditions) have demonstrated that phonological decoding has a neuronal correlate in the upper posterior region of the left temporal lobe, including the HG and PT (Rasmussen & Milner, 1977). However, clinical studies have been fraught with the disadvantage of brain lesions, which have confounded the examination of underlying principles and mediating factors. We adopted the simple behavioral technique of DL to study the asymmetry of speech perception in the left hemisphere in healthy subjects (see Hugdahl & Andersson, 1984; Hugdahl et al., 2009). DL involves the presentation of two different syllables at the same time, in the right and left ear, respectively. CV syllables are the most common stimuli used today, building the dichotic pairs from the six stop consonants paired with the vowel /a/, thus presenting pairs of CV syllables such as /ba/ – /pa/ and /da/ – /ka/ and using every possible combination of the six basic syllables (originally introduced by Studdert-Kennedy & Shankweiler, 1970).

The Right-Ear Advantage (REA)

Despite its simplicity, the DL task causes a strong bottom-up stimulus-driven advantage in healthy subjects to report the right-ear stimulus with greater accuracy than the left-ear stimulus. This right-ear advantage (REA) is caused by the preponderance of the contralateral auditory pathways, the asymmetry of speech processing (which favors the left hemisphere), and the right-ear stimulus. Figure 3.2 illustrates the principles behind the REA in DL (see also Hugdahl, 2011; Kimura, 1967, 2011).

The DL paradigm developed in Bergen, Norway, has been translated into nearly 10 different languages. The paradigm is available for interested users either as a CD or as a PC program (run in E-prime), and comes together with a manual in English and with norms for different age groups,

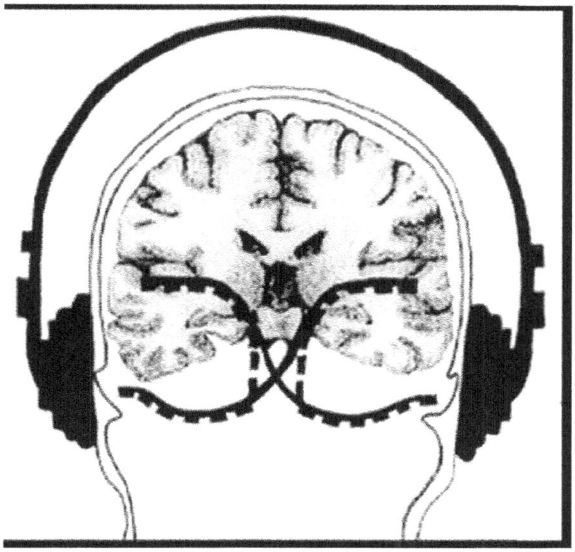

Figure 3.1. Schematic drawing of the major auditory neural pathways from the ear to the processing areas in the upper posterior parts of the temporal lobe.

gender, and handedness. The interested researcher or clinician may obtain the test by sending an e-mail to hugdahl@psybp.uib.no. In 2011, the test was launched as an iPhone app that may be downloaded for free from the App Store and run from an iPhone, iPod, or iPad. The app is listed under the "Education" category and can also be searched for under the name "iDichotic." After taking the test, the results can be submitted to a secure FTP server at the University of Bergen after approval by the individual subject. An updated version is available to allow the researcher to download data directly from the smartphone device.

THE BERGEN DL DATABASE

Over the years, we have collected data from the Bergen version of the DL paradigm, originally developed by Hugdahl and Andersson (1986). Today, the database consists of results sent in from other laboratories and clinics where the same Bergen paradigm has been used and includes 1,800 healthy male and female, right- and left-handed subjects aged 7–89. Because the data were collected from different countries, laboratories, and clinics, substantial noise also entered into the database. This may however be considered as a strength of the DL database, as the effects of the REA "survived" the interference factors that were entered when the data were collected from the different sites. Figure 3.3 shows a graphic scatter plot based on 383 adult subjects from the baseline condition, that is, nonforced (NF) attention, where the subjects were not given any instructions related to focusing their attention on either the right or left side. The x- and y-axes denote the percentage of correct reports from the right and left ears, respectively, and the 45° diagonal line divides the response space into an REA region (below the line) and a left-ear advantage (LEA) region (above the line).

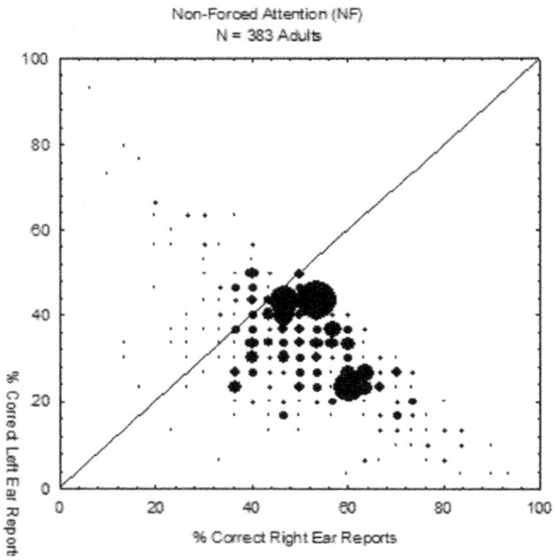

Figure 3.3. Scatter plot of scores from 651 adults (between 20 and 80 years old) on the standard version of the dichotic listening paradigm. The x-axis shows the percentage of correct reports from the right ear (0%–100%), and the y-axis shows the percentage of correct reports from the left ear (0%–100%). The larger the "ink blob," the more subjects occupying the same x and y coordinates in the response space, that is, showing similar right and left ear performance results, respectively. The diagonal line shows the 45° "symmetry line," that is, the subjects whose scores fall on the line and therefore show neither a right-ear advantage (REA) nor a left-ear advantage (LEA). All of the individuals below the line show an REA, and all of the individuals above the line show an LEA.

Table 3.1 shows data from 1,294 healthy subjects, with means and standard deviations, separated for age and gender.

Table 3.1. Descriptive Statistics of Left and Right Ear Scores for Right-Handed Female and Male Participants as a Function of Experimental Condition and (*N* = 1294). Standards Deviations in Parenthesis

Males		NON-FORCED		FORCED-RIGHT		FORCED-LEFT	
Age	N	RE	LE	RE	LE	RE	LE
<10	328	46.49 (10.75)	36.65 (9.81)	54.70 (13.27)	30.64 (10.86)	40.69 (13.01)	44.59 (14.11)
10-19	100	43.30 (9.14)	33.43 (9.17)	45.23 (10.56)	29.83 (9.38)	40.20 (10.16)	34.73 (10.90)
20-29	134	48.33 (10.94)	33.03 (9.21)	57.76 (14.70)	26.44 (10.50)	35.40 (13.83)	46.02 (14.94)
30-39	29	51.49 (10.75)	30.69 (8.65)	59.66 (12.92)	24.94 (10.60)	37.24 (16.14)	45.63 (17.32)
40-49	13	53.08 (17.18)	33.08 (15.84)	67.69 (14.23)	21.54 (11.83)	42.82 (16.82)	44.87 (17.41)
50-59	22	49.24 (19.08)	33.33 (15.63)	56.06 (18.96)	26.97 (12.68)	41.21 (16.15)	41.21 (16.92)
60-69	23	52.75 (17.60)	31.59 (14.63)	61.74 (13.78)	24.49 (13.13)	37.97 (16.48)	41.01 (16.56)
70-89	15	51.11 (16.27)	24.67 (10.97)	58.89 (20.84)	20.44 (15.16)	48.00 (23.83)	31.33 (25.19)
	664	**47.14 (11.70)**	**34.55 (10.40)**	**54.74 (14.37)**	**28.68 (11.11)**	**39.53 (13.75)**	**42.91 (15.08)**

Females		NON-FORCED		FORCED-RIGHT		FORCED-LEFT	
Age	N	RE	LE	RE	LE	RE	LE
<10	264	47.80 (12.01)	33.98 (9.45)	58.21 (14.00)	28.06 (11.51)	37.54 (14.00)	47.22 (15.75)
10-19	99	41.89 (10.46)	33.67 (8.21)	44.41 (10.94)	28.01 (8.82)	37.24 (11.13)	34.28 (10.16)
20-29	142	51.39 (9.07)	34.79 (9.56)	62.02 (13.16)	25.96 (10.11)	35.66 (15.69)	50.70 (16.54)
30-39	15	51.56 (9.75)	39.33 (9.28)	64.00 (10.71)	25.33 (9.24)	38.00 (13.08)	50.89 (17.52)
40-49	24	53.19 (12.26)	34.31 (12.72)	68.19 (16.71)	23.19 (15.40)	36.94 (16.15)	50.42 (18.37)
50-59	41	47.89 (18.62)	37.80 (18.63)	61.30 (20.03)	27.72 (18.76)	33.25 (15.48)	54.23 (17.29)
60-69	23	53.04 (14.10)	29.13 (11.34)	60.00 (21.67)	27.54 (17.87)	40.72 (22.27)	43.04 (18.64)
70-89	22	48.03 (15.79)	21.21 (9.12)	62.27 (17.10)	14.55 (7.46)	46.52 (25.29)	26.52 (21.95)
	630	**48.18 (12.31)**	**33.88 (10.67)**	**57.83 (15.58)**	**26.81 (11.97)**	**37.21 (15.13)**	**45.76 (17.15)**

Validation of the REA

Neuroimaging Studies

A critical question related to the REA in healthy individuals is the degree to which it reflects a true left-hemisphere processing advantage. This question can be addressed by validating the behavioral REA scores against parallel data acquired via functional neuroimaging (PET, fMRI) and brain lesion studies. Neuroimaging studies (Hugdahl et al., 1999; van den Noort, Specht, Rimol, Ersland, & Hugdahl, 2008) have revealed a similar response structure to that of the behavioral REA, with increased neuronal activation observed in the left HG and PT regions compared with homologous regions in the right hemisphere. Thus, these studies have essentially validated the left-hemisphere neuronal basis for the behavioral REA, showing stronger activation to dichotic presentations of CV syllables in the left temporal lobe while the subject is in the MR scanner (see Hugdahl et al., 1999; Tervaniemi & Hugdahl, 2003; van den Noort et al., 2008). Figure 3.4 shows the fMRI data related to repeated dichotic presentations of CV syllable pairs in axial slices.

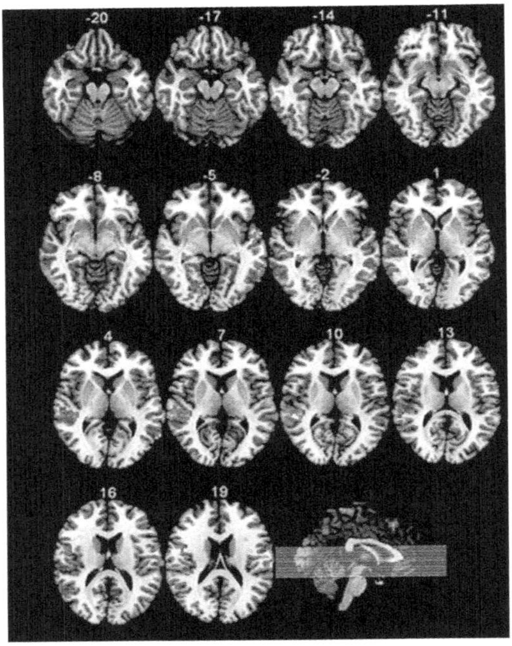

Figure 3.4. The functional magnetic resonance imaging (fMRI) results of healthy individuals who performed the standard version of the dichotic listening task. The results are calculated as intraclass correlations > .85, which means that only the voxels with correlations greater than .85 activated across three repetitions of the task are shown. The data were taken from a study by van den Noort et al. (2008) with the permission of the authors.

Lesion Studies

Lesion studies also validate the REA. Patients with circumscribed brain lesions perform the DL task, and their scores are recorded separately for the right- and left-ear CV syllables. Two lesion studies that used the Bergen paradigm include one conducted at the University of Leipzig and the Max-Planck Institute for Cognitive Neuroscience in Leipzig, Germany (Pollmann, Maertens, von Cramon, Lepsien, & Hugdahl, 2002) and another carried out at the Östra Hospital in Gothenburg, Sweden (Hugdahl, Carlsson, Uvebrant, & Lundervold, 1997). The German study investigated DL performance in patients with cerebrovascular lesions affecting the corpus callosum, which connects the two hemispheres. The hypothesis was that patients with lesions in the posterior part of the corpus callosum, where the auditory fibers cross over, would only have input from the right-ear CV syllable because no transfer of the left-ear syllable would occur due to the lesion. These patients were thus expected to show an enhanced REA compared with patients with a more anterior lesion and with healthy controls. The results confirmed the hypothesis by indicating an almost 100% REA in the patients, with the most posterior lesions affecting the isthmus and particularly the splenium region of the corpus callosum. The Swedish study investigated the REA in adolescent subjects before surgery for epilepsy. One standard test for language asymmetry before epilepsy surgery, and especially before temporal lobe resection on the left side, involves performing a sodium-amytal test, also known as a Wada test after its originator Juhn Wada. Sodium-amytal is a barbiturate that temporarily sedates one hemisphere at a time for about 7–8 minutes when injected into the bloodstream to the brain. By investigating language function while sedating the left and right hemispheres separately, the lateralization of speech and language may be determined on an individual basis. The Wada test is the "gold-standard" to determine language asymmetry, and other measures could thus be validated against the Wada method. The patients who participated in the study in Gothenburg, Sweden, also underwent the DL test after first determining the side of speech representation with the Wada test, making their DL performance comparable with the Wada test outcomes. The results are shown in Figure 3.5 and reveal that the DL procedure correctly classified every left-hemisphere speech dominant subject except one and all three of the right-hemisphere dominant subjects. Taken together, neuroimaging and brain lesion studies (Hugdahl et al., 1999, 1997; Pollmann et al., 2002; van den Noort et al., 2008) have corroborated the behavioral REA as a valid and robust indicator of speech lateralization.

MODULATIONS OF THE REA

Intensity Shifts

The REA is sensitive to a range of modulations, from perceptual to cognitive parameters (see Hugdahl et al., 2009; Rimol, Eichele, & Hugdahl, 2006; see also Westerhausen, Helland, Ofte, & Hugdahl, 2010). In terms of the perceptual parameters, changing the saliency of the right- or left-ear syllable relative to the other affects the magnitude of the REA and ultimately shifts it to an LEA. An example of manipulating relative saliency is to increase the intensity of the syllable in one ear relative to the other. This was done by Hugdahl et al. (2008); see also Westerhausen, Moosmann et al., 2010), who gradually increased the intensity in the right ear from 70 dB to +21 dB in steps of 3 dB at a time and did similarly for the left-ear stimulus. These manipulations produced a linear increase in the number

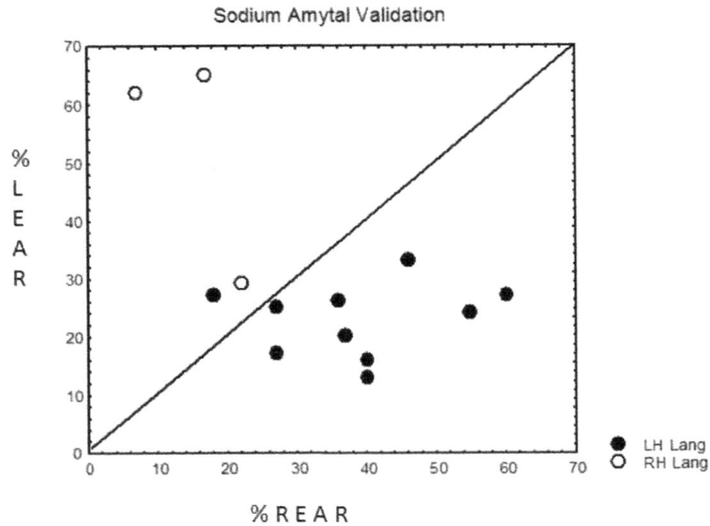

Figure 3.5. Validating performance on the dichotic listening task with performance on a sodium-amytal (Wada) test in 11 adolescent individuals before surgical treatment for epilepsy. The data were taken from a study by Hugdahl et al. (1997) with permission from the authors and the publisher.

of correctly reported items from the right or left ear as the intensity was linearly increased in either the right or left ear, relative to the other ear.

By systematic varying the interaural intensity differences between the ears, it is possible to express a cognitive construct (the REA) in physical terms (dB), thus creating a psychophysics situation in which a complex mental concept could be operationally defined in objective dB terms. The effects of relative intensity shifts on the REA for the right- or left-ear syllables are shown in Figure 3.6 (in 3-dB increments.)

Clinical Studies

We have now begun studying how various clinical groups cope with using top-down processes to modulate a bottom-up perceptual effect when the task gradually becomes more and more difficult due to the difference in

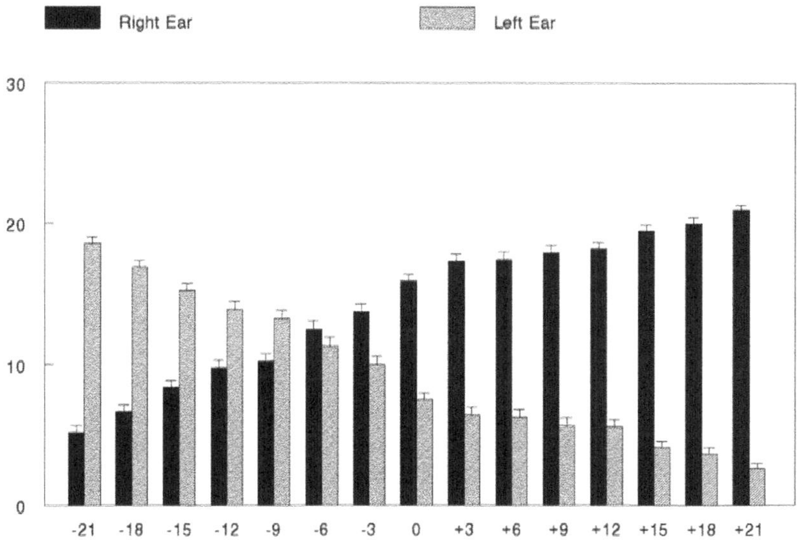

Figure 3.6. Mean percentage of the correct reports on the y-axis for the right- and left-ear syllables with an intensity increased in steps of 3 dB. The increased right-ear intensity is shown to the right on the x-axis (+dB), and the increased left-ear intensity is shown to the left on the x-axis (-dB).

interaural intensity. So far we have preliminary data from patients with schizophrenia which show that these patients seems to be vulnerable to the intensity manipulation and that this correlates with positive symptoms, in particular auditory hallucination. The latter would make sense if it is assumed that auditory hallucinations are speech-like ("hearing voices") perceptions without an acoustic source signal, and moreover, if auditory hallucinations originated in the same brain regions as ordinary speech perceptions (Hugdahl et al., 2009; see also Jones, 2010 for a discussion of different theoretical models for the origin of auditory hallucinations). If auditory hallucinations in schizophrenia originate from the same brain regions in the left temporal lobe, including the HG and PT, it could be predicted that the schizophrenia patient's experience of "hearing voices" will interfere with hearing real voices, that is, that the perception of CV syllables spoken by a real voice is compromised by the simultaneous presence of hallucinatory "voices." Preliminary data from our laboratory supports this prediction, as patients with schizophrenia were less sensitive to the intensity manipulation then the healthy control subjects (see also recent meta-analysis by Kompus et al., 2011).

A second set of predictions indicates that children with reading and other language-related problems and children experiencing delayed language development are especially vulnerable to intensity manipulation in the sense that they fail to use attention to overcome the intensity increase at relatively low levels of interaural differences compared with adults and children without reading problems.

A final set of predictions indicates that bilingual individuals and particularly professional interpreters working in environments such as the UN and European Parliament should be better than monolingual individuals at coping with increasing interaural intensity differences in right- and left-ear DL stimuli, as they should have an enhanced capacity for executive functioning and the ability to switch between the two syllables of dichotic pairs despite one being of greater intensity. The ability of bilingual individuals to switch to an LEA when instructed to focus on and report from the left ear in the standard top-down situation with equal intensity between the two stimuli was recently shown in a study by Soveri, Laine, Hämäläinen, and Hugdahl (2011), which also showed significantly enhanced reports from the left ear in bilinguals compared with monolinguals.

Voicing and Voice Onset Time

A second class of REA modulation involves the systematic variation of voiced versus unvoiced syllable pairs, where the right- and left-ear stimuli exhibit different voicing features for the syllables. "Voicing" is a phonetics term denoting the difference in onset time from the onset of the consonant segment for the pulsing of the glottals when pronouncing a stop-consonant syllable. Unvoiced CV syllables such as /pa/, /ta/, and /ka/ have long voice onset times (VOTs, 75–80 ms) compared with voiced CV syllables such as /ba/, /da/, and /ga/ (20–25 ms). Combining an unvoiced syllable in the right ear and a voiced syllable in the left ear of the dichotic pair produces a large REA. The reversed combination, an unvoiced syllable in the left ear and a voiced syllable in the right ear, produces an LEA, that is, better performance for the left-ear stimulus. The two conditions with equally voiced syllables, either unvoiced-unvoiced or voiced-voiced in the left and right ear, respectively, produce intermediate-sized REAs. The effects of voicing and systematically combining syllable pairs with different or equal VOTs for the individual syllables in a dichotic pair is seen in Figure 3.7.

The ability to modulate the size and direction of the ear advantage in DL can therefore be considered a marker of basic phonological "awareness." The VOT effect could also be considered a subphonetic manipulation of a signal's acoustic features, for example, the slope of a syllable's consonant segment onset in its initiation. Seen as an acoustic manipulation, the VOT effect could be considered a prerequisite for phonetic processing. Figure 3.8 shows the development of the ability to modulate the REA as a function of voicing or VOT (data taken from Westerhausen, Helland et al., 2010) in children who were tested repeatedly from ages 5 to 8.

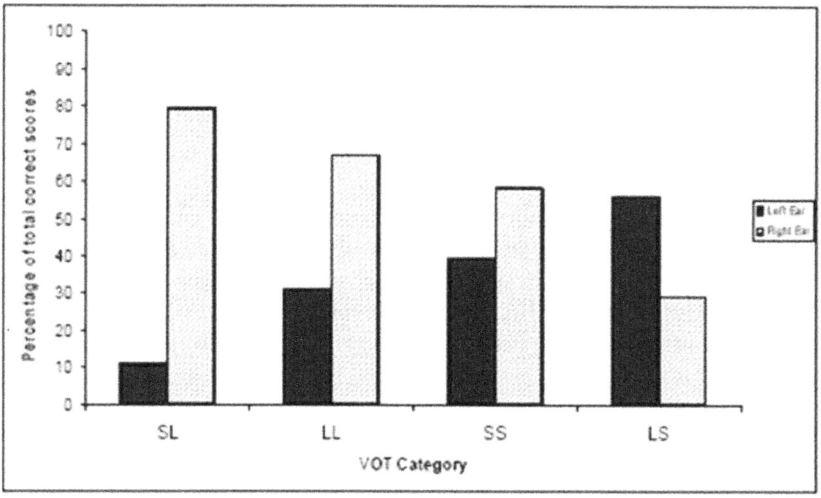

Figure 3.7. The effect of VOT on the correct right- and left-ear reports. VU = voiced CV in the left ear and unvoiced CV in the right ear; VV = voiced CV in both ears; UU = unvoiced CV in both ears; UV = unvoiced CV in the left ear and voiced CV in the right ear.

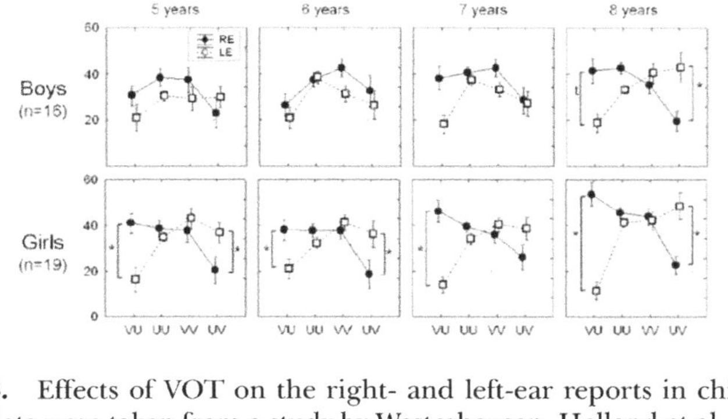

Figure 3.8. Effects of VOT on the right- and left-ear reports in children aged 5–8. The data were taken from a study by Westerhausen, Helland et al. (2010) with permission from the authors and the publisher.

Developmental Effects

As Figure 3.8 shows, there is a clear developmental effect across ages in terms of the children's ability to modulate the REA to an unvoiced-voiced combination for the right- and left-ear stimuli, respectively (seen to the left in the graphs), with a full effect initially seen at the age of 8. Perhaps of greater interest, when the data are split between the boys and the effect seen in the upper panel was mainly driven by the girls' earlier maturation, with the boys lagging by about 2 years in comparison. These results may explain why girls are more advanced in acquiring reading skills compared with boys, especially at ages 6–7. Thus, by studying the ability to modulate the REA in the DL task, which is a low-level perceptual/phonetic task, it is possible to unravel underlying mediating mechanisms required for literacy and reading ability.

At Risk for Dyslexia

Unpublished data from our laboratory have indicated that children at risk of developing dyslexia failed to show an LEA to the syllable combination with an unvoiced syllable in the left ear and voiced syllable in the right ear as the control subjects did, even at the age of 8. Thus, the VOT data showed that (a) dyslexia involves an inability to decode the phonological structures of syllables and words and (b) this may be a risk factor for dyslexia if identified at an early age. The data failed, however, to reveal an expected VOT effect in the dichotic situation at an early age before literacy. Although other phonological tests assess VOT properties, no available test simultaneously assesses VOT in relation to hemispheric asymmetry and laterality, as the DL procedure does.

ATTENTION-FOCUS INSTRUCTIONS

The perception of the CV syllables in the dichotic pair may also be manipulated by selectively instructing the subject to explicitly pay attention to and report from only the right or left ear, inducing a kind of top-down cognitive modulation of the REA while keeping the stimulus parameters constant. By instructing the subjects to pay attention to and explicitly report either the right or left ear stimulus, top-down driven modulation of the bottom-up stimulus-driven REA can be studied, thus revealing how cognitive factors modulate a built-in perceptual REA.

The study of how cognitive factors such as attention modulate the REA is an important extension of traditional approaches to speech perception. It provides an experimental analog to the real-life everyday situation of more than one stimulus source being presented simultaneously, as in the well-known "cocktail party" situation. Speech perception would be chaotic for the brain if it did not have a mechanism to filter out irrelevant sources and focus on relevant aspects of the acoustic input. This mechanism comprises attentional focus and the ability to refocus attention to a competing input source. When a subject is instructed to pay attention to the right side in auditory space in the DL situation and focus on the right-ear stimulus, the REA increases because the bottom-up ear advantage and top-down instruction act in concordance. However, when the subject is instructed to focus attention on the left-ear stimulus, the REA is reduced, and in many instances is shifted to an LEA. This last situation could be considered an executive or cognitive control situation with a processing conflict between the bottom-up tendency to report the right-ear stimulus and the top-down tendency to report the left-ear stimulus. Such a conflict would require cognitive resources for effective input inhibition, that may be unequally distributed among subjects and among clinical groups.

The Forced-Attention Paradigm

Figure 3.9 shows the scatter plots of 651 adults in the Bergen DL database for the three attention-instruction conditions. They include a nonforced (NF) attention condition with no instruction related to forcing attention focus to either side, which establishes a bottom-up lateralized REA; a forced-right (FR) condition with attention focused on the right-ear stimulus and a forced-left (FL) condition with attention focused on the left-ear stimulus. The left-hand panel shows the data for the NF attention condition (also shown in Figure 3.2), the middle panel shows the data for the FR attention condition, and the right-hand panel shows the data for the FL attention condition.

As Figure 3.9 shows, instructing the subjects to pay attention to either the right- or left-ear stimulus had profound effects on the REA. The NF condition could be considered a nonforced baseline because attention is not forced to either side through explicit instructions. Thus, it reflects a hemispheric asymmetry for CV syllables in the absence of explicit cognitive manipulations. The data for the FR condition showed that the REA was dramatically enhanced with almost the entire sample showing an REA, also supported by significantly more correct reports from the right-ear stimulus. This condition could be considered a nonexecutive attention condition, as the stimulus-driven baseline REA and the attention focus acted synergistically to produce an even larger REA. The right-hand panel in Figure 3.9 shows that when instructed to pay attention to and report from the left ear, the majority of the healthy adult subjects reversed the REA to an LEA. However, the number of subjects who continued to show an REA was much greater than the number of subjects who showed an LEA in the

FR condition. The spread of the scatters is also larger for the FL condition compared with the FR condition, indicating increased individual variability in the former condition. The individual variability indicates in turn that the task was more difficult for some subjects in the FL attention-instruction condition.

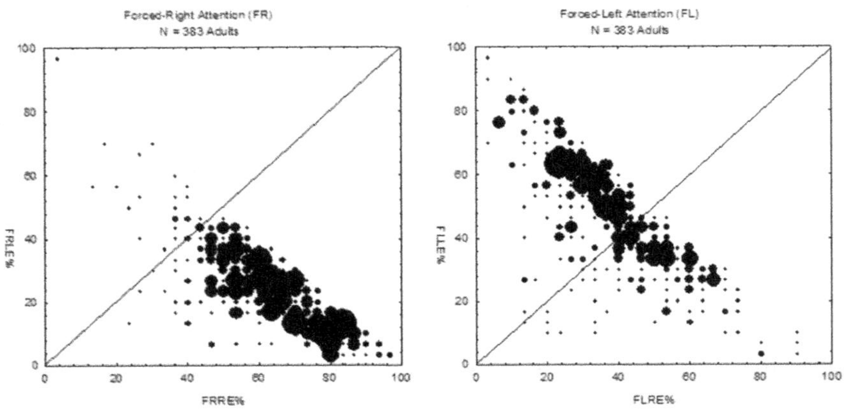

Figure 3.9. Scatter plots of the percentages of correct reports for the right- (x-axis) and left-ear (y-axis) CV syllables when the subjects were instructed to pay attention and explicitly report the right- or left-ear CV syllable. NF = nonforced attention instruction; FR = forced-right attention instruction; FL = forced-left attention instruction.

A Separate Cognitive Process

After going through the available evidence Hugdahl et al. (2009) concluded that the FL attention condition is an executive, cognitive control condition, wherein it is important to inhibit the bottom-up REA and refocus attention to the left-ear stimulus, which requires executive cognitive resources.

Over the years, the dichotic forced-attention paradigm originally developed by Hugdahl and Andersson (1986) has been applied to a number of clinical conditions and states and produced remarkably similar findings across diagnostic categories. These studies have been conducted in numerous laboratories and clinics worldwide, and only a brief summary of the findings is given here. Patients with psychosis such as schizophrenia have failed to reverse the REA to an LEA when instructed to pay attention to left-ear stimuli (FL instruction condition), which could be understood as a failure of executive control caused by deficient prefrontal lobe functioning. The same effect has interestingly been seen in patients with post-traumatic stress disorder (PTSD), Alzheimer's disease, and attention-deficit hyperactivity disorder (ADHD), to name a few examples. Figure 3.10 illustrates the failure of several clinical groups to use cognitive control to reverse an REA to an LEA in the FL attention condition.

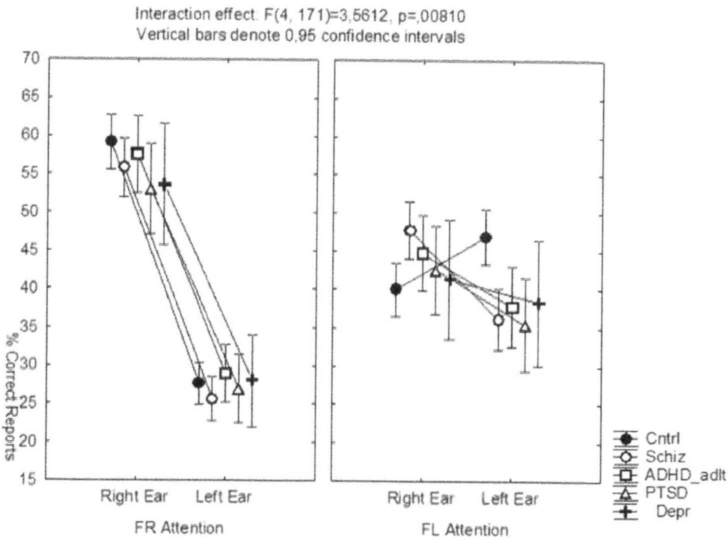

Figure 3.10. Percentage of correct right- and left-ear reports made by the healthy control subjects and patients with various psychiatric disorders for the FR and FL attention instruction conditions.

Common Cognitive Deficits Across Diagnoses

Although the aforementioned disorders have very little if anything in common when it comes to their etiology and diagnostic criteria, they may share a commonality in terms of prefrontal executive cognitive deficits. A commonality of impairment in a cognitive function across diagnostic labels such as schizophrenia and PTSD could reveal a commonality in the pathology of the underlying cognitive structure that stretches beyond clinical symptoms and diagnostic criteria. Although schizophrenia and PTSD do not show commonalities in terms of their clinical symptoms and etiologies, they share a common cognitive dysfunction in terms of their cognitive control and executive functions. In other words, although the clinical manifestations of these disorders show no clinical comorbidity, their cognitive dysfunctions do. This may have implications for theories of underlying mechanisms for these disorders, emphasizing a dimensional rather than a normative approach to diagnostics and treatment.

It has long been known that cognitive impairments in schizophrenia may persist despite symptom reductions after medical treatment (Green, 1996; Green, Kern, Braff, & Mintz, 2000). It has also been shown that schizophrenia patients with preserved secondary verbal memory and executive function impairment even after successful symptom reductions have poor social adjustment and community functioning (Buchanan, Holstein, & Breier, 1994; Green, 1998; Johnstone, Macmillan, Frith, Benn, & Crow, 1990), a finding that has interestingly also applied to PTSD patients (Azarnow et al., 1999; Walter, Palmierei, & Gunstad, 2010).

Dyslexia and Language Disorders

Child language disorders such as dyslexia, specific language impairment (SLI), and possibly also auditory processing deficit (APD) each indicate an inability to reveal an LEA when instructed to attend to left-ear stimuli. Again, this is understood as an impairment of executive control. In all of these groups, the lateralized bottom-up perceptual REA dominates despite the patients receiving instructions to disengage their attention from the right-ear stimuli and to report the left ear stimulus. The forced-attention DL paradigm has the advantage of experimental simplicity and simple task demands, which makes it possible to compare patients from many different clinical conditions on the same paradigm and yields directly comparable results. This overcomes the general disadvantage of traditional neuropsychological and linguistic tests. Such tests differ by degree in their processing demands and task difficulty. Both of these factors make it difficult to interpret the testing failure of a demented patient, which may result simply from the patient's failure to understand a task.

Several studies have shown that children with dyslexia experience problems with tasks that require executive and control functions, such as working memory (Beneventi, Tønnessen, Ersland, & Hugdahl, 2010; Helland & Asbjørnsen, 2000; Jeffres & Everatt, 2004). Thus, it is reasonable to expect children with dyslexia to be impaired on the report-left but not the report-right condition in the forced-instruction dichotic task. Such an outcome contributes to a more fine-grained characterization of cognitive impairments in dyslexia, independent of the general difficulty of the tests used or the metacognitive abilities of the subjects being tested. Because the nonexecutive attention demands in the report-right condition and the executive demands in the report-left condition are tested in the same experimental setup, with only a single word in the instruction differing between the two conditions, any difference in performance between the two conditions must be caused by the differences in the underlying cognitive structure of the two subtasks. This provides strong support for a specific executive and cognitive control deficit in dyslexia, independent of a general attention deficit that is not seen in this disorder. Previous studies hinting at a general attentional deficit in dyslexia might therefore have been the result of differences in the tests used to address attentional and executive functions.

Robustness of the FL Effect

The clinical data shown in Figure 3.10 reveal statistically significant group differences for the FL condition where the clinical groups are compared with the healthy controls (cntrl). This should be compared with the FR condition, which shows overlapping results for the groups being compared. In some cases, the differences between the groups and graphs are almost invisible for the FR condition. An advantage with the forced-attention DL paradigm applied to clinical comparisons is that there are two kinds of experimental control built into the data by default. The first is the within-group comparison between the FR and FL conditions and across the studies, with the hypothesis that there should be a clear difference in performance in the FR and FL conditions. The second is the between-group comparison between the clinical and healthy control groups for the FR and FL conditions. The groups should not differ in the FR condition but show clear differences in the FL condition.

The Evolution of an Explanation

This section presents collected citations from three articles that our group has published over the last 25 or so years in an attempt to explain the different effects observed for the FR and FL attention conditions. The length of time it took us to realize that the instruction to focus attention on either the right- or left-ear stimulus induces fundamentally different cognitive processes may seem odd in retrospect. It is also obvious from the different citations that we approached the view that we hold today gradually. However, it was not until we began examining patient groups that the full scope of the studies emerged. In our defense, during the 1980s, the focused-attention manipulation that resulted from instructions to only report right- or left-ear stimuli was used to control for the unwanted effects of attention that would "confound" a true laterality effect (cf. Bryden, Munhall, & Allard, 1983). Thus, when we more or less accidentally observed the differential FR and FL effects in 1986 (Hugdahl &

Andersson, 1986), we did not consider it particularly interesting beyond an explanation as a control condition, as most hemisphere asymmetry theories at the time considered laterality differences to be results of the nature of the stimuli. We moreover originally thought that the "instruction effect" was solely the result of attention and did not consider that it could be tapping executive functions. The respective citations below are taken from studies by Hugdahl and Andersson (1986), Asbjørnsen and Hugdahl (1995) and Hugdahl et al. (2009), and illustrate how our thinking on the top-down modulation of the REA evolved over a 15-year period:

> A few recent investigators have argued that the REA-effect may be brought about by a bias to selectively attend to the right side.... The argument is that when subjects are left free to report the items, they may chose the order in which they report, and ... attend to the right and left ear stimulus. Bryden (1982) has argued that it should be easier to focus attention on items from the right ear. Although it is somewhat unclear why it should be easier to "listen" to the right ear, it is obviously important to control for effects of attention. (Hugdahl & Andersson, 1986, p. 418)

In 1995 (Asbjørnsen & Hugdahl, 1995), we advanced our understanding of the FL attention effect by one step and realized that there may be different cognitive processes behind the performance of the FR and FL conditions. However, it had not yet struck us that this really was the case. Instead, we were puzzled that the difference was caused by an inhibition of responses to the contralateral ear rather than the enhancement of responses to the ipsilateral ear. The following is a quotation from our 1995 article:

> Although there seems to be some consensus among researchers ... that attentional factors modulate a structurally based ear advantage, there seems to be little, or no, consensus as to the basis of the attentional effect.... Generally speaking, attentional effects in DL can be the result of two processes: facilitation of correct reports from the attended ear or inhibition of intrusions from the unattended ear ... (or) both processes being present.... [T]hese results are surprising from both structural ... and attentional ... models of dichotic listening. One would predict enhancement of ear advantages during forced attention ... to be mediated by facilitation of correct reports from the attended ear, rather than inhibition of reports from the non-attended ear. (Asbjørnsen & Hugdahl, p. 198)

However, by 2009, the nature of the underlying cognitive mechanisms for the FR and FL conditions was apparent, and we made the following claim:

> We now believe that instructions to focus attention on the right or left ear stimulus induces different degrees of cognitive conflict and a corresponding

> need for (executive) cognitive control strategies.... It was found that patients with schizophrenia could not modulate the REA when instructed to focus attention and reporting the left ear stimulus while they were able to modulate the REA when ... focus[ing] on ... [the] right ear stimulus. Considering that the ... task is easy to perform it should not be more difficult to report the left ear stimulus, than to report ... [the] right ear stimulus.... [T]he FL situation ... involves ... cognitive conflict and [the] need for inhibitory control to counteract a bottom-up right ear response tendency ... [and] the ability to maintain focus in the presence of competing or interfering stimuli. (Hugdahl et al., 2009, p. 14)

FUTURE PERSPECTIVES

An interesting perspective for future studies would be to combine bottom-up and top-down experimental manipulations to conduct more fine-grained examinations of both laterality for speech perception and cognitive modulation via attention factors. Such an approach could combine the intensity-modulation paradigm with the forced-attention paradigm. Westerhausen, Helland et al. (2010) did so when they showed that the REA could withstand an intensity increase of the left-ear stimulus of about 6–9 dB before it yielded to an LEA. Researchers at the Max Planck Institute for Human Development in Berlin, Germany, similarly applied the intensity-modulated paradigm to study cognitive declines in the elderly (Passow et al., 2012). Their hypothesis was that as the task in the FL condition became increasingly difficult due to the gradual increase of the stimulus intensity in the right ear when instructed to focus attention to and report from the left ear, the differences in performance on the task would gradually increase between younger and older participants. Their results confirmed the decreased ability in the elderly to use cognitive control to compensate for the increase in intensity in the right ear when instructed to report from the left ear.

Using a new method of calculating the scores based on a combination of the laterality index and an interaural intensity difference index, Passow and colleagues (2012) found that older subjects lacked the flexibility of the younger subjects to use cognitive control to compensate for the gradual increase in task difficulty due to increasing interaural intensity differences. The researchers later continued using the intensity-modulated paradigm and studied the differences between younger (< 10 years) and older (> 10 years) children in terms of cognitive control and mental flexibility. Their findings showed a similar structure of cognitive inflexibility in young children, as seen in older adults. Thus, it seems that the mental flexibility provided by the use of cognitive control and executive processes is subject to a developmental trajectory that follows an inverted U-shape.

SUMMARY AND CONCLUSIONS

This chapter provides a selective review of our DL research at the University of Bergen over the last 25 years, highlighting bottom-up and top-down interactions in terms of processing simple speech sounds such as CV syllables. Because the wiring of the auditory pathways and the asymmetry of speech perception favor the left hemisphere, the dichotic signal input provides an ideal experimental situation for studying bottom-up and top-down interaction. The influence of top-down cognitive factors such as attention and executive functions has often been ignored in speech perception and sound processing theories and models, which have instead argued that such low-level processing is devoid of cognitive influence. As reviewed in this chapter, our research has shown that this is not the case, but rather that attention profoundly influences low-level acoustic-phonetic processes. I furthermore show how clinical group studies could combine a bottom-up and top-down perspective. Both child and adult disorders have revealed striking similarities in terms of mental flexibility impairment and lack of cognitive control in early childhood and late adulthood.

ACKNOWLEDGMENT

The chapter partly overlaps with a talk and following chapter given at the YLMP Conference on Language and Language Disorders in Poznan, Poland in 2010.

REFERENCES

Asbjørnsen, A., & Hugdahl, K. (1995). Attentional effects in dichotic listening. *Brain and Language, 49*, 189–201.

Azarnow, J., Glynn, S., Pynoss, R. S., Nahum, J., Guthrie, D., Cantwell, D. P., & Franklin, B. (1999). When the earth stops shaking: Earthquake sequelae among children diagnosed for pre-earthquake psychopathology. *Journal of the American Academy of Child and Adolescence Psychiatry, 38*, 1016–1023.

Beneventi, H., Tønnessen, F. E., Ersland, L., & Hugdahl, K. (2010). Executive working memory processes in dyslexia: Behavioral and fMRI evidence. *Scandinavian Journal of Psychology, 51*, 192–202.

Bryden, M. P., Munhall, K., & Allard, F. (1983). Attentional biases and the right-ear effect in dichotic listening. *Brain and Language, 18*, 236–248.

Buchanan, R. W., Holstein, C., & Breier, A. (1994). The comparative efficacy and long-term effect of clozapine treatment on neuropsychological test performance. *Biological Psychiatry, 36*, 717–725.

Dorsaint-Pierre, R., Penhune, V. B., Watkins, K. E., Neelin, P., Lerch, J. P., Bouffard, M., & Zatorre, R. J. (2006). Asymmetries of the planum temporale and Heschl's gyrus: Relationship to language lateralization. *Brain, 129*, 1164–1176.

Gannon, P. (2010). Evolutionary depth of human brain language areas. In K. Hugdahl & R. Westerhausen (Eds.), *The two halves of the brain* (pp. 37–64). Cambridge, MA: MIT Press.

Gannon, P. J., Holloway, R. L., Broadfield, D. C., & Braun, A. R. (1998). Asymmetry of chimpanzee planum temporale: Humanlike pattern of Wernicke's brain language area homolog. *Science, 279*, 220–222.

Geschwind, N., & Levitsky, W. (1968). Left-right asymmetries in temporal speech region. *Science, 161*, 186–187.

Green, M. F. (1996). What are the functional consequences of neurocognitive deficits in schizophrenia? *American Journal of Psychiatry, 153*, 321–330.

Green, M. F. (1998). *Schizophrenia from a neurocognitive perspective*. Boston, MA: Allyn and Bacon.

Green, M. F., Kern, R. S., Braff, D.-L., & Mintz, J. (2000). Neurocognitive deficits and functional outcome in schizophrenia: Are we measuring "the right stuff"? *Schizophrenia Bulletin, 26*, 119–136.

Helland, T., & Asbjørnsen, A. (2000). Executive functions in dyslexia. *Child Neuropsychology, 6*, 37–46.

Hugdahl, K. (2011). Fifty years of dichotic listening research—Still going and going and ... *Brain and Cognition, 76*, 211–213.

Hugdahl, K., & Andersson, B. (1984). A dichotic listening study of differences in cerebral organization in dextral and sinistral subjects. *Cortex, 20*, 135–141.

Hugdahl, K., & Andersson, L. (1986). The "forced-attention paradigm" in dichotic listening to CV-syllables: A comparison between adults and children. *Cortex, 22*, 417–432.

Hugdahl, K., Brønnick, K., Kyllingsbæk, S., Law, I., Gade, A., & Paulson, O. B. (1999). Brain activation during dichotic presentations of consonant-vowel and musical instruments stimuli: A 15O-PET study. *Neuropsychologia, 37*, 431–440.

Hugdahl, K., Carlsson, G., Uvebrant, P., & Lundervold, A. J. (1997). Dichotic-listening performance and intracarotid injections of amobarbital in children and adolescents: Preoperative and postoperative comparisons. *Archives of Neurology, 54*, 1494–1500.

Hugdahl, K., & Westerhausen, R. (2009). What is left is right: How speech asymmetry shaped the brain. *European Psychologist, 14*, 78–89.

Hugdahl, K., & Westerhausen, R. (2010). *The two halves of the brain*. Cambridge, MA: MIT Press.

Hugdahl, K., Westerhausen, R., Alho, K., Medvedev, S., Laine, M., & Hämäläinen, H. (2009). Attention and cognitive control: Unfolding the dichotic listening story. *Scandinavian Journal of Psychology, 50*, 11–22.

Jeffres, S., & Everatt, J. (2004). Working memory: Its role in dyslexia and other reading difficulties. *Dyslexia, 10*, 196–214.

Johnstone, E. C., Macmillan, J. F., Frith, C. D., Benn, D. K., & Crow, T. J. (1990). Further investigation of the predictors of outcome following first schizophrenic episodes. *British Journal of Psychiatry, 157*, 182–189.

Jones, S. R. (2010). Do we need multiple models of auditory verbal hallucinations? Examining the phenomenological fit of cognitive and neurological models. *Schizophrenia Bulletin*, *36*(3), 566–575.

Kimura, D. (1967). Functional asymmetry of the brain in dichotic listening. *Cortex*, *3*, 163–168.

Kimura, D. (2011). From ear to brain. *Brain and Cognition*, *76*, 214–217.

Kompus, K., Westerhausen, R., & Hugdahl, K. (2011). The "paradoxical" engagement of the primary auditory cortex in patients with auditory verbal hallucinations: A meta-analysis of functional neuroimaging studies. *Neuropsychologia*, *49*, 3361-3369.

Moncrieff, D. (2010). Hemispheric asymmetry in pediatric development disorders: Autism, attention-deficit hyperactivity disorder and dyslexia. In K. Hugdahl & R. Westerhausen (Eds.), *The two halves of the brain* (pp. 561–602). Cambridge, MA: MIT Press.

Musiek, F., Reeves, A., & Baran, J. (1985). Release from central auditory competition in the split-brain patient. *Neurology*, *35*, 983–987.

Obrzut, J., & Mahoney, E. B. (2011). Use of dichotic listening technique with learning disabilities. *Brain and Cognition*, *76*, 323–331.

Passow, S., Westerhausen, R., Wartenburger, I., Hugdahl, K., Heekeren, H. R., Lindenberger, U., & Li, S.-C. (2012). Human aging compromises attentional control of auditory perception. *Psychology and Aging*, *27*, 99–105.

Pollmann, S., Maertens, M., von Cramon, D. Y., Lepsien, J., & Hugdahl, K. (2002). Dichotic listening in patients with splenial and nonsplenial callosal lesions. *Neuropsychology*, *16*, 56–64.

Rasmussen, T., & Milner, B. (1977). The role of early left-brain injury in determining lateralization of cerebral speech function. *Annals of the New York Academy of Science*, *229*, 355–369.

Rimol, L. M., Eichele, T., & Hugdahl, K. (2006). The effect of voice-onset-time on dichotic listening with consonant-vowel syllables. *Neuropsychologia*, *44*(2), 191–196.

Sininger, Y. S., & Bhatara, A. (2012). Laterality of basic auditory perception. *Laterality*, *17*, 129–149.

Soveri, A., Laine, M., Hämäläinen, H., & Hugdahl, K. (2011). Bilingual advantage in attentional control: Evidence from the forced-attention dichotic listening paradigm. *Bilingualism: Language and Cognition*, *14*, 371–378.

Studdert-Kennedy, M., & Shankweiler, D. (1970). Hemispheric specialization for speech perception. *Journal of the Acoustical Society of America*, *48*, 579–594.

Tervaniemi, M., & Hugdahl, K. (2003). Lateralization of auditory-cortex functions. *Brain Research Reviews*, *43*, 231–246.

Toga, A. W., & Thompson, P. M. (2003). Mapping brain asymmetry. *Nature Reviews Neuroscience*, *4*, 37–48.

van den Noort, M., Specht, K., Rimol, L. M., Ersland, L., & Hugdahl, K. (2008). A new verbal reports fMRI dichotic listening paradigm for studies of hemispheric asymmetry. *Neuroimage*, *40*, 902–911.

Walter, K. H., Palmierei, P. A., & Gunstad, J. (2010). More than symptom reduction: Changes in executive function over the course of PTSD treatment. *Journal of Traumatic Stress*, *23*, 292–295.

Westerhausen, R., Helland, T., Ofte, S., & Hugdahl, K. (2010). A longitudinal study of the effect of voicing on the dichotic ear advantage in boys and girls at age 5 to 8. *Developmental Neuropsychology, 35*, 752–761.

Westerhausen, R., Moosmann, M., Alho, K., Belsby, S. O., Hämäläinen, H., Medvedev, S., et al. (2010). Identification of attention and cognitive control networks in a parametric auditory fMRI study. *Neuropsychologia, 48*, 2075–2081.

Yakovlev, P. I., & Rakic, P. (1996). Patterns of decussation of bulbar pyramids and distribution of pyramidal tracts on two sides of the spinal cord. *Transactions of the American Neurological Association, 91*, 366–367.

Zatorre, R. J., Evans, A., Meyer, E., & Gjedde, A. (1992). Lateralization of phonetic and pitch discrimination in speech processing. *Science, 256*, 846–849.

CHAPTER 4

CLINICAL ASSESSMENT OF AUDITORY PROCESSING DISORDER IN CHILDREN

Piers Dawes

Although it is not recognized by mainstream diagnostic classification systems, such as DSM-IV (APA, 2000) or ICD-10, APD is diagnosed in the United States (Emanuel, Ficca, & Korczak, 2011), Australasia (Cameron & Dillon, 2005) and interest the United Kingdom and elsewhere is increasing (Hind, 2006; Hind et al., 2011). APD is conceptualized as impairment in processing of information in the auditory central nervous system with difficulties identifying or discriminating sounds, despite normal peripheral hearing sensitivity. APD in children is a topic of interest because it is suggested that a disorder of auditory processing has a causal relationship with reading, language, and listening difficulties (e.g., Tallal, 2004). Treatments for these difficulties involve modifying the acoustic environment, teaching compensatory strategies, or attempting to address the presumed contribution of auditory processing by training auditory skills directly (Bellis, 2003).

The typical clinical presentation is of a school-aged child, a complaint of "listening difficulties" despite normal hearing sensitivity and poor academic achievement (Chermak & Musiek, 1997). Dawes and Bishop (2010) carried out a psychometric evaluation of children who had received

Understanding Developmental Disorders of Auditory Processing, Language and Literacy Across Languages: International Perspectives, pp. 67–90

a diagnosis of APD and found a highly heterogeneous group; some children would have fit a diagnosis of dyslexia, some SLI, some ADHD, and some may fit a diagnosis of Asperger's syndrome or high functioning autism. Other researchers from independent groups have come to similar conclusions (Ferguson, Hall, Riley, & Moore, 2011; Miller & Wagstaff, 2011; Sharma, Purdy, & Kelly, 2009). A suspicion raised by these studies was that the type of diagnosis may depend on the profession of the consulting clinician; those who had seen an audiologist would be diagnosed with APD, while those who had seen a speech-language therapist, educational psychologist, or pediatrician may receive a diagnosis of dyslexia, SLI, or ADHD. Co-occurrence of language difficulties in those with APD has long been recognized (Chermak & Musiek, 1997). The issue is whether auditory processing problems contribute to the child's academic/listening difficulties or whether these difficulties may be better explained in terms of established developmental disorders and thus may also be more appropriately addressed with different treatment and management approaches.

APD is therefore a controversial diagnosis. In this chapter, it is suggested that a focus on assessment of APD may be a way of addressing this controversy. We will begin with a discussion of the definition of APD and how this impacts upon assessment, then an overview of current APD assessments along with their advantages and shortcomings, some examples of recent studies that illustrate difficulties with APD assessment, and finally some recommendations for elucidating APD with a focus on assessment.

Definition of APD

The latest report by the American Speech-Language-Hearing Association (ASHA, 2005a) defines auditory processing, auditory processing disorder, and relevant areas of assessment. Auditory processing is described as involving the following skills:

- Sound localization and lateralization
- Auditory discrimination
- Auditory pattern recognition
- Temporal aspects of audition, including temporal integration, temporal ordering, and temporal masking
- Auditory performance in competing acoustic signals
- Auditory performance with degraded acoustic signals

APD is defined as a deficit on one or more of the above, with a basis in impaired processing of auditory perceptual information within the CNS.

APD is seen as a deficit in the neural processing of sound not due to higher order language, cognitive or related factors. The behavioral consequences of APD are taken to include misunderstanding rapid speech and difficulties following directions, listening in noisy environments, singing or appreciating music, and determining the location of sound.

Criticisms of the ASHA definition include (a) it simply being a list of symptoms rather than a coherent syndrome, with a likely overlap between the skills listed in terms of their dependence on a common set of more basic auditory skills (Chermak, 2001; McFarland & Cacace, 1995), and (b) the problematic distinction between a specifically auditory disorder and the contribution of global mechanisms such as attention and memory (Bellis & Ferre, 1999; Cacace & McFarland, 2005).

In practice, there is considerable variability in clinician and researchers' understanding of what is meant by "auditory processing disorder." The broadest conceptions characterize auditory processing as "what you do with what you hear," and this is taken by some to include sequencing and integration of any information through the auditory modality, including language comprehension. Impairments in auditory memory and inability to focus and sustain attention on the auditory signal may also be included in the conception of APD (e.g., the Test of Auditory Processing Skills; Martin & Brownell, 2005; also see Moore, 2012). Note that this definition would not fit with the ASHA conception of APD, which specifically excludes higher order language, cognitive or related factors.

Others include impairments of phonology and phonological awareness (awareness of sounds composing speech) as part of APD and include phonology as part of formal assessment and diagnostic subtyping of APD. At least in the field of psychology and psycholinguistics, phonology is typically considered to be a linguistically based skill (Wagner & Torgesen, 1987). A conception of APD that includes phonological processing would therefore be at odds with the ASHA definition of APD that excludes linguistic factors. One example of a conception of APD that involves phonological processing is the Buffalo model (Katz, 1992).[1] This model is based on patterns of performance on three tests; the Staggered Spondaic Word test (SSW; Katz, 1962), a phonemic synthesis test and a speech-in-noise test. In the SSW, overlapping two syllable (spondaic) words are presented to each ear via headphones, and the task is to repeat the word directed to a target ear. The phonemic synthesis test involves blending individual sounds to make a word, such as N-O-Z → "nose." Katz (1992) described four categories of performance, with associated treatment recommendations for each. For example, the "Decoding" category is characterized by a poor right-competing[2] score on the SSW, with a breakdown at the level of phonemic processing, possibly because of poorly specified phonological representations. The Buffalo model's test battery[3] relies on linguistically based tests and so may be readily affected by poor language skills. The inclusion of phonological processing as part of the definition of auditory processing suggests that any child with a phonological impairment (in other words, most cases of SLI and dyslexia) would be diagnosed with APD. Note that there has not yet been any experimental validation of any system of classification and treatment for APD.

The ASHA (2005a) definition of APD and the recent American Academy of Audiology (AAA) statement (2010) on APD both assert that APD is a sensory processing impairment due to disordered processing of sound in the central auditory nervous system. Both the ASHA and the AAA documents explicitly exclude a top-down, cognitive contribution to APD. In contrast, the British Society of Audiology (BSA) recently issued a position statement that said, "APD presents as impaired perception of both non-speech and speech sounds, and is *closely associated with impaired top-down, cognitive function. There is no evidence that it is produced by a primary, sensory disability*" (2010; my italics). This followed the findings of a large U.K. population-based study whose conclusion was that "listening difficulties" were associated with cognitive deficits (specifically, in attention). Although present in the general population, impairments in auditory processing were only very weakly associated with listening difficulties (Moore, Ferguson, Edmonson-Jones, Ratib, & Alison, 2010). Cognitive scores—not auditory processing skills—were the best predictors of listening, communication, and speech-in-noise performance (for a similar study in the United States, see Waston & Kidd, 2002; Watson et al., 2003). The marked discrepancy in conception of APD between the BSA and ASHA and the AAA underscores the lack of agreement about that APD is.

In summary, clinician and researchers' conception of APD varies, with significant disagreement even between national professional bodies such as the BSA, ASHA, and the AAA. An absence of consensus about what APD is has serious implications for both research and clinical practice: If there is no agreed definition, what should be measured, and how should the validity of assessment be established?

APD Diagnosis

If there is uncertainty about what APD actually is, reliable diagnosis seems elusive. ASHA's (2005b) recommendation is that diagnosis should be made by a multidisciplinary team, minimally a speech-language therapist working together with an audiologist. Peripheral hearing should be tested first using hearing thresholds, immittance measures, and otoacoustic emissions to rule out a peripheral hearing impairment. ASHA then recommends administration of an APD test battery in order to tap various aspects of auditory processing. ASHA does not recommend a specific test battery, although it does describe various categories of tests (based on the AHSA definition of APD), described in Table 4.1 (adapted from Dawes & Bishop, 2009, with permission).

Table 4.1. Descriptions of Common APD Tests

Description	*Example*
Temporal resolution: Ability to discriminate different durations of auditory stimuli or detect silent gaps between stimuli.	Random Gap Detection Test (Keith, 2000a)[ns]
Temporal Ordering: Perception and processing of the order of two or more auditory stimuli over time.	Pitch Patterns Sequence Test (Pinhiero, 1977)[ns]
Perception of artificially degraded speech: Speech may be time compressed, filtered, interrupted, or competing with background noise.	Filtered Words and Auditory Figure Ground subtests from the SCAN (Keith, 2000b)[s]
Dichotic listening: Two auditory stimuli are presented simultaneously, one to each ear. Listener is asked to attend to and report one or both stimuli.	Competing Words and Competing Sentences subtests from the SCAN (Keith, 2000b)[s] Staggered Spondiac Word Test (Katz, 1962)[s]
Binaural interaction, Localization, and Lateralization: Processing involving signals from both ears, dependent on interaural time and intensity differences.	The Listening in Spatialized Noise test (Cameron, Dillon, & Newall, 2006b)[s]
Electrophysiological measures. Recording of electrical brain responses to auditory stimuli.* Timing and shape of components of the recorded signal are thought to represent sequential stages of processing by different components of the auditory CNS.	Auditory Brainstem Response Middle Latency Response Late Evoked Response

Source: categories adapted from ASHA (2005a).

ns: nonspeech stimuli; s: speech stimuli
* Speech or nonspeech stimuli can be used to elicit responses. See "electrophysiological studies" below.

The ASHA guidelines (ASHA, 2005a) recommend that APD diagnosis be made on the basis of comparison with normative data, with performance greater than two standard deviations below the mean the (albeit arbitrary) cut-off, or with reference to specific patterns of deficit on intra- or intertest performance. A test battery approach may seem sensible in order to address various aspects of auditory processing. However, note that as the number of tests increases, so does the possibility of a child doing poorly merely by chance and so the possibility of mistaken diagnosis of APD (Binder, Iverson, & Brooks, 2009). ASHA (and the AAA, 2010) guidelines suggest that assessment should be individualized in order to take into account such things as age, cultural background, motor skill, visual acuity, memory, and language skill, although exactly how this should be done is not specified.

Various researchers have suggested appropriate test batteries for APD, and these are shown in Table 4.2 (adapted from Dawes & Bishop, 2009, with permission). The suggested test batteries are all different from each other, in terms of both selection of specific tests and the categories of performance addressed. All the suggested batteries include at least one dichotic listening test, although no battery contains a test in each of ASHA's test categories. Some batteries have more than one test per category, and only one (Jerger & Musiek, 2000) includes an electrophysiological test as a main measure. Jerger & Musiek's (2000) battery also seems the most comprehensive in terms of tapping the greatest number of test categories. This test battery was the result of a consensus meeting between a group of APD experts, although it was subsequently severely criticized by a rival group (Katz et al., 2002).

In terms of how diagnosis currently proceeds in clinical settings, surveys of clinical practice in the United States (Emanuel, 2002; Emanuel et al., 2011) and the United Kingdom (Hind, 2006) suggest that APD is diagnosed on the basis of responses to a questionnaire (either a commercially available one or a self-developed one) and an APD test battery, which varies depending on availability of particular tests. The SCAN (reviewed below) was one of the most commonly used APD tests. Different clinics appear to be using different test batteries and thus different criteria for diagnosing APD. If criteria for APD diagnosis vary between clinics and clinicians, it may be possible for a child to receive a diagnosis of APD at one clinic with one clinician but have APD excluded as a diagnosis at another.

APD Assessments

APD assessments include behavior rating scales, electrophysiological tests, and behavioral tests. Each category of tests is reviewed as follows.

Table 4.2. Suggested APD Test Batteries

Test Category	*Test Name*	*Test Battery*[a]				
		1.	*2.*	*3.*	*4.*	*5.*
Temporal resolution	Temporal gap detection	√ √				
	Tallal tests*		√			
	Backward masking				√ √	
Temporal Ordering	Duration pattern sequence test	√ √			√ √	
	Frequency patterns test	√ √			√ √	√ √
	Tests of temporal patterning			√ √		
Perception of artificially degraded speech.	Words in noise				√ √	
	Sentences in noise				√ √	
	Monaural low redundancy speech			√ √		
	Compressed speech		√			
	Filtered speech				√ √	
Dichotic listening	Dichotic digits	√ √	√ √	√ √	√ √	√ √
	Competing sentences		√ √			√ √
	Staggered Spondiac Word Test		√			√ √
Binaural interaction, Localization, and Lateralization	Binaural interaction tasks			√ √		
	Binaural fusion				√ √	

(Table continues on next page)

Table 4.2. (Continued)

		Test Battery[a]				
Test Category	*Test Name*	*1.*	*2.*	*3.*	*4.*	*5.*
Electro-physiological measures	Auditory brainstem response	√ √				
	Middle latency response	√ √	√ √			
	Cortical ERPs	√				
Other	Auditory vs. visual continuous performance	√				
	Questionnaire				√ √	

[a]Key: (1) Jerger & Musiek, 2000; (2) Musiek & Chermak, 1994; (3) Bellis & Ferre, 1999; (4) Neijenhuis, Stollman, Snik, & Van der Broek, 2001; (5) Musiek, Geurkink, & Kietel, 1982.
√√ main test: √ supplementary test
* Also known as the Repetition Test. See Tallal and Piercy (1973) for a description.

Behavior Rating Scales

Commonly used rating scales include Fisher's auditory problems checklist (Fisher, 1976), the Children's Auditory Performance Scale (CHAPS; Smoski, Brunt, & Tannahill, 1998), the Screening Identification for Targeting Educational Risk (SIFTER; Anderson, 1989), and the Scale of Auditory Behaviors (Schow & Seikel, 2006). Parents or teachers are asked to respond to questions about the child that relate to behaviors thought to be indicative of APD. For example, items from Fisher's (1976) checklist include "misunderstands or misinterprets what is said," "has difficulty following conversation," "has difficulty following spoken directions," "has difficulty with phonics," and "has a short attention span." Some rating scales (but not all) provide comparison with a normative sample so that a judgment can be made about the degree to which a child's behavior is typical of his or her peers or not.

One drawback with behavioral rating scales is that they are not specific to APD. For example, listening difficulties may indicate an auditory processing disorder, although they may alternatively be due to peripheral hearing loss, a memory or attention deficit, a social/pragmatic deficit, weak language skills, low general ability, or low motivation.[4] Rating scales do not typically have a strong basis in research but rather are informal, descriptive instruments. They may be useful in providing a description of a child's behavior in home and school settings, though they should be used with caution. Wilson and colleagues (2011) examined the relation between APD rating scales (the CHAPS and the SIFTER) and a battery of four diagnostic behavioral tests of APD in 104 children who attended a University-based APD clinic. A regression analysis showed poor ability of the rating scales to predict performance on the APD tests. The authors concluded that rating scales may be used to highlight concerns about a child's performance, but they should not be used to determine whether APD assessment is required, and they certainly should not be used to base a diagnosis of APD on by themselves.

Behavioral Tests

A wide range of behavioral APD tests are available, and some examples are briefly described in Table 4.3 (adapted from Dawes & Bishop, 2009, with permission). Behavioral tests require the child respond to a standardized presentation of an auditory stimulus. The child's responses are scored for accuracy, and scores may then be compared against normative data (where available) to determine whether performance is within the normal range or not. All of the tests mentioned in Table 13.3 are available commercially, and many have only minimal requirements for administration, such as good quality headphones and a CD player.

A significant problem with all APD tests, however, is that if there is no consensus on a definition for APD and thus no "gold standard" for APD diagnosis, then it is logically impossible to determine the validity of any test for diagnosis of APD. This issue is returned to in the discussion of future research directions, at the end of the chapter. Other criticisms of APD tests do not inspire confidence. Cacace and McFarland (1995, 1998) and Dawes and Bishop (2009) outlined concerns about reliability and validity. First, some APD tests (such as the SSW) were originally developed as neuropsychological tests for adults and have subsequently been applied for use with children. These tests are somewhat abstract, procedurally demanding and tedious, and so may not be appropriate for use with children. Second, children's auditory processing performance tends to improve with age (Werner, 1996), although some APD tests lack age-based performance norms that are appropriate for children. Third, the majority of APD tests lack information about their psychometric properties, and when available, reliability is often poor (Friberg & McNamara, 2010). This is unsurprising; children's psychophysical performance is notoriously variable (Werner, 1992). Fourth, APD tests are cognitively demanding in terms of memory and attention, and this may represent a confound between auditory processing and general cognitive abilities (Lum & Zarafa, 2010). Additionally, many APD tests use speech stimuli, and this may represent a confound between auditory processing and language (as reviewed further below). For example, some APD tests require repetition of words and sentences, and difficulties with this have been shown to be a reliable marker of language impairment (Conti-Ramsden, Botting, & Faragher, 2001).

Table 4.3. Descriptions of Common APD Tests

Description	*Example*
Temporal resolution: Ability to discriminate different durations of auditory stimuli or detect silent gaps between stimuli.	Random Gap Detection Test (Keith, 2000a)[ns]
Temporal Ordering: Perception and processing of the order of two or more auditory stimuli over time.	Pitch Patterns Sequence Test (Pinhiero, 1977)[ns]
Perception of artificially degraded speech: Speech may be time compressed, filtered, interrupted, or competing with background noise.	Filtered Words and Auditory Figure Ground subtests from the SCAN (Keith, 2000b)[s]
Dichotic listening: Two auditory stimuli are presented simultaneously, one to each ear. Listener is asked to attend to and report one or both stimuli.	Competing Words and Competing Sentences subtests from the SCAN (Keith, 2000b)[s] Staggered Spondiac Word Test (Katz, 1962)[s]
Binaural interaction, Localization, and Lateralization: Processing involving signals from both ears, dependent on interaural time and intensity differences.	The Listening in Spatialized Noise test (Cameron et al., 2006b)[s]

Source: categories adapted from ASHA (2005a).

ns: nonspeech stimuli; s: speech stimuli

In order to illustrate the concern over APD test reliability, we shall take as an example the SCAN-3C (Keith, 2009), intended for use with children aged between 5 and 12 years. Earlier versions of the SCAN-3C are the SCAN-C (Keith, 2000b) and the SCAN (Keith, 1986). The main differences between the SCAN-3C and the earlier SCAN-C are (a) the addition of a compressed sentences test, (b) the auditory-figure ground subtest is presented at three different signal-to-noise ratios rather than one, and (c) a screening test of gap detection, which was included in order to address criticisms that the SCAN lacked a temporal processing measure. The SCAN is the most commonly used test for auditory processing (Emanuel, 2002; Hind, 2006) for understandable reasons; it is readily available commercially, relatively inexpensive, can be administered with minimal equipment (headphones and a CD player, no sound-treated booth required), and has a manual with U.S. population-based performance norms. The SCAN-3C has four screening, five diagnostic, and three supplementary subtests that reportedly tap low-redundancy speech perception, dichotic speech perception, and temporal processing. In all subtests (except the gap detection screening test), the test-taker is required to repeat target words or sentences and scored for accuracy. Accuracy scores are then compared against age-based performance norms to provide a standard score that may be categorized as "normal," "borderline," or "disordered." The SCAN-3C provides information about its psychometric properties, as follows:

Reliability[5]

Split-half reliability is a measure of internal consistency of a test. To estimate split-half reliability, test items are divided in two and the scores for each half of the test compared with the other. For the Composite score from the whole SCAN-3C, split-half reliability varied between .89 and .93, depending on age group; the Composite score has adequate internal consistency. The internal consistency of SCAN-3C subtests is more variable, however, and ranged between .52 and .94. Split-half reliabilities are used to construct confidence intervals for scaled, normative scores. A confidence interval is an estimate of the reliability of an individual's score. For subtests with low split-half reliability, confidence intervals are so large that one cannot be say with confidence where the "true" score would be. Test-retest reliability is the extent to which a test gives the same result with repeated administration. For SCAN-3C subtests, retest reliability of scores ranged from .54 to .73, while retest reliability for the composite SCAN-3C score was .77. Retest reliabilities for both the composite and subtest scores are not sufficient for diagnostic decision-making purposes. By way of comparison, retest reliabilities for *subtests* of the CELF-4 (Semel, Wiig, & Secord, 2003), a commonly used diagnostic test for language impairment, range between .88 and .92.

Validity[6]

The SCAN-3C appears to have good content validity; subtests purport to measure the sorts of auditory skills described in the ASHA (2005a) definition of APD. However, validity of the various subtests seems uncertain; although there are eight subtests (composed of five diagnostic and three supplementary subtests) on which patterns of scores may be interpreted according to the SCAN-3C manual, a factor analysis by Canivez (2010) suggested that these eight SCAN-3C subtests map onto only two psychometric dimensions (similar to the psychometric structure reported for the SCAN-C and the SCAN; Dawes & Bishop, 2007; Domitz & Schow, 2000). In other words, the SCAN-3C appears to measure only two performance variables. Canivez (2010) suggested that because the reliability of most individual SCAN-3C subtest scores were inadequate for individual decision making, factor scores might provide more valid and reliable alternative.

The sensitivity and specificity of the SCAN-3C was determined with reference to a subset of the standardization sample and a clinical sample, composed of children who had been determined by audiological experts to have APD. The SCAN-3C manual does not provide much detail on APD diagnosis; APD diagnosis was made by an audiologist or a speech-language therapist, or a composite score of < –1 SD from the mean on "a test of auditory processing" (p. 73). Note that diagnosis by an expert is not a gold standard and, as discussed above, there is no consensus on the definition or diagnosis of APD. Attempts to examine the sensitivity/specificity of an APD test using a clinically referred sample have the problem of circularity if the same tests are used to identify the clinical sample. On average, the clinical group scored significantly worse than the standardization sample on all subsets (except Filtered Words) as well as the composite score. However, diagnostic accuracy (ability of the SCAN-3C to correctly classify clinical cases) was below the suggested threshold for diagnostic purposes (Landau, Milich, & Widiger, 1991).

There is also research evidence that the SCAN-3C is open to confound with language and memory skills. Dawes and Bishop (2007) compared the performance of 100 U.K. mainstream schoolchildren aged 6 to 10 years to the U.S. population-based norms with the previous (2000) version of the SCAN-3C (the SCAN-C). U.K. children scored nearly one standard deviation worse than the U.S. sample, with the difference ascribed to mishearing the U.S. accent with which the SCAN-C (and SCAN-3C) stimuli are recorded. Applying U.S. norms to the U.K. sample would result in at least a doubling of the proportion of children identified by the SCAN-C as being within the clinical range. The SCAN-C purports to measure the pre-cognitive, perception stage of auditory processing (Keith, 2000b), though Rosen (2005) asserts that perception of phonetic differences does depend on language experience. Any test that uses speech stimuli must therefore draw on phonological processing, which is shaped by language experience. Given the requirement for listening and responding to single word and sentence stimuli, the SCAN-C/3C is also likely to be impacted by semantic and syntactic skill. It is problematic that a test of auditory processing may be sensitive to language and phonological skills, particularly because language and reading problems are thought to co-occur with auditory processing problems. Dawes and Bishop (2007) recommended that nonspeech tests should be used in conjunction with speech-based tests in diagnosis of APD, and this fits with a BSA recommendation that nonspeech tests be used in order to avoid the confound with language skill (BSA, 2005, 2011).

The SCAN is a demanding test in terms of attention and memory skills. One might expect that memory demands would be particularly high for subtests involving sentence repetition. Lum and Zafara (2010) examined the extent to which verbal working memory impacted on SCAN-C (2000) performance by comparing a group of school-aged children with SLI to an age-matched group of typically developing (TD) children. The SLI group scored significantly worse than the TD group on the SCAN-C, although this difference was no longer significant when differences in verbal working memory were taken into account. The authors concluded that SCAN-C performance was impacted by verbal working memory.

The SCAN recommends presentation of stimuli at a comfortable listening level. Indeed, it would not be possible to ensure a particular intensity level of the stimuli using the standard mode of presentation via headphones and a CD player. However, SCAN performance varies with presentation level (Lovett & Johnson, 2011), and this may be further threat to the reliability of the SCAN.

In summary, the SCAN-C/3C is the most widely used and well-developed APD test, although there are significant concerns over reliability, validity, and confound with language, memory, and attention. Formal reviews concluded that although the SCAN-3C is improved compared to previous versions of the test, the psychometric properties of the SCAN-3C are not satisfactory and that it should not be used for diagnostic purposes (Canivez, 2010; Lovett, 2011; Lovett & Johnson, 2010; although see England, 2010 for a contrasting view).

Electrophysiological Tests

Electrophysiological tests involve recording of electrical brain responses to auditory stimuli, which may be either speech or nonspeech. The timing and shape of the components of the recorded signal are thought to represent sequential stages of processing by different parts of the central auditory nervous system. Electrophysiological measures are appealing as a means to complement or validate behavioral APD tests because they may avoid confound with attention and/or motivation. Examples of "obligatory" electrophysiological responses—those that can be elicited without active attention by the child—include the auditory brainstem response (ABR) and frequency following response (FFR), middle latency response (MLR), and late evoked response potential (ERP). A particularly promising ERP measure is the mismatch negativity (MMN) (Näätänen, 1995). Briefly, the mismatch negativity involves recording ERPs to a series of standard stimuli. At random intervals, a deviant stimuli is inserted, and the ERP to the deviant shows a characteristic change in morphology compared to the ERP to the standard. If the ERP to deviants differs significantly from that of standards, this may be taken as an objective measure of the brain's ability to discriminate between sounds. The advantages of the MMN are that the deviant can differ from the standard in one or more perceptual features, such as loudness, duration, pitch, or location, so that sensitivity to a variety of acoustic parameters may be assessed. The MMN can also be elicited without conscious attention to the stimuli, for example, while watching a silent movie.

There have been attempts to develop electrophysiological measures for use as diagnostic tests of APD (e.g., Liasis et al., 2002), however they are currently not routinely used in clinical practice (Emanuel, 2002; Emanuel et al., 2011; Hind, 2006). Reasons for this may be partly due to the expense of specialized electrophysiological equipment and the expertise required to administer and interpret electrophysiolgical tests, but also that electrophysiological measures have not lived up to their initial promise. A common flaw with electrophysiological measures such as the MMN is the wide variation of response within both typically developing and clinical populations so that although there may be significant differences at group level, differences in electrophysiological responses are not reliable at individual level (Bishop, 2007; McFarland & Cacace, 2012), and this limits clinical applicability. However, electrophysiological research is ongoing, and these measures may have future potential if reliable and informative electrophysiological indices can be identified.

Reliability of APD Diagnosis

Given the concerns outlined above regarding instruments for APD assessment and diagnosis, one may question the reliability of clinical diagnosis of APD. There is some research evidence to suggest that this concern is justified. Dawes, Bishop, Sirimanna, and Bamiou (2008) conducted a review of the medical case notes of children referred to a large hospital-based APD clinic in the United Kingdom. Children had been diagnosed with APD (or had APD excluded as a diagnosis) on the basis of (a) complaint of "listening difficulties" despite normal peripheral hearing, (b) poor performance on the SCAN-C plus poor performance on at least one other nonspeech APD test (Gap detection, pitch patterns, duration patterns). Some 32 children were identified with APD and 57 non-APD, with listening difficulties ascribed to other causes. Dawes et al. were interested to see whether there were any differences in the patterns of symptoms reported or in etiological factors that may be associated with APD. Table 4.4 shows mean scores on parent-completed Fishers auditory problems checklist (Fisher, 1976) and the Children's Auditory Performance Scale (CHAPS; Smoski et al., 1998). Scores on the two checklists were not significantly different for the APD versus the non-APD group; both groups exhibited similar listening difficulties.

Table 4.4. Average Auditory Checklist Scores by Group

	Group	*N*	*Mean*	*Standard Deviation*
Fishers %*	APD	8	48.0	26.4
	Non-APD	21	47.8	16.9
Total CHAPS#	APD	10	–2.1	1.0
	Non-APD	21	–2.0	2.9

*A score of 72% or lower (close to –1sd) on Fisher's checklist is the recommended cut-off score for referral for APD examination.

#Total scores lower than –0.05 should be referred for APD investigation, according to CHAPS guidelines.

Table 4.5 shows the type and frequency of report of symptoms in the APD and the non-APD group. Difficulties with speech in noise, difficulties with spoken instructions, reading, and spelling difficulties were the most common symptoms. Neither the type nor frequency of symptoms differed between the APD and the non-APD group. No etiological factor (including history of otitis media, adverse obstetric history, or familial history of listening problems) predicted APD group membership. Overall, there were no differences between the APD and the non-APD group in terms of symptoms or etiology. The only distinction between groups was on the performance of APD tests. One conclusion was that auditory processing problems may contribute to the listening difficulties of some children, but not others. An alternative conclusion was that APD assessment is unreliable, and so it may have been at least partly a matter of chance whether APD had been diagnosed or not.

Finally, Miller and Wagstaff (2011) compared the psychometric profiles of a group of children diagnosed with APD (n = 35) with those of a group with SLI (n = 29) and a typically developing group (n = 20). As well as a psychometric test battery assessing reading, language, and general ability, they administered an APD test battery, which included the Frequency Patterns Test, Duration Patterns Test, Dichotic Digits, and the Staggered Spondaic Word test. Criterion for identification of APD was based on ASHA (2005a) recommendations, that is, children were identified with APD if they scored lower than two standard deviations from the mean on two or more of the APD tests. Miller and Wagstaff found that 74% (26/35) of the APD group failed the APD test battery. It is surprising that 100% of the

Table 4.5. Incidence and Type of Reported Symptoms for Children Diagnosed With APD and Those for Whom APD has Been Excluded

Symptom	*APD (N = 32)*	*Non-APD (N = 57)*
Difficulties with speech in noise	20 (66%)	42 (76%)
Reading problems	15 (47%)	18 (32%)
Difficulties with spoken instructions	11 (34%)	28 (49%)
Spelling problems	12 (37%)	17 (30%)
Concentration problems	7 (22%)	12 (21%)
Memory problems	7 (22%)	14 (25%)
Hyperacusis	6 (19%)	13 (23%)
Needs TV loud	6 (19%)	3 (5%)
Pragmatic/social problems	4 (13%)	11 (19%)
Average number of symptoms reported	3.4 (1.8)	3.8 (1.8)

APD group did not fail the APD test battery, although this might perhaps be because the original clinical diagnosis of APD had been based on a different APD test battery to the one used in the research study. Of the SLI group, 86% (25/29) failed the APD test battery, which might suggest high comorbidity of SLI with APD. Most surprisingly however, 50% (10/20) of the typically developing group failed the APD test battery. Such a high rate of positive identification in the typically developing group suggests a high false positive rate, with an APD test battery composing commonly used APD tests and based on ASHA-recommended guidelines for identification of APD.

In summary, there is currently no consensus over the definition or diagnosis of APD. Psychometric information is often unavailable for commonly used APD tests, and when available, it tends to be unsatisfactory. APD tests may be confounded with language, memory, and attention skills. All of this points to significant concerns over the reliability of APD assessment.

Future Recommendations

The key questions concerning APD are (a) What is APD? (b) What is the relation between auditory processing difficulties, listening difficulties, and learning disabilities? (c) What are the appropriate diagnostic methods? and (d) What are appropriate treatment and management strategies?

The conception of APD may depend on utility of the diagnostic category. If APD is to be a useful clinical diagnostic category, it would seem necessary that auditory processing problems have a key role in the communication or academic problems for affected children. It does seem plausible that an impairment in the low-level processing of sound could affect language and reading development, social interaction, and listening in challenging acoustic environments (Tallal, 2004). However, although there is evidence that auditory processing impairments do occur in a substantial minority of children with reading and language problems, there is no evidence to support either a strong causal role for auditory processing impairments in reading and language problems or listening difficulties that could not be accounted for by weak language or other cognitive skills (Bailey & Snowling, 2002; McArthur & Bishop, 2001; Ramus, 2003, 2004; Rosen, 1999, 2003).

A large population-based study involving 1,650 U.K. school children tested auditory processing as well as a psychometric test battery (Moore et al., 2010). The study concluded that auditory processing difficulties were weakly associated with poor academic performance, but contribution of auditory processing difficulties was minimal. Overall, attention and cognitive factors were most strongly associated with academic difficulties and reports of "listening difficulties." The study concluded that APD may be better seen as a disorder of attention or other cognitive skills, because these skills were more strongly associated with functional difficulties. However, it seems odd to posit an "auditory processing disorder" that involves cognitive contributions when the disorder may be more accurately be named as "language impairment" or "attention deficit disorder," both well-recognized established diagnoses. Further, if APD is seen primarily as a disorder of attention or other higher-order cognitive skill, then some children may fit a diagnosis of "Auditory Processing Disorder," even if they have no demonstrable impairment in auditory processing on psychophysical tests. However, it may be that cognitive factors, especially the contribution of focused and sustained auditory attention, deserve further investigation rather than attempting to control or exclude them from studies of APD (Moore, 2012). Such a move would reflect a growing trend in audiology to recognize the importance of cognitive factors in listening performance.

A focus on reliable tests of auditory processing is a necessary prerequisite for progress in understanding APD. Reliable APD tests need to be clinically applicable, appropriate for children, and resistant to nonauditory effects such as attention and memory. Caution is warranted in the use of speech-based tests, as they may be susceptible to confound with language skills. This is a challenging, though tractable, problem for the audiological community. Electrophysiological measures and novel test designs, such as those based on within-subject difference such as the IMAP (Moore et al., 2010) and LISN test (Cameron, Dillon, & Newall, 2006a) hold promise for the future. Electrophysiological measures are appealing as they may avoid confound with attention, memory, language, and motivation. Tests based on within-subject difference are potentially useful because in theory they minimize confounds with attention, memory, and language skill by subtracting performance in two conditions with identical procedures but different stimuli in order to provide an estimate of auditory performance. Similar within-subject designs might be applicable in testing a range of auditory skills. Other powerful and informative study designs could include genetic studies and treatment studies (Dawes & Bishop, 2009).

A general difficulty in both assessment and in elucidating the nature of APD is that the same symptom, that is, listening difficulties may have a range of different and perhaps overlapping causes. Listening difficulties may be due to an auditory processing impairment, though may alternatively (or additionally) be due to linguistic or cognitive impairment. The challenge is to identify the primary reason for the difficulty. Much debate has centred on the validity of "APD" as a diagnostic category. In reality, while it may be necessary in order to satisfy a need for a "diagnosis" and perhaps bureaucratic demands, for example, for eligibility for support services, a categorical conceptualization of learning disability may not be realistic and may actually limit both research and clinical practice.

Learning disabilities tend to be frequently comorbid with each other. Individuals are not either impaired or unimpaired, but rather show a spectrum of ability, and there is a wide range of individual difference (Hulme & Snowling, 2009). Causes of learning disability are multifactorial and complex (Bishop, 2006). Patterns of impairment within an individual tend to change character over time, so that a child may be labeled with one disability at one age, perform within normal range at another age, and fit a different diagnostic category at a still later age (Bishop, 1997). Thus a simple categorical conceptualization such as "APD," "ADHD," "dyslexia," or "SLI" may limit research because it is inaccurate. A categorical conceptualization may also limit clinical practice if it focuses treatment and management efforts on a certain aspect of performance to the neglect of others.

Future research and clinical work to clarify the identity and significance of APD and in studying learning disabilities generally must adopt a multifactorial, developmental approach in which the aim is to describe patterns of impairment, interrelations between impairments, and change over time. This is a challenging task, and will involve multidisciplinary collaboration between audiologists, speech-language therapists, educational psychologists, paediatricians, and teachers. The challenge for researchers is to explain the significance of auditory impairments and their relation with learning disabilities.

For clinicians and those working with children, those presenting with "listening difficulties" are a highly heterogeneous group and may include those with attention deficits, dyslexia, language impairment, autistic spectrum disorder, and auditory impairments. The significance of auditory processing difficulties is currently unknown, although the listening difficulties of these children are real and do have a significant impact on social and academic performance. The challenge for clinicians is to identify an individual child's strengths and weaknesses, and to tailor intervention appropriately.

NOTES

1. Bellis and Ferre (1999) suggested a similar, though somewhat expanded classification system.
2. The test-taker is instructed to ignore the words presented to the right ear and repeat the words presented to the left ear. "Right-competing score" refers to the number of words correctly identified in this test condition.
3. As well as that recommended by Belis and Ferre (1999).
4. At the time of writing, Dr Johanna Barry at the Institute of Hearing Research was endeavoring to develop a rating scale that may reliably identify specific behavioral profiles; see www.ihr.mrc.ac.uk/app/webroot/downloads/research/EPIC.pdf
5. Reliability statistics range between .00 and 1, with those closer to 1 being stronger. Tests are considered reliable enough for clinical decision making if the reliability statistic is equal to or greater than .90 (Salvia, Ysseldyke, & Bolt, 2007).
6. Validity is the extent to which the test actually measures what it claims to measure.

REFERENCES

American Academy of Audiology (AAA). (2010). *Diagnosis, treatment and management of children and adults with auditory processing disorder.* Retrieved December 2010, from http://www.audiology.org/resources/documentlibrary/Documents/CAPD%20Guidelines%208-2010.pdf

American Psychiatric Association (APA). (2000). *Diagnostic and statistical manual of mental disorders* (4th ed., text rev. ed.). Washington, DC: American Psychiatric Association.

American Speech-Language Hearing Association (ASHA). (2005a). *(Central) auditory processing disorders*. Retrieved from http://www.asha.org/docs/html/TR2005-00043.html

American Speech-Language Hearing Association (ASHA). (2005b). *(Central) auditory processing disorders—The role of the audiologist*. Anderson, K. L. (1989). *SIFTER: Screening identification for targeting educational risk in children identified by hearing screening or who have known hearing loss*. Tampa, FL: Educational Audiology Association. Retrieved from http://www.asha.org/policy/PS2005-00114.htm

Bailey, P. J., & Snowling, M. J. (2002). Auditory processing and the development of language and literacy. *British Medical Bulletin, 63*, 135–146.

Bellis, T. J. (2003). *Assessment and management of central auditory processing disorders in the educational setting: From science to practice* (2nd ed.). Clifton Park, NY: Delmar Learning.

Bellis, T. J., & Ferre, J. M. (1999). Multidimensional approach to the differential diagnosis of central auditory processing disorders in children. *Journal of the American Academy of Audiology, 10*, 319–328.

Binder, L. M., Iverson, G. L., & Brooks, B. L. (2009). To err is human: "Abnormal" neuropsychological scores and variability are common in healthy adults. *Archives of Clinical Neuropsychology, 24*, 31–46.

Bishop, D. V. M. (1997). *Uncommon understanding*. Hove, UK: Psychology.

Bishop, D. V. M. (2006). What causes specific language impairment in children? *Current Directions in Psychological Science, 15*(5), 217–221.

Bishop, D. V. M. (2007). Using mismatch negativity to study central auditory processing in developmental language and literacy impairments: Where are we and where should we be going? *Psychological Bulletin, 133*(4), 651–672.

British Society of Audiology (BSA). (2005). Working definition of APD. Retrieved September 20, 2005, from http://www.thebsa.org.uk/apd/Home.htm#working%20def;2005

British Society of Audiology (BSA). (2011). *Position statement. Auditory Processing Disorder.* Retrieved from http://www.thebsa.org.uk/index.php?option=com_content&view=category&layout=blog&id=21&Itemid=29

Cacace, A. T., & McFarland, D. J. (1995). Opening Pandora's box: The reliability of CAPD tests [Comment]. *American Journal of Audiology, 4*(2), 61–62.

Cacace, A. T., & McFarland, D. J. (1998). Central auditory processing disorder in school-aged children: A critical review. *Journal of Speech, Language and Hearing Research, 41*, 355–373.

Cacace, A. T., & McFarland, D. J. (2005). The importance of modality specificity in diagnosing central auditory processing disorder. *American Journal of Audiology, 14*, 112–123.

Cameron, S., & Dillon, H. (2005). Three case studies of children with auditory processing disorder. *The Australian and New Zealand Journal of Audiology, 27*(2), 97–112.

Cameron, S., Dillon, H., & Newall, P. (2006a). Development and evaluation of the listening in spatialized noise test. *Ear and Hearing, 27*, 30–42.

Cameron, S., Dillon, H., & Newall, P. (2006b). The listening in spatialized noise test: An auditory processing disorder study. *Journal of the American Academy of Audiology, 17*(4), 306–320.

Canivez, G. L. (2010). Review of the SCAN-3 for children: Tests for auditory processing disorders. In K. F. Geisinger & R. A. Spies (Eds.), *The eighteenth mental measurements yearbook* (pp. 500–504). Lincoln, NE: Buros Institute of Mental Measurements.

Chermak, G. D. (2001). Auditory processing disorder: An overview for the clinician. *The Hearing Journal, 54*(7), 10–22.

Chermak, G. D., & Musiek, F. E. (1997). *Central auditory processing disorders*. San Diego, CA: Singular.

Conti-Ramsden, G., Botting, N., & Faragher, B. (2001). Psycholinguistic markers for specific language impairment (SLI). *Journal of Child Psychology and Psychiatry and Allied Disciplines, 42*(6), 741–748.

Dawes, P., & Bishop, D. V. M. (2007). The SCAN-C in testing for auditory processing disorder in a sample of British children. *International Journal of Audiology, 46*(12), 780–786.

Dawes, P., & Bishop, D. V. M. (2009). Auditory processing disorder in relation to specific learning disabilities: A review and critique. *International Journal of Language and Communication Disorders, 44*(3), 440–465.

Dawes, P., & Bishop, D. V. M. (2010). Psychometric profile of children with auditory processing disorder (APD) and children with dyslexia. *Archives of Disease in Childhood, 95*, 432–436.

Dawes, P., Bishop, D. V. M., Sirimanna, T., & Bamiou, D. E. (2008). Profile and aetiology of children with auditory processing disorder (APD). *International Journal of Pediatric Otorhinolaryngology, 72*(4), 483–489.

Domitz, D. M., & Schow, R. L. (2000). A new CAPD battery-multiple auditory processing assessment: Factor analysis and comparisons with SCAN. *American Journal of Audiology, 9*, 1–11.

Emanuel, D. C. (2002). The auditory processing battery: Survey of common practices. *Journal of the American Academy of Audiology, 13*, 93–117.

Emanuel, D. C., Ficca, K. N., & Korczak, P. (2011). Survey of the diagnosis and management of auditory processing disorder. *American Journal of Audiology, 20*, 48–60.

England, C. T. (2010). Review of the SCAN-3 for children: Tests for auditory processing disorders. In K. F. Geisinger & R. A. Spies (Eds.), *The eighteenth mental measurements yearbook* (pp. 504–506). Lincoln, NE: Buros Institute of Mental Measurements.

Ferguson, M. A., Hall, R. L., Riley, A., & Moore, D. R. (2011). Communication, listening, cognitive and speech perception skills in children with auditory processing disorder (APD) or specific language impairment (SLI). *Journal of Speech, Language and Hearing Research, 54*, 211–227.

Fisher, L. (1976). *Fisher's auditory problems checklist*. Bemidji, MN: Life Products.

Friberg, J. C., & McNamara, T. L. (2010). Evaluating the reliability and validity of (central) auditory processing tests: A preliminary investigation. *Journal of Educational Audiology, 16*, 4–17.

Hind, S. (2006). Survey of care pathway for auditory processing disorder. *Audiological Medicine*, *4*(1), 12–24.

Hind, S., Haines-Bazrafshan, R., Benton, C. L., Brassington, W., Towle, B., & Moore, D. R. (2011). Prevalence of clinical referrals having hearing thresholds within normal limits. *International Journal of Audiology*, *50*(10), 708–716.

Hulme, C., & Snowling, M. J. (2009). *Developmental disorders of language learning and cognition*. Chichester, UK: Wiley-Blackwell.

Jerger, J., & Musiek, F. E. (2000). Report of the consensus conference on the diagnosis of auditory processing disorders in school-aged children. *Journal of the American Academy of Audiology*, *11*, 467–474.

Katz, J. (1962). The use of staggered spondiac words for assessing the integrity of the central auditory nervous system. *Journal of Auditory Research*, *2*, 327–337.

Katz, J. (1992). Classification of auditory processing disorders. In J. Katz, N. Stacker, & J. Henderson (Eds.), *Central auditory processing: A transdisciplinary view* (pp. 81–91). St Louis, MO: Mosby.

Katz, J., Johnson, C., Tillery, K. L., Bradham, T., Brander, S., Delagrange, T., et al. (2002). *Clinical and research concerns—Regarding Jerger & Musiek (2000) APD recommendations*. Retrieved February 10, 2008, from http://audiologyonline.com/articles/pf_article_detail.asp?article_id=341

Keith, R. W. (Ed.). (1986). *SCAN: A screening test for auditory processing disorders in children*. San Antonio, TX: Psychological Corporation.

Keith, R. W. (2000a). *Random Gap Detection test*. St Louis, MO: AUDiTEC.

Keith, R. W. (Ed.). (2000b). *SCAN-C test for auditory processing disorders in children—Revised*. San Antonio, TX: Psychological Corporation.

Keith, R. W. (2009). *SCAN3-C*. Oxford, UK: Pearson Assessments.

Landau, S. R., Milich, R., & Widiger, T. A. (1991). Predictive power methods may be more helpful in making a diagnosis than sensitivity and specificity. *Journal of Child and Adolescent Psychopharmacology*, *1*, 343–351.

Liasis, A., Bamiou, D. E., Campbell, P., Sirimanna, T., Boyd, S., & Towell, A. (2002). Auditory event-related potentials in the assessment of auditory processing disorders: A pilot study. *Neuropediatrics*, *34*, 23–29.

Lovett, B. J. (2011). Auditory processing disorder: School psychologist beware? *Psychology in the Schools*, *48*(8), 855–867.

Lovett, B. J., & Johnson, T. L. (2010). Test review: SCAN-3 for adolescents and adults: Tests for auditory processing disorders. *Journal of Psychoeducational Assessments*, *28*(6), 603–607.

Lovett, B. J., & Johnson, T. L. (2011). The impact of presentation level on SCAN—A test performance. *Contemporary Issues in Communication Sciences and Disorders*, *38*, 135–139.

Lum, J. A. G., & Zarafa, M. (2010). Relationship between verbal working memory and the SCAN–C in children with specific language impairment. *Language, Speech and Hearing Services in School*, *41*, 521–530.

Martin, N. A., & Brownell, R. (2005). *TAPS-3 test of auditory processing skills*. Novato, CA: Academic Therapy.

McArthur, G. M., & Bishop, D. V. M. (2001). Auditory perceptual processing in people with reading and oral language impairments: Current issues and recommendations. *Dyslexia*, *7*, 150–170.

McFarland, D. J., & Cacace, A. T. (1995). Modality specificity as a criterion for diagnosing central auditory processing disorders. *American Journal of Audiology, 4*, 36–48.

McFarland, D. J., & Cacace, A. T. (2012). Questionable reliability of the speech-evoked auditory brainstem response (sABR) in typically developing children. *Hearing Research, 287*(1/2), 1.

Miller, C. A., & Wagstaff, D. A. (2011). Behavioral profiles associated with auditory processing disorder and specific language impairment. *Journal of Communication Disorders, 44*(6), 745–763.

Moore, D. R. (2012). Listening difficulties in children: Bottom-up and top-down contributions. *Journal of Communication Disorders*, in press.

Moore, D., Ferguson, M., Edmonson-Jones, A., Ratib, S., & Alison, R. (2010). The nature of auditory processing disorder in children. *Pediadtrics, 126*, e382–e390.

Musiek, F. E., & Chermak, G. D. (1994). Three commonly asked questions about central auditory processing disorders: Assessment. *American Journal of Audiology, 3*, 23–27.

Musiek, F. E., Geurkink, N. A., & Kietel, S. A. (1982). Test battery assessment of auditory perceptual dysfunction in children. *Laryngoscope, 92*(3), 251–257.

Näätänen, R. (1995). The mismatch negativity: A powerful tool for cognitive neuroscience. *Ear & Hearing, 16*(1), 6–18.

Neijenhuis, K. A., Stollman, M. H., Snik, A. F., & Van der Broek, P. (2001). Development of a central auditory test battery for adults. *Audiology, 40*(2), 69–77.

Pinhiero, M. L. (1977). Tests of central auditory function in children with learning disabilities. In R. W. Keith (Ed.), *Central auditory dysfunction* (pp. 223–256). New York, NY: Grune and Stratton.

Ramus, F. (2003). Developmental dyslexia: A specific phonological deficit or general sensorimotor dysfunction? *Current Opinion in Neurobiology, 13*, 212–218.

Ramus, F. (2004). Neurobiology of dyslexia: A reinterpretation of the data. *Trends in Neurosciences, 27*(12), 720–726.

Rosen, S. (1999). Language disorders: A problem with auditory processing? *Current Biology, 9*, R698–R700.

Rosen, S. (2003). Auditory processing in dyslexia and specific language impairment: Is there a deficit? What is its nature? Does it explain anything? *Journal of Phonetics, 31*, 509–527.

Rosen, S. (2005). "A riddle wrapped in a mystery inside an enigma": Defining central auditory processing disorder. *American Journal of Audiology, 14*, 139–142.

Salvia, J., Ysseldyke, J. E., & Bolt, S. (2007). *Assessment: In special and inclusive education* (10th ed.). Boston, MA: Houghton Mifflin.

Schow, R. L., & Seikel, J. A. (2006). Screening for (central) auditory processing disorder. In G. D. Chermak & F. E. Musiek (Eds.), *Handbook of central auditory processing disorder* (Vol. 1). San Diego, CA: Plural.

Semel, E., Wiig, E. H., & Secord, W. A. (2003). *Clinical evaluation of language fundamentals (CELF-4)* (4th ed.). Toronto, Canada: Psychological Corporation.

Sharma, M., Purdy, S. C., & Kelly, A. S. (2009). Co-morbidity of auditory processing, language, and reading disorders. *Journal of Speech, Language and Hearing Research, 52*, 706–722.

Smoski, W. J., Brunt, M. A., & Tannahill, J. C. (1998). *Children's Auditory Performance scale*. Tampa FL: Educational Audiology Association.

Tallal, P. (2004). Improving language and literacy is a matter of time. *Nature Neuroscience, 5*, 1–8.

Tallal, P., & Piercy, M. (1973). Deficits of non-verbal auditory perception in children with developmental aphasia. *Nature, 241*, 468–469.

Wagner, R. K., & Torgesen, J. K. (1987). The nature of phonological processing and its causal role in the acquisition of reading skills. *Psychological Bulletin, 101*(2), 192.

Watson, C. S., & Kidd, G. R. (2002). On the lack of association between basic auditory abilities, speech processing and other cognitive skills. *Seminars in Hearing, 23*(1), 85–95.

Watson, C. S., Kidd, G. R., Horner, D. G., Connell, P. J., Lowther, A., Eddins, D. A., et al. (2003). Sensory, cognitive, and linguistic factors in the early academic performance of elementary school children: The Benton-IU Project. *Journal of Learning Disabilities, 36*(2), 165–197.

Werner, L. A. (1992). Interpreting developmental psychophysics. In L. A. Werner & E. W. Rubel (Eds.), *Developmental psychophysics* (pp. 47–89). Washington, DC: American Psychological Association.

Werner, L. A. (1996). The development of auditory behavior (or what the anatomists and physiologists have to explain). *Ear & Hearing, 17*(5), 438–446.

Wilson, W. J., Jackson, A., Pender, A., Rose, C., Wilson, J., Heine, C., et al. (2011). The CHAPS, SIFTER, and TAPS–R as predictors of (C)AP skills and (C)APD. *Journal of Speech, Language and Hearing Research, 54*, 278–291.

CHAPTER 5

THE CHALLENGES AND IMPLICATIONS OF ASSESSING AUDITORY PROCESSING IN DIVERSE COMMUNITIES BASED ON CURRENT GUIDELINES

Jenny H. Y. Loo

Auditory processing disorder (APD) is being diagnosed more widely in the United States, the United Kingdom, and Australia (Cameron & Dillon, 2005; Emanuel, 2002; Hind, 2006) despite the lack of universal agreement on its nature and how it should be diagnosed (Keith, 2007; Rosen, 2005). While most APD studies have been conducted predominantly on native English speaking (monolingual) populations, little is known about the effect of different language backgrounds on auditory processing (AP). This issue comes to the fore when considering how to diagnose APD in multilingual populations, such as those in most Asian countries.

In this chapter, I review the diagnostic criteria and controversies of APD and provide a brief overview of the AP tests that are commonly used in clinical diagnosis. This should allow readers to better understand the

Understanding Developmental Disorders of Auditory Processing, Language and Literacy Across Languages: International Perspectives, pp. 91–112

current issues surrounding APD and AP assessment. Further, I discuss a study that examined the effect of language background on different AP test performances. My aim is to raise awareness among audiology professionals of the needs of diverse, multilingual communities when selecting AP test batteries for use in clinics.

The study reported here focused on a large group of Singaporean children who presented with listening complaints. Most of the children (about two thirds) were multilingual and came from a diverse community, and the rest were monolingual children whose native language was English (Loo, Bamiou, & Rosen, 2013). The study compared the performances of the two groups on a variety of AP tests and examined the extent to which other language-related disorders (LRDs) were present, and whether they had an effect on AP test performance.

DIAGNOSTIC CRITERIA AND CONTROVERSIES OF APD

The clinical diagnosis of APD remains a challenge. There has been a long-standing debate on the nature of APD and its diagnostic criteria. A few consensus statements on APD have emerged over the years (ASHA, 1996, 2005; BSA, 2007). Despite the clarity of the current definition, APD remains controversial among different professional groups and at the international level. There are two major controversial issues surrounding the clinical diagnosis of APD: (a) the modular-specificity nature of APD and its differential diagnosis and (b) AP test batteries.

Modular-Specificity Nature of APD and Its Differential Diagnosis

APD was originally vaguely defined and diagnosed in any case involving overlapping symptoms such as other learning disorders and LRDs (e.g., language impairment [LI], specific reading disorder [SRD]), making differential diagnosis very difficult (Bellis, 2007). This led to criticism by McFarland and Cacace (1995) and Cacace and McFarland (1998) that APD should be considered distinct from other attention, language, and more generalized higher order dysfunctions and that it should be more precisely defined as an auditory-modality-specific perceptual dysfunction. Cacace and McFarland (2005) further contended that achieving a clear conceptualization of APD as a useful clinical construct requires a multimodality testing approach, as such testing would demonstrate poor performance in a battery of auditory tasks in the presence of age-appropriate normal performance in comparable tasks in other sensory domains (e.g., vision). Cases with comparable auditory and visual task deficits (e.g., auditory frequency pattern tasks versus visual color pattern tasks) would indicate a more global disorder or the influence of attention/cognition deficits.

The auditory-modality-specificity concept of APD and the diagnostic criteria proposed by Cacace and McFarland (2005) were criticized by others (Katz & Tillery, 2005; Musiek, Bellis, & Chermak, 2005; Rosen, 2005). For instance, Rosen (2005) questioned the practicality of a multimodal testing approach, as it may prevent a close match between two tasks in the two modalities. Others, such as Katz and Tillery (2005), argued that intra- and intertest comparisons in an auditory test battery (i.e., the unimodal approach) work well in disassociating APD from other supramodal factors (i.e., attentional influence). The ASHA Working Group (2005), while recognizing the auditory nature of the disorder, concluded that complete modality specificity is neurophysiologically untenable as a diagnostic criterion for APD because the interactive nature of brain functions is nonmodular. The nonmodularity of the brain is demonstrated by the complex shared neuroanatomic substrates, multisensory neural interfaces, convergence, and divergence of sensory "tracts" and the interdependence of bottom-up and top-down factors (ASHA, 2005; Bellis, 2007).

Another major point of criticism is the extent to which AP deficits are causally linked to language and reading disorders. Tallal's (1976, 1980) "rapid auditory processing deficit" theory explicitly claims that an auditory temporal processing deficit is the underlying cause of LI and SRD. This view posits that the inability to perceive rapidly changing or transient sound leads to poor phonological representation and processing, which consequently hinders the development of typical language and reading abilities. Although this theory has received support from some studies (e.g., Merzenich et al., 1996; Tallal et al., 1996; Wright et al., 1997), it has not been universally accepted. A growing body of evidence has shown that auditory temporal processing deficits do not necessarily underpin LI or SRD in every individual (Bishop, Carlyon, Deeks, & Bishops, 1999; Griffiths, Hill, Bailey, & Snowling, 2003; McArthur & Hogben, 2001; Rosen, Adlard, & van der Lely, 2009; see Rosen, 2003 for a review).

The validity of APD as a distinct clinical construct has recently been questioned. The APD consensus statement by the ASHA Working Group (2005) clearly indicates that APD may be associated with, but is not consequent upon, difficulties in higher order language, cognitive, or related communicative functions. In other words, APD is considered a distinctive clinical disorder. As cited by the American Academy of Audiology (AAA, 2010, p. 3), a substantial body of literature (e.g., Hugdahl et al., 2003; Moncrieff, McColl, & Black, 2008; Musiek & Lee, 1998) also supports the existence of APD. However, the questioning of APD as a distinct clinical entity surfaced when recent studies reported that the clinical diagnoses of APD and LI are indistinguishable, based on laboratory-test-based classifications. For example, Ferguson, Hall, Riley, and Moore (2011) found that children in the United Kingdom who received a clinical diagnosis of APD or LI performed very similarly on some of the most commonly used behavioral test measures (i.e., verbal and nonverbal IQ, digit span, nonsense word repetition, spoonerisms, reading, grammar, sentence, and VCV nonword intelligibility). Neither clinical group showed any deficits in speech intelligibility when placed in quiet or noisy conditions. The parental reports based on questionnaires related to the children's communication, listening, and behavior did not differ significantly between the APD and LI groups. The observed behavioral and parental report profiles lead us to suggest that these children were differentially diagnosed on the basis of their referral routes rather than on their actual differences.

Miller and Wagstaff (2011) further reported that whereas the behavioral profiles (in terms of spoken language, AP, reading, memory, and motor speed) of a group of American children with *a priori* APD or LI diagnoses were very similar, the laboratory-test-based classifications of APD and LI did not correspond closely to the clinical diagnoses. The authors suggested that to prove that APD and LI are distinct constructs, behavioral measures that target a specific cognitive process with minimal influence of other factors (e.g., nonspeech auditory processing tests) should be devised. In the speech-language pathologist community, some researchers (e.g., Fey et al., 2011; Kamhi, 2011) have strongly opposed treating APD as a distinct clinical entity due to the lack of evidence that auditory interventions provide unique benefits to auditory, language, or academic outcomes compared with language interventions. Therefore, it has been suggested that APD may be more appropriately viewed as a processing deficit that commonly occurs with other developmental disorders (e.g., LI, SRD). The recently published BSA Position Statement on APD stated that APD may be one symptom of a broader neurodevelopmental problem that is closely linked with other LRDs (BSA, 2011).

Auditory Processing Test Batteries

To date, no "gold standard" test battery has been produced for APD diagnosis, and no minimal set of AP tests has been universally agreed upon. While both speech and nonspeech AP tests are currently used for APD diagnosis, as recommended by the ASHA Working Group (2005), some authors have advocated the use of nonspeech AP tests only to identify APD (Hall & Johnston, 2007; Moore, 2006). The position published by the British Society of Audiology (BSA, 2007) explicitly stated that APD should only be diagnosed using nonspeech tasks to minimize the confounding influence of language and other cognitive factors.

However, a contrasting view has emerged from the belief that the central auditory nervous system (CANS) has different processing mechanisms for speech and nonspeech signals (AAA, 2010). This view has been supported by neurophysiologic studies that have shown that atypical neural responses or hemispheric asymmetries occur in a CANS function when tested with speech stimuli as opposed to nonspeech stimuli (e.g., AAA, 2010, p. 14; Jerger, Moncrieff, Greenwald, Wambacq, & Seipel, 2000; Song, Banai, Russo, & Kraus, 2006). Nonetheless, the AAA (AAA, 2010) has recognized the need to develop nonspeech AP tests that could be applied internationally to facilitate consistency and uniformity in APD diagnosis.

In summary, there are two contrasting views on the types of test used for AP assessment. One view limits APD to a disorder that is strictly related to the processing of low-level acoustic-phonetic features of speech and therefore demands that nonspeech AP tests be used. Another view holds that speech tasks remain an important component in APD assessment because CANS dysfunction is likely to have more of an effect on speech than nonspeech signal processing.

AUDITORY PROCESSING TESTS

In the absence of a clear "gold standard" test battery for APD, most audiologists refer to the guidelines published by professional organizations when diagnosing APD (e.g., AAA, 2010; ASHA, 2005; BSA, 2007, 2011). In these guidelines (AAA, 2010, pp. 16–22; ASHA, 2005, pp. 12–13), five auditory processes (as seen in Table 5.1) have been identified as appropriate for assessment in diagnosing APD, and a variety of test options have been recommended to assess each process. It has been recommended that an individualized test battery approach be adopted (AAA, 2010; ASHA, 2005). This means that the selection of AP tests should be based on the individual's case history and relevant information provided to the audiologist.

However, a survey conducted by Emanuel, Ficca, and Korczak (2011) revealed that the majority of U.S. audiologists (n = 155/199; 81%) remain driven by a minimum test battery approach of four to six different AP tests for every patient, with additions based on individual case histories and ages. The most commonly used tests are the dichotic listening, temporal processing, and patterning tests, in addition to the monaural low redundancy speech tests (highlighted with asterisks in Table 5.1). At this point, no minimal set of AP tests has been universally agreed upon. Hind (2006) reported that different types of direct and indirect AP tests (e.g., language, cognitive and memory tests, and questionnaires) were being used in different clinics in the United Kingdom. These studies reflect a lack of consistency and uniformity in APD diagnoses among audiology professionals at both the national and international levels.

Table 5.1. Categorization of Central Auditory Tests and the Types of Measures

Auditory Domains	*Test Function*	*Types of Test Measures*
Auditory discrimination tests	Assess the ability to differentiate similar acoustic stimuli that differ in frequency, intensity, and duration	• Difference limen for frequency • Difference limen for intensity • Phoneme discrimination
Auditory temporal processing and patterning tests	Assess the ability to analyze acoustic events over time	• *Frequency patterns • *Duration patterns • *Gap detection thresholds • Fusion discrimination • Forward and backward masking
Dichotic listening (speech) tests	Assess the ability to separate (i.e., binaural separation) or integrate (i.e., binaural integration) disparate acoustic stimuli presented to each ear simultaneously	• *Dichotic digits • Dichotic Consonant Vowels (CVs) • *Competing sentences • Competing words
Monaural low redundancy speech tests	Assess the recognition of degraded speech stimuli presented to one ear at a time	• *Speech in noise • Speech in competition • *Filtered speech • Compressed speech
Binaural interaction tests	Assess the binaural (i.e., dichotic) processes dependent on the intensity of or time differences in acoustic stimuli across both ears	• Masking level difference • Localization and lateralization • Interaural intensity difference

Source: adapted from ASHA (2005).

* Commonly used for clinical diagnostic purposes.

As shown in Table 5.1, some of the AP measures are nonspeech and others are speech-based tests. The basis on which an audiologist would determine a certain type of test over another remains in question. Clinical groups in countries where English is the official language have conveniently often adopted both speech and nonspeech AP tests developed in the United States with reference to native (American) English-speaking populations. However, although it has not been thoroughly investigated thus far, practicing audiologists should be cautious that different language experiences may affect the assessment of AP and thus the interpretation of the test results.

Speech Test or Nonspeech Test?

Evidence has shown that language experience has an effect on the performance of speech-based tests of the kind used in APD batteries. For example, Tabri, Chacra, and Pring (2011) showed that bilingual/trilingual individuals with normal hearing have poorer speech perception of their second language than monolingual native speakers under unfavorable conditions (e.g., with competing noise), despite performing equally well under quiet conditions. Other researchers (e.g., Crandell & Smaldino, 1996; Shi, 2009; von Hapsburg, Champlin, & Shetty, 2004) have reported similar results. It has also been found that speech perception deficits in noise persist for speakers who are highly proficient in their second language (Tabri et al., 2010). Therefore, AP tests that use degraded speech (e.g., presented in background noise or after low-pass filtering) may require careful interpretation. A test failure may reflect either a disordered AP or the effects of the individual's language background.

What are the solutions to applying speech-based AP tests more generally? One possibility is to develop a test in the native language or dialects used in the community. However, this may not be viable in a polyglot country with several minority subgroups due to the expense and effort required for each language or dialect (Lew & Canon, 2010). Furthermore, it is uncertain whether specific speech-based AP tests translated into other languages would still be assessing the same auditory processes, as different languages have different neurophysiological representations in the brain (Valaki et al., 2004).

An alternative involves renorming the speech-based AP tests. While this may seem more achievable, it may not address the problem of accent differences and word familiarity effects in diverse communities. For example, Dawes and Bishop (2007) found that primary school children in the United Kingdom scored significantly worse than the U.S. norms in SCAN-C (a speech-based screening test for APD), primarily due to the difference in accent. Marriage, King, Briggs, & Lutman (2001) reported a similar problem in an earlier study when using the SCAN test. These authors (Dawes & Bishop, 2007; Marriage et al., 2001) recognized the desirability of rerecording the test with a British speaker, but also observed that this would not solve the possible problem of regional accent variations influencing performance.

An additional factor affecting the use of speech-based AP tests is the potential confounding influence of LRDs such as LI and SRD on performance. This was an earlier concern highlighted by the UK's audiology community that led to the requirement for the use of nonspeech-based AP tests in APD assessment and diagnosis. (Readers may to refer to the interim position statement on APD published by the BSA in 2007.) The use of speech-based AP tests may add to the difficulties involved in making a differential diagnosis, as APD has often been reported as comorbid LI (Bamiou, Musiek, & Luxon, 2001; Ferguson et al., 2011; Miller & Wagstaff, 2011; Sharma, Purdy, & Kelly, 2009) and SRD (Dawes, Bishop, Sirimanna, & Bamiou, 2008; Iliadou, Bamiou, Kaprinis, Kandylis, & Kaprinis, 2009; King, Lombardina, Crandell, & Leonard, 2003). Evidence has also shown that LI itself may lead to poor performance in some of the typical speech tasks used for diagnosing APD. In particular, Conti-Ramsden, Botting, and Faragher (2001) found performance in a sentence repetition task under quiet conditions to be the best of four applied LI predictors. In short, children with LRDs may be more likely to underperform in speech-based tasks.

In summary, the use of speech-based AP tests in the clinical diagnosis of APD may prove to be a challenge, especially in diverse multilingual societies. In the following section, I discuss the recent findings from a retrospective study that lends further support to the need for nonspeech AP tests in diagnosing APD from international and multicultural perspectives.

Recommendations for Test Interpretation

The ASHA Technical Report (2005) proposed interpreting AP test results on the bases of norms and patients. A *norm-based interpretation* involves comparing an individual's performance to normative data, in which a performance score that falls below two standard deviations from the mean on two or more tests in the battery are considered indicative of deficits in AP. In contrast, a *patient-based interpretation* involves comparing an individual's test scores to his or her own baseline by comparing the respective performance scores of the two ears within a given test (intratest analysis) or comparing the overall results across the diagnostic test battery (intertest analysis). Another approach for patient-based interpretation is cross-discipline comparison, in which AP test results are compared with language, psycho-educational, and related cognitive test findings.

It is worth highlighting that in some circumstances, an APD diagnosis may not be warranted despite a child meeting the performance criteria. For instance, poor or inconsistent performance across all of the tests may be indicative of other nonauditory factors such as higher order cognitive, memory, or motivational issues confounding the results. An APD diagnosis should also be considered carefully in cases wherein poor performance is found on only one test, unless the performance was at least three standard deviations below the mean and there was a manifestation of functional auditory difficulty related to the demonstrable auditory deficit. To confirm the initial findings, a readministration of the same test or a similar test assessing the same process is required (ASHA, 2005).

PERFORMANCE OBSERVED IN AP TESTS: MULTILINGUAL VERSUS MONOLINGUAL CHILDREN

My colleagues (Professor Stuart Rosen and Dr. Doris Bamiou from the University College London) and I studied the performance of a group of multilingual and monolingual children who were referred for AP assessment between January 2008 and December 2009 at a hearing center in Singapore. Our aim was to examine whether the two groups of children performed differently in some of the commonly used speech and nonspeech AP tests for clinical diagnostic purposes. As most children referred for AP assessment also present with LI and/or SRD, we further examined the extent to which these LRDs affected the children's AP test performances.

Demographic Information on the Study Groups

The studied population consisted of 133 children from multilingual backgrounds and 71 from monolingual backgrounds. The multilingual group comprised Singaporean children who were attending mainstream government schools and came from different ethnic groups across a range of socioeconomic backgrounds. All of these multilingual children were English speakers, as English is the official language of instruction in every Singaporean school. However, their home language(s) could have been English, another language (typically Mandarin, Malay, or Tamil), a Chinese dialect, or a mixture of languages/dialects. The monolingual group consisted of nonlocal children whose first language was English and who attended international schools in Singapore (e.g., the Singapore American School, Canadian International School, Australian International School, Tanglin Trust British International School). These monolingual children generally came from families who had relocated to Singapore for employment and thus tended to have higher socioeconomic backgrounds than the multilingual children. Most of the children had been living in Singapore for fewer than 5 years, and only a minority were born there. The histograms in Figure 5.1 show the age distribution of the children.

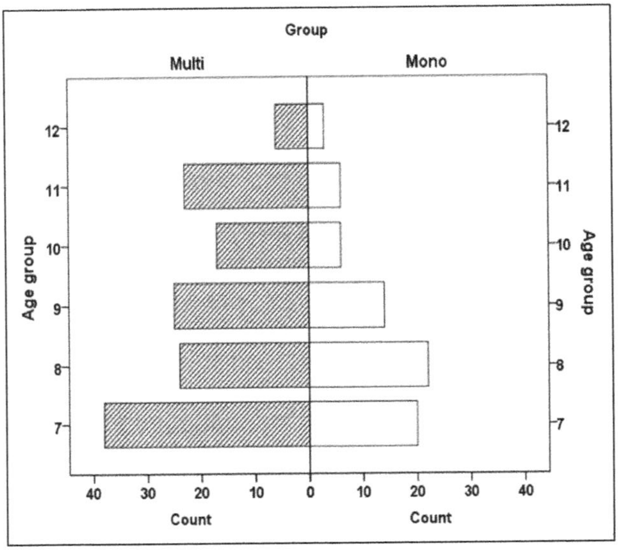

Source: Loo et al. (2013)

Figure 5.1. Histograms of the age distribution of children in the multilingual (n = 133) and monolingual (n = 71) groups. All of the children were between 7 and 12 years old.

Table 5.2 shows the number of children with prior LI, SRD, and LI/SRD diagnoses and indicates that no comorbid disorders were found in the study population. The diagnoses of language or reading impairments in the multilingual Singaporean children were performed in accordance with published guidelines, accounting for the different language development expectations for children acquiring English as an additional language (Brebner, McCormack, & Rickard-Liow, 2004) or on the basis of personal clinical experience (Lew & Cannon, 2010). The LI and SRD diagnoses in the monolingual population were based on general guidelines. LI was diagnosed when a child experienced significant language difficulty (receptive or expressive) despite having normal hearing sensitivity and nonverbal intelligence and showing no other physical or emotional difficulties (Bishop, 1992). SRD was diagnosed when the child experienced a deficit in reading fluency and spelling in the presence of adequate hearing and general intelligence (Castles & Coltheart, 1993).

Table 5.2. Number and Proportion of Children With a Provisional Diagnosis of a Language-Related Disorder in the Referred Population Split by Language Background (*n* = 204)

Study Groups	*LI*	*SRD*	*LI and SRD*	*No Other LRD*
Multilingual (*n* = 133)	55 (41.4%)	9 (6.8%)	12 (9.0%)	57 (42.9%)
Monolingual (*n* = 71)	20 (28.2%)	6 (8.5%)	3 (4.2%)	42 (59.2%)

Source: Loo et al. (2013)

LI = language impairment; SRD = specific reading disorder; LRD = language-related disorder.

Statistical Analysis and Results

Different statistical models (i.e., logistic regression, univariate general linear, linear mixed model) were applied to study the effects of individual factors (i.e., age, language background [multi- versus monolingual] and comorbid LRD [i.e., LI, SRD, LI/SRD and none]) and their interactions on each AP test. Detailed analyses have been provided elsewhere (Loo et al., 2013).

Nonspeech Tests

The following summarizes the conclusions that can be drawn from the results of the nonspeech tests.

1. *Frequency Pattern Test* (FPT): Children improved significantly with age, and their language background had no effect. However, having LI and/or SRD led to a somewhat lower performance.
2. *Random Gap Detection Test* (RGDT): Language background had no effect on performance, and the failure to perform RGDT decreased with age regardless of LRD. However, the presence of a comorbid condition led to higher failure rates overall.
3. *Masking Level Difference* (MLD): Language background and a comorbid LRD did not affect the size of the MLD, and age had no effect on performance.

Speech-Based AP Tests

The following summarizes the conclusions that can be drawn from the results of the speech-based tests.

1. *Low Pass Filtered Words* (LPFWs): LPFW performance improved with age. The multilingual children performed more poorly than the monolingual children (by about 12%), and the presence of LI affected their performance (again, by about 12%). However, the presence of SRD did not seem to exert any influence.
2. *Dichotic Digits Test* (DDT): Performance changed with age differently within the groups defined by comorbidity, and the effect depended on the language group. The scatterplots in Figure 5.2 show that in the absence of any LRDs, performance improved with age similarly in both language groups. Whereas the monolingual children did not seem to improve with age in the presence of comorbid conditions, the multilingual children did improve. Of the children who had no comorbid disorder, their language group had no significant effect. In fact, the multilingual group performed only slightly better on average (by 2 percentage points) than the monolingual group. Comparing the groups with comorbid disorders was complicated due to the clear interaction between language background and age. However, the performance of the multilingual group was at least as good as, and occasionally somewhat better than, that of the monolingual group (Figure 5.2).
3. *Competing Sentences* (CS): CS performance improved with age in all of the groups. The monolingual children had a bigger magnitude of right ear advantage (REA) than the monolingual children, irrespective of comorbid conditions (nearly 10 percentage points). There was no group difference (monolingual versus multilingual children) in the left ear, regardless of whether a comorbid LRD was present. In the right ear, however, the monolingual children with comorbid LRDs significantly outperformed the multilingual children with comorbid LRDs by about 12 percentage points. Of the children without any other LRDs, the group difference just missed significance at $p = 0.051$. Even so, the monolingual children scored about 10 percentage points higher (Figure 5.3).

Discussion

This study clearly showed that certain AP tests are influenced by an individual's language experience and the presence of any comorbid conditions such as LI and SRD. Such effects must influence the interpretation of the test results.

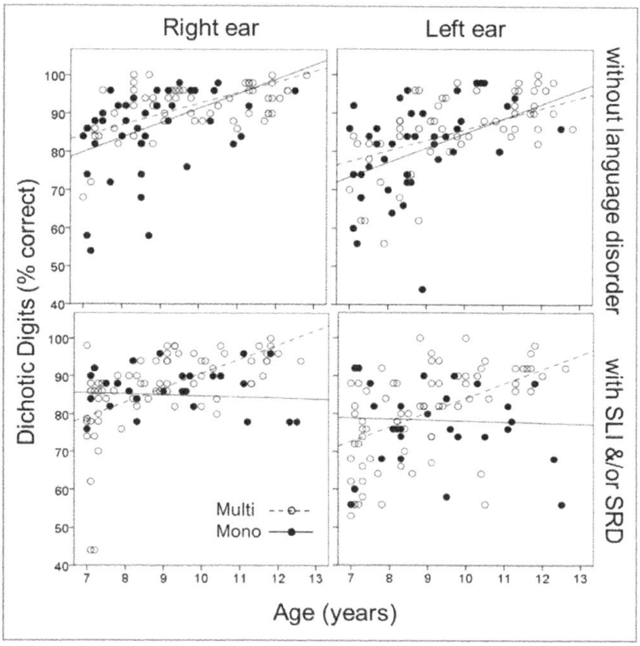

Source: Loo et al. (2013).

Figure 5.2. Performance in the Dichotic Digits Test (DDT) as a function of language background and the presence/absence of a comorbid condition. The open circles/dotted lines and filled circles/solid lines represent multilingual and monolingual children, respectively (from Loo, Bamiou, & Rosen, 2013).

Effect of Language Background on AP Performance

As hypothesized, nonspeech tasks such as FPT, RGDT, and MLD were less influenced by an individual's language background. When evaluating the AP performances of children using speech stimuli, language experience is clearly an important factor when it comes to interpreting the test results. However, tests differ substantially in terms of the extent to which such performance is affected. The most straightforward situation was found in the LPFW test, where the multilingual children performed worse than their monolingual counterparts.

Ample evidence has shown that listeners whose second language is English perform worse than monolingual listeners in English-based speech tasks such as monosyllabic word recognition, speech-in-noise, or repetition of computer-synthesized sentences (Axmear et al., 2005; Stuart, Zhang, & Swink, 2010; Tabri et al., 2011). Further, nonnative listeners have been found to be less able to make use of acoustic and linguistic cues that are

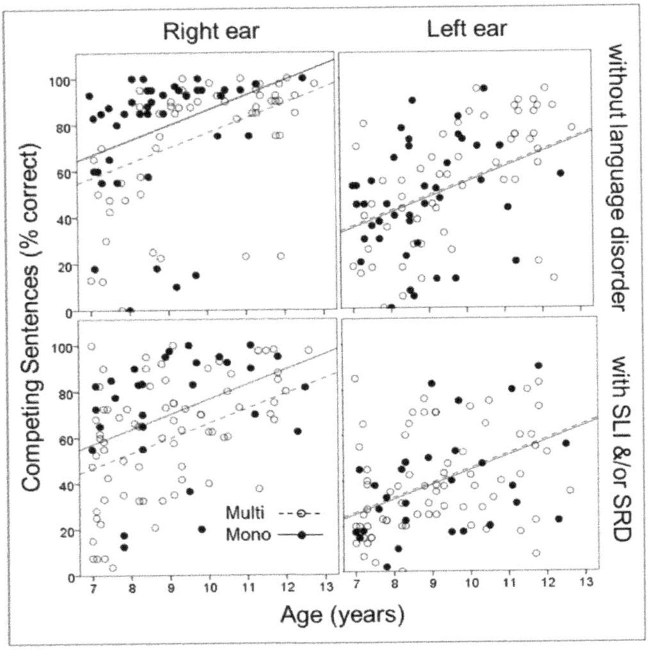

Source: Loo et al. (2013).

Figure 5.3. Performance in the Competing Sentences (CS) test as a function of language background and the presence/absence of a comorbid condition. The open circles/dotted lines and filled circles/solid lines represent multilingual and monolingual children, respectively (from Loo, Bamiou, & Rosen, 2013).

readily accessible to native English listeners (Mayo, Florentine, & Buus, 1997). Taken together, these results indicate that LPFWs test linguistic competence in terms of guessing the composition of a whole based on limited information rather than testing *auditory sensory* processing. It is therefore easy to understand why the multilingual children performed worse in this task.

The results for the two dichotic speech tasks (CS and DDT) were rather more complex. In the CS test, performance was not only affected by language experience but also dependent on any comorbid condition. The magnitude of the REA was smaller in the multilingual group than in the monolingual group. The two groups performed similarly in the left-ear tests, but their performances differed significantly in the right-ear tests. This may be related to the finding that monolingual and late-bilingual individuals (i.e., those who acquired their second language later than age 6) show a left hemisphere (LH) functional dominance for language processing. However, early bilingual individuals (i.e., those who acquire a second language before age 6), who predominantly composed the multilingual group in this study, use both hemispheres for language processing (Hull & Vaid, 2006, 2007). Less hemispheric asymmetry is likely to lead to smaller REAs. However, this explanation may not be adequate, as even the multilingual children had REAs. Perhaps more importantly, the strongest evidence of LH dominance in the Hull and Vaid (2006, 2007) studies came from dichotic tests of single words. However, the magnitude of the REA in the DDTs, which involved single words, did not depend on language background. In fact, the DDT performances of the two language groups in the absence of a comorbid disorder were indistinguishable.

An alternative explanation is that while the CS test depends more on linguistic competency, the DDT, which requires little language expertise, depends as much as or more than the CS test on auditory attention and memory. The CS test considers directed attention with a reasonably heavy linguistic (and memory) load, and its findings are broadly in keeping with Hull and Vaid's (2007) study. The DDT, on the other hand, consists only of a small set of overlearned digits and is thus less likely to depend on language background. However, the working memory load involved is high, as two digits from each ear must be reported. Perhaps the study's most surprising finding was that whereas the monolingual children with comorbid conditions did not seem to improve with age in their DDT performance, the multilingual children did. Bilingualism is a form of sensory enrichment that may lead to gains in cognitive ability (Bialystok, Craik, & Luk, 2012; Carlson & Meltzoff, 2008). One may postulate that exposure to multilingualism in the pediatric group led to attention improvements that were reflected in the improvements with age. However, further study is required to explain the interaction of bi- and monolingualism in the presence of an LRD and how this interaction affects dichotic listening across ages.

In summary, language experience has little effect, if any, on the development of the AP skills assessed by the kind of nonspeech tests used in this study. This means that establishing specific population-based norms (i.e., establishing different norms in different countries) is not necessary for the application of these nonspeech tests in the clinical diagnosis of APD. However, while an individual's language background affects his or her AP performance on some speech-based tasks, it does not always do so in a straightforward way. An important caveat relates to the particular multilingual population studied here. All of the child participants had had, as a minimum, complete immersion in English once they started school. Their skills in English were thus relatively high. It is likely that participants with less fully developed language skills would be even more severely affected in their speech tasks.

Effect of LRDs on AP Performance

The presence of a comorbid condition such as LI or SRD appears to have a broader effect on performance in AP tests than language background, insofar as it appears to affect performance even in some nonspeech tests. The children with comorbid conditions performed worse than those without such conditions in the majority of the speech and nonspeech AP tests. Insofar as the LPFW test could be considered more a test of language ability than AP, it makes sense that the children with LRDs performed worse than those without LRDs. The CS test similarly taps higher cognitive functions, particularly short-term auditory memory and linguistic processing. Evidence suggests that children with language and reading deficits suffer short-term verbal memory deficits (Baird, Slonims, Simonoff, & Dworynski, 2011; Ellis-Weismer, Evans, & Hesketh, 1999; Hutchinson, Bavin, Efron, & Sciberras, 2012; Martinez Perez, Majerus, Mahot, & Poncelet, 2012; Nickisch & von Kries, 2009). Of particular relevance to the CS task, children with LI have been shown to perform significantly worse than typically developing children in sentence repetition tasks under quiet conditions (Conti-Ramsden et al., 2001). It is therefore hardly surprising that children with LRDs would perform poorly in the CS task, which requires sentence repetition.

What is quite unexpected is that the performance in tests with low linguistic demands like the DDT and two of the nonspeech AP tests (i.e., FPT and RGDT) were affected by the presence of comorbid LRDs. Cognitive factors such as memory and attention in children with comorbid LRDs may have played a part. As mentioned, the working memory of the children with comorbid LRDs may have been impaired. To perform well in a test like the DDT, the children had to recall four digits presented concurrently in both ears. A more plausible explanation for the lower performance among children with LRDs on the FPT and RGDT may thus be attentional problems. Although both of these tests could be considered temporal processing tests, the findings seem to favor the theory of temporal processing deficits promulgated most notably by Tallal (1976, 1980), as there were no auditory temporal processing deficits underpinning LI or SRD in any of the children (see Rosen, 2003 for a review).

In fact, numerous studies have shown that children with language and reading deficits have a decreased capacity for sustained attention in the absence of clinically significant attention deficits compared with those without (Finneran, Francis, & Leonard, 2009; Marzocchi, Ornaghi, & Barboglio, 2009; Noterdaeme, Amorosa, Mildenberger, Sitter, & Minow, 2001). In these AP tasks, children must focus their attention on the auditory stimuli and recall either the order of the tones presented (FPT), indicate whether one or two sounds were heard (RGDT), or repeat all four of the digits heard simultaneously in both ears (DDT). Although these tasks make minimal or no linguistic demands, they may present a greater challenge to children with LRDs than to those without comorbid conditions. In this case, one may argue that the attentional and memory problems associated with LRDs should also affect the MLD. However, in this study, the MLD did not differ between the children with and without LRDs. Note that the MLD is the only test in which the outcome measure is derived from the *subtraction* of two listening conditions. We may thus expect the effects of attention and memory to be factored out, and for this measure to represent sensory processing more purely. This point of view is in line with the findings of Moore, Ferguson, Edmondson-Jones, Ratib, and Riley (2010), who found that their derived measures (i.e., temporal resolution and frequency resolution), all of which involved subtraction to factor out cognitive determinants, did not correlate with other cognitive abilities despite the component measures doing so.

In a nutshell, the effect of LRDs on AP test performance appears to be substantially more wide-ranging than the effects of language background, insofar as the majority of speech and nonspeech AP tests are significantly affected by the presence of a comorbid condition.

CONCLUSIONS

Linguistic tasks remain an important component in the APD test battery, but it is believed that the CANS has different processing mechanisms for speech and nonspeech signals (AAA, 2010), and thus the practicality of using speech-based AP tests in a diverse community with separate norms to cater to different language backgrounds is questionable. In view of the absence of a universally acceptable AP test battery, the need to assess individuals using APD, DDT, and nonspeech AP tests such as those mentioned in this chapter seems more appropriate for clinical use, particularly in a multicultural context. However, the presence of comorbid LRDs has a somewhat wide-ranging effect on the majority of AP tests, even nonspeech tests. A multidisciplinary team assessment that involves language, cognitive, and AP measures is therefore essential. It would help to determine an individual's primary learning difficulty, whether predominantly a language, cognitive, or AP-based deficit, and subsequently help in the design of an individual-based intervention. Further well-controlled research that considers the effect of bilingualism is necessary to arrive at an international consensus on the definition of APD and its diagnostic criteria.

REFERENCES

American Academy of Audiology (AAA). (2010). *Practice guidelines for the diagnosis, treatment, and management of children and adults with central auditory processing disorder (CAPD)*. Retrieved from http://www.audiology.org/resources/documentlibrary/Documents/CAPD%20Guidelines%208-2010.pdf

American Speech-Language-Hearing Association (ASHA). (1996). Central auditory processing: Current status of research and implications for clinical practice. *American Journal of Audiology, 5*(2), 41–54.

American Speech-Language-Hearing Association (ASHA). (2005). *Technical report—(Central) auditory processing disorders*. Retrieved from http://www.asha.org/docs/pdf/TR2005-00043.pdf

Axmear, E., Reichle, J., Alamsaputra, M., Kohnert, K., Drager, K., & Sellnow, K. (2005). Synthesized speech intelligibility in sentences: A comparison of monolingual English-speaking and bilingual children. *Language, Speech, and Hearing Services in Schools, 36*, 244–250.

Baird, G., Slonims, V., Simonoff, E., & Dworzynski, K. (2011). Impairment in non-word repetition: A marker for language impairment or reading impairment? *Developmental Medicine and Child Neurology, 53*(8), 711–716.

Bamiou, D. E., Musiek, F. E., & Luxon, L. M. (2001). Aetiology and clinical presentations of auditory processing disorders—A review. *Archive of Diseases in Childhood, 85*, 361–365.

Bellis, T. J. (2007). Historical foundations and the nature of (central) auditory processing disorders. In D. Cacace, & D. J. McFarland (Eds.), *Controversies in central auditory processing disorder* (pp. 119–136). San Diego, CA: Plural.

Bialystok, E., Craik, F. I. M., & Luk G. (2012). Bilingualism: Consequences for mind and brain. *Trends in Cognitive Sciences, 16*(4), 240–250.

Bishop, D. V. M. (1992). The underlying nature of specific language impairment. *Journal of Child Psychology and Psychiatry, 33*, 3–66.

Bishop, D. V. M., Carlyon, R. P., Deeks, J. M., & Bishops, S. J. (1999). Auditory temporal processing impairment: Neither necessary nor sufficient for causing language impairment in children. *Journal of Speech, Language and Hearing Research, 42*, 1295–1310.

Brebner, C., McCormack, P., & Rickard-Liow, S. J. (2004). The acquisition of the morphology and syntax English spoken in Singapore. In B. Murdoch (Ed.), *Proceedings of the 26th World Congress of the International Association of Logopeadics and Phoniatrics, Melbourne, Australia*.

British Society of Audiology (BSA). (2007). *Interim position statement on APD*. Retrieved from http://www.thebsa.org.uk/apd/

British Society of Audiology (BSA). (2011). *Position statement—Auditory processing disorder (APD)*. Retrieved from http://www.thebsa.org.uk/images/stories/docs/BSA_APD_PositionPaper_31March11_FINAL.pdf

Cacace, A. T., & McFarland, D. J. (1998). Central auditory processing disorder in school-aged children: A critical review. *Journal of Speech, Language and Hearing Research, 51*, 355–373.

Cacace, A. T., & McFarland, D. J. (2005). The importance of modality specificity in diagnosing central auditory processing disorder. *American Journal of Audiology, 14*, 112–123.

Cameron, S., & Dillon, H. (2005). Auditory processing disorder—From screening to diagnosis and management—A step by step guide. *Audiology Now, 21*, 47–55.

Carlson, S. M., & Meltzoff, A. N. (2008). Bilingual experience and executive functioning in young children. *Developmental Science, 11*(2), 282–298.

Castles, A., & Coltheart, M. (1993). Varieties of developmental dyslexia. *Cognition, 47*, 149–180.

Conti-Ramsden, G., Botting, N., & Faragher, B. (2001). Psycholinguistic markers for specific language impairment (SLI). *Journal of Child Psychiatry, 42*(6), 741–748.

Crandell, C. C., & Smaldino, J. J. (1996). Speech perception in noise by children for whom English is a second language. *American Journal of Audiology, 5*, 47–51.

Dawes, P., & Bishop, D. V. (2007). The SCAN-C in testing for auditory processing disorder in a sample of British children. *International Journal of Audiology, 46*, 780–786.

Dawes, P., Bishop, D. V., Sirimanna, T., & Bamiou, D. E. (2008). Profile and aetiology of children diagnosed with auditory processing disorder (APD). *International Journal of Pediatric Otorhinolaryngology, 72*, 483–489.

Ellis-Weismer, S., Evans, J., & Hesketh, L. J. (1999). An examination of verbal working memory capacity in children with specific language impairment. *Journal of Speech, Language, and Hearing Research, 42*, 1249–1260.

Emanuel, D. C. (2002). The auditory processing battery: Survey of common practices. *Journal of the American Academy of Audiology, 13*, 93–117.

Emanuel, D. C., Ficca, K. N., & Korczak, P. (2011). Survey of the diagnosis and management of auditory processing disorder. *American Journal of Audiology, 20*(1), 48–60.

Ferguson, M. A., Hall, R. L., Riley, A., & Moore, D. R. (2011). Communication, listening, cognitive and speech perception skills in children with auditory processing disorder (APD) or specific language impairment (SLI). *Journal Speech, Language, and Hearing Research, 54*(1), 211–227.

Fey, M. E., Richard, G. J., Geffner, D., Kamhi, A. G., Medwetsky, L., Paul, D., & Schooling, T. (2011). Auditory processing disorder and auditory/language interventions: An evidence-based systematic review. *Language, Speech, and Hearing Service in Schools, 42*(3), 246–264.

Finneran, D. A., Francis, A. L., & Leonard, L. B. (2009). Sustained attention in children with specific language impairment (SLI). *Journal Speech, Language, and Hearing Research, 52*(4), 915–912.

Griffiths, Y. M., Hill, N. I., Bailey, P. J., & Snowling, M. J. (2003). Auditory temporal order discrimination and backward recognition masking in adults with dyslexia. *Journal of Speech, Language and Hearing Research, 46*, 1352–1366.

Hall, J. W., & Johnston, K. N. (2007). Electroacoustic and electrophysiologic auditory measures in the assessment of (central) auditory processing disorder. In F. E. Musiek, & G. D. Chermak (Eds.), *Handbook of (central) auditory processing disorder: Auditory neuroscience and diagnosis* (Vol. 1, pp. 287–317). San Diego, CA: Plural.

Hind, S. (2006). Survey of care pathway for auditory processing disorder. *Audiological Medicine, 4*, 12–24.

Hugdahl, K., Heiervang, E., Ersland, L., Lundervold, A., Steinmetz, H., & Smievoll, H. (2003). Significant relation between MR measures of planum temporale area and dichotic processing of syllables in dyslexic children. *Neuropsychologia, 41*(6), 666–675.

Hull, R., & Vaid, J. (2006). Laterality and language experience. *Laterality: Asymmetries of Body, Brain & Cognition, 11*(5), 436–464.

Hull, R., & Vaid, J. (2007). Bilingual language lateralization: A meta-analytic tale of two hemispheres. *Neuropsychologia, 45*, 1987–2008.

Hutchinson, E., Bavin, E., Efron, D., & Sciberras, E. (2012). A comparison of working memory profiles in school-aged children with specific language impairments, attention deficit/hyperactivity disorder, comorbid SLI and ADHD and their typically developing peers. *Child Neuropsychology, 18*(2), 190–207.

Iliadou, V., Bamiou, D. E., Kaprinis, S., Kandylis, D., & Kaprinis, G. (2009). Auditory processing disorders in children suspected of learning disabilities—A need for screening? *International Journal of Pediatric Otorhinolaryngology, 73*, 1029–1034.

Jerger, J., Moncrieff, D., Greenwald, R., Wambacq, I., & Seipel, A. (2000). Effect of age on interaural asymmetry of event-related potentials in a dichotic listening task. *Journal of the American Academy of Audiology, 11*(7), 383–389.

Kamhi, A. G. (2011). What speech-language pathologists need to know about auditory processing disorder. *Language, Speech, and Hearing Services in School, 42*(3), 265–272.

Katz, J., & Tillery, K. L. (2005). Can central auditory processing tests resists supramodal influences? *American Journal of Audiology, 14*, 124–127.

Keith, R. W. (2007). Controversies in standardization of auditory processing tests. In D. Cacace & D. J. McFarland (Eds.), *Controversies in central auditory processing disorder* (pp. 169–186). San Diego, CA: Plural.

King, W. M., Lombardina, L. J., Crandell, C. C., & Leonard, C. M. (2003). Comorbid auditory processing disorder in developmental dyslexia. *Ear and Hearing, 24*, 448–456.

Lew, J., & Canon, A. (2010). SLT practices in a multilingual context: The challenges of educational, social and language policies for children with language disorders in Singapore. In M. Cruz-Ferreira (Ed.), *Multilingual norms* (pp. 251–277). Frankfurt am Main, Germany: Peter Lang.

Loo, H. J., Bamiou, D., & Rosen, S. (2013). The impacts of language background and language-related disorders in auditory processing. *Journal of Speech, Language, and Hearing Research, 56*(1), 1–12.

Marriage, J., King, J., Briggs, J., & Lutman, M. E. (2001). The reliability of the SCAN test: Results from a primary school population in the UK. *British Journal of Audiology, 35*, 199–208.

Martinez Perez, T., Majerus, S., Mahot, A., & Poncelet, M. (2012). Evidence for a specific impairment of serial order short-term memory in dyslexic children. *Dyslexia, 18*(2), 94–109.

Marzocchi, G. M., Ornaghi, S., & Barboglio, S. (2009). What are the causes of the attention deficits observed in children with dyslexia? *Child Neuropsychology, 15*(6), 566–581.

Mayo, L. H., Florentine, M., & Buus, S. (1997). Age of second-language acquisition and perception of speech in noise. *Journal of Speech, Language, and Hearing Research, 40*, 686–693.

McArthur, G. M., & Hogben, J. H. (2001). Auditory backward recognition masking in children with specific language impairment and children with specific reading disability. *The Journal of the Acoustical Society of America, 109*, 1092–1100.

McFarland, D. J., & Cacace, A. T. (1995). Modality specificity as a criterion for diagnosing central auditory processing disorders. *American Journal of Audiology, 4*, 36–48.

Merzenich, M. M., Jenkins, W. M., Johnston, P., Schreiner, C., Miller, S. L., & Tallal, P. (1996). Temporal processing deficits of language-learning impaired children ameliorated by training. *Science, 271*, 77–81.

Miller, C. A., & Wagstaff, D. A. (2011). Behavioural profiles associated with auditory processing disorder and specific language impairment. *Journal of Communication Disorders, 44*(6), 745–763.

Moncrieff, D., McColl, R. W., & Black, J. R. (2008). Hemodynamic differences in children with dichotic listening deficits: Preliminary results from an fMRI study during a cued listening task. *Journal of the American Academy of Audiology, 19*(1), 33–45.

Moore, D. (2006). Auditory processing disorder (APD): Definition, diagnosis, neural basis, and intervention. *Audiological Medicine, 4*(1), 1651–3835.

Moore, D. R., Ferguson, M. A., Edmondson-Jones, A. M., Ratib, S., & Riley, A. (2010). Nature of auditory processing disorder in children. *Pediatrics, 126*(2), 382–390.

Musiek, F. E., & Lee, W. W. (1998). Neuroanatomical correlates to central deafness. *Scandinavian Audiology, 27*, 18–25.

Musiek, F. E., Bellis, T. J., & Chermak, G. D. (2005). Nonmodularity of the central auditory nervous system: Implications for (central) auditory processing disorder. *American Journal of Audiology, 14*, 128–138.

Nickisch, A., & von Kries, R. (2009). Short-term memory constraints in children with specific language impairment (SLI): Are there differences between receptive and expressive SLI? *Journal of Speech, Language, and Hearing Research, 52*, 578–595.

Noterdaeme, M., Amorosa, H., Mildenberger, K., Sitter, S., & Minow, F. (2001). Evaluation of attention problems in children with autism and children with a specific language disorder. *European Child and Adolescent Psychiatry, 10*(1), 58–66.

Rosen, S. (2003). Auditory processing in dyslexia and specific language impairment: Is there a deficit? What is its nature? Does it explain anything? *Journal of Phonetics, 31*, 509–527.

Rosen, S. (2005). "A riddle wrapped in a mystery inside an enigma": Defining central auditory processing disorder. *American Journal of Audiology, 14*, 139–142.

Rosen, S., Adlard, A., & Van der Lely, H. K. J. (2009). Backward and simultaneous masking in children with grammatical specific language impairment: No simple link between auditory and language abilities. *Journal of Speech, Language and Hearing Research, 52*, 396–411.

Sharma, M., Purdy, S. C., & Kelly, A. S. (2009). Comorbidity of auditory processing, language, and reading disorders. *Journal of Speech Language and Hearing Research, 52*, 706–722.

Shi, L. F. (2009). Normal hearing English-as-a-second language listeners' recognition of English words in competing signals. *International Journal of Audiology, 48*, 260–270.

Song, J., Banai, K., Russo, N., & Kraus, N. (2006). On the relationship between speech- and non-speech-evoked brainstem responses in children. *Audiology and Neurotology, 11*(4), 233–241.

Stuart, A., Zhang, J., & Swink, S. (2010). Reception thresholds for sentences in quiet and noise for monolingual English and bilingual Mandarin-English listeners. *Journal of American Academy Audiology, 21*(3), 239–248.

Tabri, D., Chacra, K. M. S. A., & Pring, T. (2011). Speech perception in noise by monolingual, bilingual and trilingual listeners. *International Journal of Language Communication Disorders, 46*(4), 411–422.

Tallal, P. (1976). Rapid auditory processing in normal and disordered language development. *Journal of Speech and Hearing, 3*, 561–571.

Tallal, P. (1980). Auditory temporal perception, phonics, and reading disabilities in children. *Brain and Language, 9*, 182–198.

Tallal, P., Miller, S. L, Bedi, G., Byma, G., Wang, X., Nagarajan, S. S., ... Merzenich, M. M. (1996). Language comprehension in language-learning impaired children improved with acoustically modified speech. *Science, 271*, 81–84.

Valaki, C. E., Maestu, F., Simos, P. G., Zhang, W., Fernandez, A., Amo, C. M., ... Papanicolaou, A. C. (2004). Cortical organization for receptive language functions in Chinese, English, and Spanish: A cross-linguistic MEG study. *Neuropsychologia, 42*(7), 967–979.

Von Hapsburg, D., Champlin, C. A., & Shetty, S. R. (2004). Reception thresholds for sentences in bilingual (Spanish/English) and monolingual (English) listeners. *Journal of the American Academy of Audiology, 15*, 88–98.

Wright, B. A., Lombardinao, L. J., King, W. M., Puranik, C. S., Leonard, C. M., & Merzenich, M. M. (1997). Deficits in auditory temporal and spectral resolution in language-impaired children. *Nature, 387*, 176–178.

CHAPTER 6

THEORY AND RESEARCH IN THE STUDY OF EARLY READING DIFFICULTIES

A Personal Odyssey

Frank R. Vellutino

Many years ago, when I was a graduate student pursuing my doctorate in clinical psychology, I became aware of children who experienced difficulties in learning to read. These children were said to perceive letters and words as reversed images, as inferred from letter and word naming errors such as calling "b" "d" or "was" "saw." Upon further inquiry, I learned that this affliction was often called "optical reversibility" and that the afflicted children were suffering from what was believed to be a neurodevelopmental disorder in visual perception called "dyslexia" ("specific reading disability"). Although I had taken an elective course in reading education that involved remedial work with struggling readers, I knew nothing about dyslexia or other types of learning disabilities. However, I remember thinking that optical reversibility was a strange and somewhat inexplicable affliction that must surely make it difficult for a young child to process all types of visual information and not just printed letters and words. Moreover, in the

Understanding Developmental Disorders of Auditory Processing, Language and Literacy Across Languages: International Perspectives, pp. 113–145

materials I read, dyslexics were typically described as children with average or above average intelligence and average or above average learning abilities in other content areas. These disparities seemed to be equally strange and inexplicable. Nevertheless, because I was working with delusional and hallucinatory psychotic patients who routinely claimed to be seeing and hearing things I did not see or hear, I tried to be open-minded about the possibility that reading difficulties in some children may be caused by optical reversibility, although I reserved the right to be skeptical.

I did not give much more thought to dyslexia or optical reversibility in graduate school because I was far too occupied with the work involved in obtaining my doctorate. After completing doctoral studies and receiving my degree, I worked for just under 3 years at a large psychiatric hospital that provided diagnostic and treatment services for psychotic patients. It soon became apparent to me that everything I had learned at graduate school had very limited utility in facilitating recovery from psychosis. I concluded at the time that the scientific community would not have a "cure" for psychosis for the foreseeable future. I was thereafter grateful for the serendipitous opportunity to begin clinical work with a small number of kindergarten and first-grade struggling learners. My work with these children piqued my interest in the causes and correlates of early learning difficulties in young children. Not long afterwards, I became aware of an opening in the position of Associate Director of the Child Research and Study Center, a research and graduate student training center sponsored by the University of Albany for the purpose of conducting research in the study of learning disabilities and other developmental disorders. The person who filled the opening would become a member of the graduate faculty in the Department of Educational Psychology at the university and possibly receive a joint appointment with the Department of Psychology. I applied for and procured this position and eventually became both the director of the center and a full professor in both departments.

One of the many responsibilities I had as director of the Child Research and Study Center was to train graduate students to determine the origin of the learning difficulties experienced by the children who were referred to the center, in the interest of helping school officials develop appropriate formats and procedures for remediating such difficulties. This enterprise required that I not only work with graduate students, but also with the children referred for learning difficulties. The most frequent referrals by far were those requesting evaluations of children experiencing difficulties in learning to read and spell. I learned a great deal about literacy development through working with such children and teaching graduate students, and these experiences became the foundation for a program of research that my students and I initiated to learn more about the causes and correlates of the difficulties involved in acquiring early literacy skills.

The remainder of this chapter summarizes the high points of this personal odyssey. It focuses on select findings that I consider to be among our most important contributions to this area of inquiry.

Visual Deficit Studies

Optical Reversibility Studies

The initial phase of our research was motivated by my interest in evaluating the idea that children who experience difficulties in acquiring early literacy skills are afflicted by optical reversibility, as manifested in naming errors made during oral reading of letters and words, such as calling "b" "d" or "was" "saw." In my reading of the dyslexia literature, I learned that this hypothesis was initially forwarded by Orton (1925), who theorized that the left and right hemispheres of the brain store "mirror image" representations of visual stimuli that compete with each other in the early stages of perceptual development and that one of these representations becomes "elided" (suppressed) during the establishment of hemispheric dominance for language. In accordance with this theory, Orton suggested that dyslexia is caused by a developmental lag in hemispheric dominance for language that adversely affects the normal process of "eliding" irrelevant representations stored in the nondominant hemisphere. A similar visual deficit theory of dyslexia was forwarded by Herman (1959), who suggested that "b/d" and "was/saw" type errors in dyslexic readers are manifestations of genetically based deficits in spatial orientation and sense of direction (see Vellutino, 1979 for other early visual deficit theories of dyslexia).

However, as indicated previously, I was skeptical that a deficit in visual perception characterized by optical reversibility was psychologically real. I strongly suspected that there might be alternative explanations for "b/d" or "was/saw" type naming errors, and the illogical nature of Orton's theory served to strengthen my suspicion. I was also skeptical of Herman's (1959) directional confusion theory of dyslexia and intuited that this theory provided no better explanation for letter reversal and letter sequencing errors than Orton's (1925) theory. As I thought more about the issue, an alternative explanation that came to mind was that they were caused by a dysfunction in name learning and retrieval processes, perhaps due to an inability to process the linguistic components of written words rather than a dysfunction in visual perception and memory. It occurred to me that deficiencies in phonological coding could impair a child's ability to establish connective bonds between printed letters and the sounds they represent, and between printed words as wholes and the words they represent in spoken language. It seemed that such deficiencies were likely to have a deleterious effect on the ability to acquire both alphabetic coding and whole-word identification skills, both of which are important for becoming literate in an alphabetically based orthography such as written English. It also seemed quite possible and even probable that more general language deficits such as vocabulary and syntactic deficits would have similar effects. Thus, we designed several studies to directly assess the visual deficit theories of dyslexia proposed by Orton (1925) and Hermann (1959).

The first study we conducted (Vellutino, Steger, & Kandel, 1972) assessed the performance of poor and normally developing readers (henceforth called "normal readers") in processing the visual components of written symbols compared with their performance in processing the verbal components of the same stimuli. We also assessed and compared the performance of the two groups in processing geometric designs. More specifically, we administered intelligence, word identification, and oral reading measures to an unstratified sample of children between the ages of 9 and 14 (grades 4–9) who were initially selected according to the exclusionary criteria typically used to identify children believed to be afflicted by a "specific learning disability," that is, an absence of sensory acuity deficits, emotional problems, extreme physical and neurological deficits, sociocultural disadvantage, and frequent absence from school. We then identified samples of poor and normal readers at each grade level using conventional criteria to identify each group. Both groups had to exhibit at least average intelligence and normal development in areas other than reading. The poor readers had to be reading well below grade level, and the normal readers had to be reading at or above grade level. (Note that similar procedures were used to identify poor and normal reader groups in all of our studies evaluating the causes and correlates of early reading difficulties). After identifying and constituting both research samples, we provided the children in both samples with pseudoword decoding measures to further evaluate the possibility that dyslexics were afflicted by phonological deficits that impaired the type of letter-sound correspondence learning involved in becoming literate.

We then presented the children in each sample with 3-, 4-, and 5-letter words (three in each set) and parallel sets of randomly ordered letters and numbers. We also presented them with two sets of geometric designs (three in each set), one consisting of 2-item designs and the other consisting of three-item designs (see Figure 6.1). All of the 33 stimuli were randomly ordered, and each stimulus was presented tachistoscopically for 600 milliseconds. (We were not equipped with personal computers at this point). The children were given paper and pencils and asked to reproduce each stimulus from visual memory immediately after presentation. After a short break, the geometric designs were removed from the tachistoscope and each child was again presented with the letter, number, and word stimuli using the same presentation procedure. However, their task for these presentations was to name each stimulus. Thus, for each word stimulus, the children were asked to name the word and then spell out its letters immediately afterwards (e.g., "LOIN," "L - O - I - N"). For the random letter and number stimuli, the children were asked to name the components in each stimulus set from left to right.

REAL WORDS

Three Letter	Four Letter	Five Letter
fly	loin	blunt
bed	form	drawn
was	calm	chair

SCRAMBLED LETTERS

Three Letter	Four Letter	Five Letter
dnv	jpyc	ztbrc
hbd	gzfs	yfpqg
mcw	qvlt	qldnr

NUMBERS

Three Digit	Four Digit	Five Digit
382	4328	96842
974	3724	31579
296	9156	86314

GEOMETRIC DESIGNS

Two Items Three Items

Figure 6.1. Verbal and nonverbal stimuli used to assess visual memory and name retrieval in the optical reversibility studies.

The performance of the poor reader group closely approximated that of the normal reader group on the visual reproduction tasks, but the two groups performed more disparately on the naming tasks. There were no statistically significant reader group differences in the visual reproduction of the geometric designs, random letters, and numbers. However, the groups began to diverge in their visual reproductions of the 5-letter words, no doubt because the normal readers could identify the words better than the poor readers and did not have to rely as heavily on visual memory. While differences in the reader groups were evident for all of the reading tasks, these differences were found to be substantially larger on the letter and word naming tasks than on the number naming task. However, the observed group differences tended to be of greater magnitude when younger children were involved. This finding was not surprising, given that the older children in the sample had more experience than the younger children with letter and word identification.

The results from this study provided initial support for our hypothesis that "b/d" and "was/saw" type errors were a manifestation of a language-based dysfunction rather than a manifestation of dysfunction in visual perception and memory. In fact, they made us more suspicious of Orton's optical reversibility and Herman's directional confusion theories of dyslexia. However, because the research sample in the study was not stratified and the reliability of the results obtained at the different grade levels was therefore in question, my colleagues and I conducted a second study with stratified samples of poor and normal readers in the second and sixth grades (ages 7–11) to further evaluate the theories (Vellutino, Smith, Steger, & Kaman, 1975). The materials and presentation procedures used in the study were identical to those used in the previous study, and the results we obtained essentially replicated those obtained in our first study. It is important to note that in both of the studies, the poor readers performed significantly worse than the normal readers on the pseudoword decoding tests, which it may be recalled were administered to both groups after the sample selection procedure was completed. This finding provided us with strong reasons to believe that poor readers as a group are afflicted with basic phonological deficits that impair their ability to acquire letter-sound correspondence rules.

However, we had to acknowledge that our interpretations of the results of these studies were tentative, especially those related to group and developmental differences in the visual reproduction of 5-letter words, wherein we attributed the advantage enjoyed by normal readers and older children to their greater reading ability. We also had to acknowledge that the results did not have wide applicability, because the materials and procedures used in both studies were identical, leaving open the question of whether similar results could be obtained with different materials or procedures. Thus, we designed several other studies using a paradigm that we believed would provide a stronger test of visual deficit theories of dyslexia.

Hebrew Word Studies

All of these studies compared the performance of poor and normal reader groups using tasks that required visual memory for words written in an alphabetic orthography with which the two groups were unfamiliar, specifically, written Hebrew. The performance of these two groups was compared with that of normal readers at the same age and grade levels who were learning to read and write Hebrew. There were several reasons for using this paradigm. First, we reasoned that presenting poor and normal readers with tasks that assessed their memory for complex visual symbols from an unfamiliar alphabetic orthography would more strongly test our belief that the difficulties they experienced in learning to read did not arise from deficiencies in visual perception and memory, because it involved memory for unfamiliar visual stimuli sharing the structural properties of words in an alphabetic writing system. This procedure also controlled for possible confounds associated with reader group differences in reading ability, which in our previous studies gave the advantage to normal readers on tasks that required visual memory for letters and words from a familiar orthography.

Second, we reasoned that by comparing the performance of poor and normal readers who were unfamiliar with written Hebrew with that of children who were familiar with written Hebrew on a task requiring visual memory for Hebrew words, we would be able to assess the effects of familiarity with both the verbal and visual components of Hebrew words on visual memory for those words. Further, we fully expected that the children who were familiar with written Hebrew would have better visual memory for Hebrew words and their component letters than the children who were unfamiliar with these stimuli, due in part to the familiarity with their names and visual characteristics. Finally, because written Hebrew is conventionally processed from right to left and written English is conventionally processed from left to right, a comparison of the directional processing strategies of the children who were familiar and unfamiliar with Hebrew facilitated a direct test of Hermann's (1952) directional confusion theory of dyslexia. Hermann's theory predicts that poor readers' processing strategies should either be erratic or more like that of children learning to read and write Hebrew. Our theory predicted that there would be no differences in the processing strategies of poor and normal readers who were unfamiliar with Hebrew and that both would process Hebrew words from left to right, in contrast to children who were learning to read and write Hebrew who were expected to process Hebrew words from right to left.

Visual memory for Hebrew words was assessed using both visual recall and recognition tasks, and we found that the poor and normal readers who were unfamiliar with Hebrew did not differ on any of the measures used to assess their visual processing abilities. However, in accordance with our expectations, neither group performed as well on these measures as the children learning to read and write printed Hebrew. These measures assessed spatial orientation and directional processing errors in addition to accuracy in reproducing Hebrew words from visual memory.

To be more specific, in the first of the studies using Hebrew word stimuli (Vellutino, Pruzek, Steger, & Mesholoum, 1973), children in grades 4–6 were presented with 3-, 4-, and 5-letter Hebrew words (see Figure 6.2) for 3, 4, and 5 seconds, respectively, and simply asked to reproduce each word from visual memory. Whereas the poor and normal readers who were unfamiliar with Hebrew letters and words performed at comparable levels on the visual reproduction task, the children in each group performed well below the children learning to read and write Hebrew on this task. The only exceptions were the 3-letter words task, on which the three groups performed equivalently.

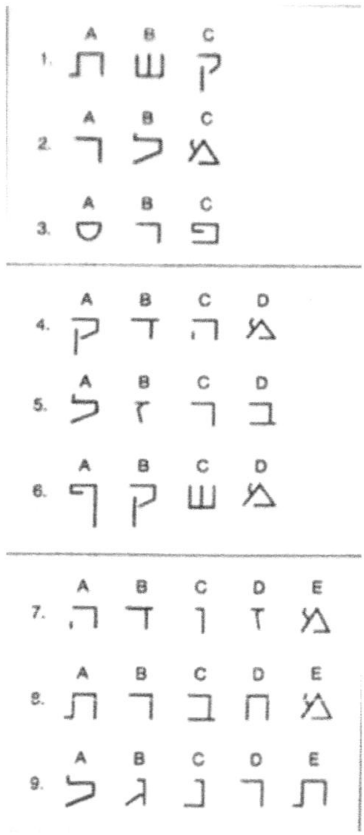

Figure 6.2. Hebrew words that were used to assess visual memory and directional processing in the Hebrew word studies.

To assess directional processing strategies, the location of omission errors was assessed in the three groups. It was found that the poor and normal readers who were unfamiliar with Hebrew made all of their omission errors at the right terminal positions of the words, suggesting that both groups were using a left-to-right processing strategy to reproduce a word's letters, consistent with conventional English. In contrast, the children who were familiar with Hebrew made all of their omission errors at the left terminal positions of the words, suggesting that they used a right-to-left processing strategy, consistent with conventional Hebrew. Finally, in terms of the Hebrew words containing letters similar in appearance to certain Roman letters used in written English (e.g., 1c, 2a, and 3c in Figure 6.2), the children who were unfamiliar with Hebrew often made spatial orientation errors that conformed to the orientation of Roman letters. However, the number of such errors made by the poor readers was no greater than that made by the normal readers relative to the children who were learning to read and write Hebrew.

We conducted two other studies that compared the performance of poor and normal readers on tasks assessing visual memory for Hebrew letters and words (Vellutino, Steger, DeSetto, & Phillips, 1975; Vellutino, Steger, Kaman, & DeSetto, 1975). The results obtained from these studies essentially replicated the results obtained from the preceding study. Moreover, in all three of the studies, the poor readers were found to perform worse than the normal readers on a pseudoword decoding test, supporting our growing belief that they suffered from basic phonological deficits that impaired their ability to acquire letter-sound correspondence rules. Combining these findings with those obtained in the first two studies evaluating the two most prominent and influential visual deficit theories of dyslexia, we became quite confident that these and similar visual deficit theories of dyslexia were invalid, and we continue to hold this view. However, there is one other visual deficit theory of dyslexia worth mentioning briefly: the "transient system deficit" theory of dyslexia initially proposed by Lovegrove and colleagues (e.g., Lovegrove, Martin, & Slaghuis, 1986; see also Stein, 2001). To better understand this theory, it is important to provide some background information.

First, note that the visual system consists of two parallel systems that complement each other: the magnocellular and parvocellular systems. The magnocellular system consists of large neurons that have high conduction velocities and are very sensitive to movement and rapid changes in the visual field. These properties have led researchers to refer to the magnocellular system as the "transient visual system." The parvocellular system consists of small neurons that are sensitive to form, color, and fine detail. This system is responsible for foveal or focused vision. In reading, the parvocellular system is operative during eye fixations. The magnocellular system is operative during saccadic movements of the eyes and is believed to be responsible for suppressing traces of the visual information processed during eye fixations.

Lovegrove et al. (1986) theorized that reading difficulties are caused by a transient system deficit that impairs the normal inhibitory function of the magnocellular neurons, thereby producing a visual trace of abnormal longevity that creates visual acuity and masking problems. Their research suggested that dyslexic and normal readers process low and high spatial frequencies differently, insofar as dyslexics (apparently) require greater luminosity than normal readers to distinguish visual stimuli with low spatial frequencies. Their findings were believed to be caused by transient system deficits.

However, there are several contraindications to the transient system deficit theory of dyslexia. First, note that in the studies conducted by Lovegrove and others, some normal readers were found to have transient system anomalies, thereby undermining any strong generalizations regarding causal relationships between such anomalies and reading difficulties. Second, the theory predicts that dyslexics should be impaired only when they are reading connected text and not when they are reading one word at a time, which is anomalous. We know that dyslexics experience as much difficulty reading individual words presented one at a time as they do reading the same words in connected text. Third, there is no clinical evidence that dyslexics experience visual acuity and masking problems under normal reading conditions. Finally, the dyslexics evaluated in the studies conducted by Lovegrove and others (e.g., Stein, 2001) were also found to be afflicted with phonological deficits such as those found to be causally related to reading difficulties (e.g., phoneme awareness and letter-sound decoding deficits), supporting similar results obtained from our own studies.

However, enough reliable and thereby suggestive evidence has been produced to show that some poor readers process low spatial frequencies differently than normal readers. Eden and Zeffiro (1998) provided one possible explanation of such findings. These investigators reviewed a large number of neurophysiological and fMRI studies, and provided evidence to suggest that dyslexics have structural and functional anomalies in adjacent regions of the brain supporting linguistic and transient system processes of the types found to be deficient in this group. They acknowledged that transient system anomalies were not causally related to reading difficulties and suggested that visual processing deficits implicating the transient system may be biological markers that could aid differential diagnosis. I consider this a plausible hypothesis that deserves further study.

Studies Assessing General Learning Deficits

As I indicated in the previous section, the results of the studies we conducted evaluating visual deficit theories of dyslexia convinced me that early reading difficulties in otherwise normal children are not caused by visual perception and visual memory deficits. These findings suggested that such difficulties could be due in some measure to language and language-based deficits of one description or another. For example, from time to time, we all find it difficult to retrieve the name of someone or something familiar. This could be a more pervasive and chronic abnormality that impairs a child's ability to learn to read, at least in some cases. This hypothesis was tentatively supported by research conducted by Denckla and Rudel (1976a, 1976b; see also Denckla, 1972), who documented deficits in the rapid naming of colors and objects in dyslexic children. It seemed that vocabulary deficits or general language deficits could similarly be the source of early reading difficulties. The logical next step was to conduct research that more directly evaluated the possibility that the difficulties experienced in learning to read may be caused by language-based deficits that impair a child's ability to integrate the visual and verbal components of printed words.

However, before discussing the seminal research we conducted to assess this possibility, other seemingly illogical theories of dyslexia that have been advanced in the literature should be discussed. I refer to theories of dyslexia that implicate deficiencies in the general learning abilities involved, not only in learning to read, but also in every new learning enterprise. For example, difficulties in learning to read have been attributed to deficiencies in selective attention (Douglas, 1972), associative learning (Brewer, 1967; Gascon & Goodglass, 1970), intersensory learning (often called cross-modal transfer; Birch, 1962), serial-order processing (Bakker, 1972), and both pattern analysis and rule learning (Blank & Bridger, 1966; Morrison & Manis, 1982). Such theories can be questioned purely on logical grounds. Given that all of these cognitive abilities are entailed on virtually all tests of intelligence and are certainly entailed in all academic learning, dysfunction in any of these rather basic and general learning abilities could seemingly be ruled out as a significant cause of the difficulties experienced by some children when learning to read, even when they have at least average intelligence and no general learning difficulties. More importantly, all of these hypotheses have been negated by empirical research (Vellutino, 1979, 1987; see also Katz, Healy, & Shankweiler, 1983). I discuss this research as follows.

Inter- and Intrasensory Learning

To further evaluate the "logical disconnect" created by theories suggesting that reading difficulties in children with no other learning difficulties could be caused by deficiencies in general learning abilities of the types mentioned in the preceding section, we conducted several other studies directly assessing this possibility beginning with two studies that assessed those theories suggesting that reading disability is caused by select deficiencies in either associative learning (Brewer, 1967; Gascon & Goodglass, 1970) or intersensory learning (Birch, 1962). Although basic deficits in associative learning would necessarily imply basic deficits in intersensory (cross-modal) learning, the latter would not necessarily imply the former. Thus, in an initial study designed to evaluate the possibility that reading difficulties are caused by deficiencies in one or both types of learning (Vellutino, Steger, & Pruzek, 1973), poor and normal readers in grades 4–7 were presented with inter- and intrasensory learning tasks that involved nonverbal paired-associate learning. The intersensory learning task required the integration of visual and auditory nonverbal (VANV) stimuli. The stimuli for this task were simple novel designs (see Figure 3) paired with simple vocalic responses, such as coughing, whistling, or humming. As a control measure, the same children were also presented with two intrasensory learning tasks: visual-visual (V-V) and auditory-auditory (A-A) paired-associate learning tasks. The stimuli used for the V-V learning task were simple designs different from those used for the VANV learning task. The stimuli used for the A-A learning task consisted of simple environmental stimuli (presented with a tape recorder) paired with simple (nonlinguistic) vocalic responses.

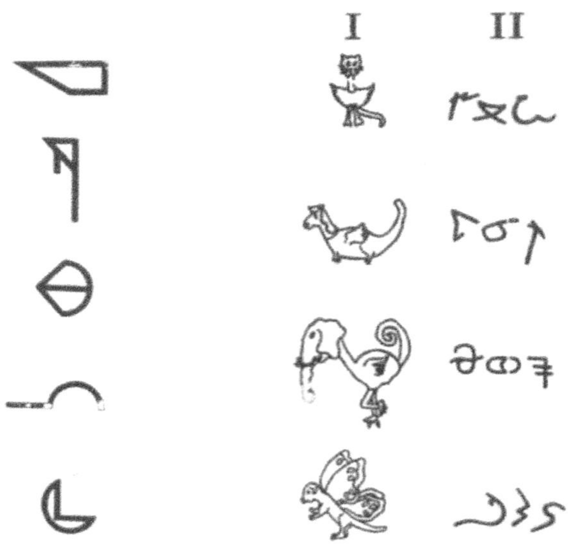

Figure 6.3. Geometric designs used to assess visual-auditory nonverbal learning (left); cartoon figures used to assess name learning (middle), and novel script used to assess sight word learning (right).

There were no statistically significant differences between the two reader groups on either the intersensory or intrasensory learning tasks. The results contradicted theories of reading disability that suggest that reading difficulties are caused by deficiencies in either associative learning or intersensory integration (i.e., cross-modal transfer). Additional evidence against such theories was provided by another study conducted at our laboratory (Steger, Vellutino, & Meshoulam, 1972) that evaluated Birch's suggestion that any intersensory learning deficits underlying reading disability would be evident in learning that involves sensory systems other than those involved in reading. To assess this hypothesis, we compared poor and normal readers on tactile-tactile and visual-tactile learning tasks and found no significant differences between the groups. We tentatively concluded from the results of these studies that reading difficulties are not caused by basic deficits in either associative or intersensory learning. Given that all of the tasks used in these studies required the utmost in focal attention, the results were also at odds with theories of dyslexia that suggest that reading difficulties in otherwise normal children may be caused by attention deficits of one description or another (Douglas, 1972). Although I do not deny that attention deficits may cause reading difficulties, I reject the idea that such difficulties may be caused by attention deficits in children who have no learning difficulties in other academic areas.

Serial Order Processing

Dysfunction in serial order processing is another hypothesized cause of reading disability that has long held great appeal for clinicians working with children who have difficulty learning to read and spell. This hypothesis has also held great appeal for a number of scholars (e.g., Bakker, 1972; Bannatyne, 1971; Johnson & Myklebust, 1967). The clinical indicators of dysfunction in serial order processing that have motivated this view include phoneme reversals such as saying "/ephelant/" rather than "elephant"; sequencing errors in reading or spelling ("was/saw"; "pot/top"); difficulty with other school learning tasks such as reciting the alphabet or ordering the days of the week and months of the year; and difficulty on more formal measures of serial order processing such as those that involve memory for words, sentences, digits, objects, and designs presented either visually or auditorily. Such difficulties have led both factions to suggest that reading disabilities are caused by a neurological dysfunction that results in modality-specific difficulties with ordering information in any of the sensory systems.

I reviewed the seminal research conducted in this area (Vellutino, 1979) and concluded that the evidence that reading disability is caused by a neurologically based deficit in serial order processing was weak and equivocal. I also pointed out that the research conducted in this area was in most instances post hoc and atheoretical. The only scholar whose research was based on a well-formulated theory was Bakker (1972), who suggested that reading disability is caused by a dysfunction in temporal order perception (TOP). This theory was based on previous work done by Hirsh and colleagues (Hirsh, 1959, 1966; Hirsh & Sherrick, 1961), who demonstrated that adults require an interstimulus interval of at least 20 milliseconds to detect a succession of two tones. Hirsh (1966) in fact suggested that speech perception is determined by the order in which phonemes occur over time and that some individuals may be impaired in making such distinctions because of dysfunction in speed of processing acoustic stimuli. Bakker's (1972) TOP theory of reading disability was based on a similar assumption. However, as pointed out in a review by Vellutino (1979), the research that Bakker conducted in support of his TOP theory was no less weak or equivocal than the research conducted by other scholars who evaluated serial-order processing in dyslexic readers.

Finally, it is worth noting that Bakker's (1972) TOP theory of reading disability appears to be the precursor to a more recently formulated theory of reading disability forwarded by Tallal (1980), who suggested that reading difficulties are caused by a deficit in the temporal resolution of rapidly changing auditory stimuli that impairs speech perception and phonological processing in general. The initial evidence for this theory came from a study conducted by Tallal, who found that poor readers performed below normal readers in making judgments as to the order in which high and low tones were presented at short (50 millisecond) interstimulus intervals. In contrast, the differences in group performance on this task were not found at long (400 millisecond) interstimulus intervals, and the combined results were taken as an indication that poor readers require more time than normal readers to process auditory stimuli.

However, the results from that study were equivocal, as only 9 out of 20 poor readers had difficulty making temporal order judgments at the short interstimulus interval. At the same time, some normal readers were found to experience such difficulties, suggesting that Tallal's (1980) findings were unreliable and quite likely attributable to measurement error. Moreover, Tallal's study, along with some other studies that provided support for her theory, did not control for attention deficit hyperactivity disorder (ADHD), and the studies that did so found no differences between poor and normal readers in performance on temporal order judgment tasks. Thus, the theory has received tenuous support at best (see an article by Vellutino, Fletcher, Snowling, & Scanlon (2004) for a comprehensive review of these and related findings).

Pattern Analysis and Rule Learning

As indicated earlier, some researchers have suggested that reading-disabled children may be afflicted with basic deficits in pattern analysis and rule learning that impair their ability to detect and represent patterned invariance (Blank & Bridger, 1966; Morrison & Manis, 1982). In theory, such deficits could impair a child's ability to acquire and represent letter-sound correspondence rules, which are critically important for learning to read in an alphabetic system such as written English. For the reasons cited earlier, I did not believe that reading problems in otherwise normal children could be caused by deficiencies in detecting and representing patterned invariance. In fact, on the strength of the possibility that reading difficulties are caused by language-based deficits, I wondered whether difficulties in acquiring letter-sound correspondence rules could be caused by verbal learning deficits rather than pattern detection deficits. To directly assess this hypothesis, my colleagues and I conducted a study that compared the performance of poor and normal readers on associative learning tasks that involved detecting patterned invariance in associating visual and verbal stimuli, relative to associative learning tasks involving the detection of patterned invariance in associating two sets of visual stimuli (Vellutino, Harding, Phillips, & Steger, 1975). In keeping with the verbal deficit explanation of reading disability, we expected that the poor readers would perform below the normal readers on the visual-verbal learning tasks, but not on the visual-visual learning tasks.

Two independent and comparably selected samples of poor and normal readers (grades 4–6) participated in this study. The children from each reader group were randomly assigned to either the visual-verbal or the visual-visual learning conditions. Both conditions employed a transfer-learning paradigm, our intent being to simulate the type of generalization learning involved in acquiring skill in reading (e.g., learn "cat," "rat," and "can"; independently decode "ran"). The stimuli on both sets of tasks were novel, complex, and in the case of the visual-visual paired associates task, provided ample opportunity for children in both groups to make the types of orientation and sequencing errors believed to be cardinal signs of spatial confusion (Hermann, 1959; Orton, 1925). Those that were paired under the training condition remained paired under the transfer condition. Thus, in the visual-verbal condition, a novel visual stimulus was paired with the first syllable of a two-syllable nonsense word, and a second visual stimulus adjacent to the first was paired with the second syllable of the same nonsense word. The children were informed of these relationships and were given practice in learning them with different stimuli. The transfer task presented reordered combinations of the visual-verbal associates presented on the training task (see Figure 6.4a). The same paired-associates format was used on the training and transfer tasks presented in the visual-visual condition, except that learning in the latter condition was assessed using a match-to-standard task (see Figure 6.4b).

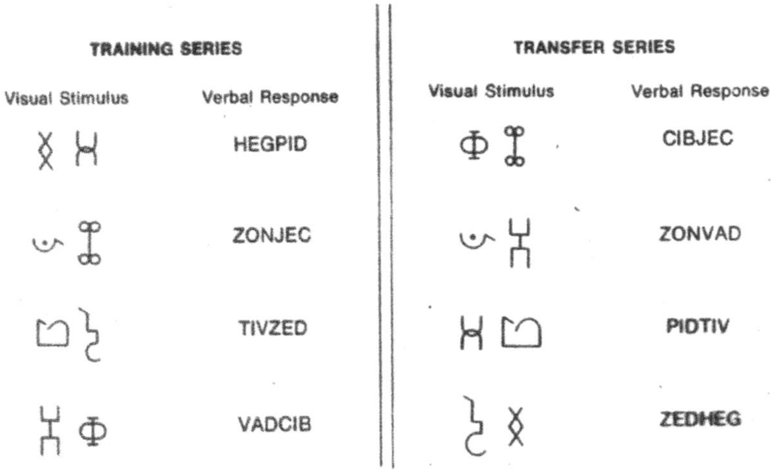

Figure 6.4a. Visual and verbal stimuli used in the training and transfer conditions to assess visual-verbal pattern analysis and rule learning.

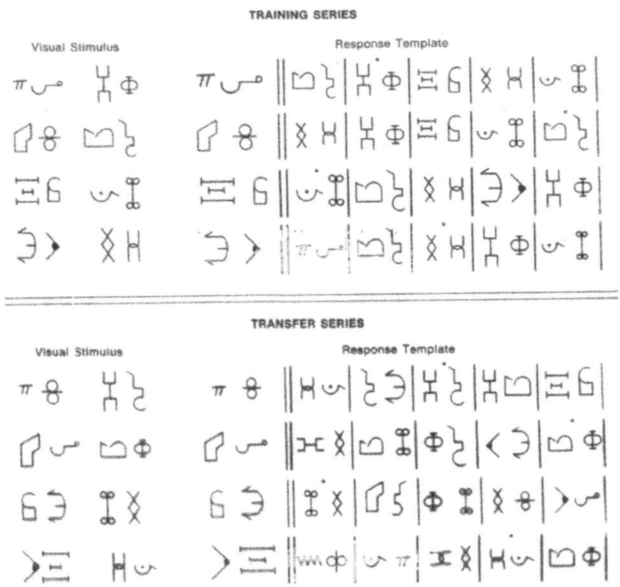

Figure 6.4b. Visual stimuli used in the training and transfer conditions to assess visual-visual pattern analysis and rule learning.

In accord with our expectations, the poor readers performed below the normal readers on the visual-verbal training and transfer-learning tasks, but as well as the normal readers on the visual-visual training and transfer-learning tasks. We concluded from these findings that "poor readers can successfully process the categorical relationships contained in patterned stimuli when such information is of a nonverbal nature, but can be expected to have difficulty in processing patterned information of a verbal nature" (Vellutino, 1979, p. 242).

Verbal Deficit Studies

The results of the studies reported in the preceding sections provided compelling evidence that reading disabilities in children with no generalized learning difficulties are not caused by either visual processing or general learning ability deficits. Moreover, the results from our visual-verbal transfer-learning study (Vellutino, Harding et al., 1975) were consistent with my suspicion that poor readers are impaired by some type of language-based deficit that makes it difficult for them to integrate the visual symbols that represent speech segments with their verbal counterparts. This suspicion was buttressed by another finding, that the poor readers in both the visual-verbal and visual-visual learning conditions performed significantly below the normal readers on a pseudoword decoding test, thereby replicating the pattern of results obtained from the previous studies that we conducted to assess this skill in the two groups. We were also made aware of the work being done by other researchers, who have suggested that many poor readers suffer from basic phoneme segmentation and awareness deficits that impair their ability to map alphabetic symbols to sounds (Downing, 1973; Elkonin, 1973; Liberman, 1971; Liberman & Shankweiler, 1978; Liberman, Shankweiler, Fischer, & Carter, 1974; Liberman, Shankweiler, Orlando, Harris, & Berti, 1971; Savin, 1972). In the case of learning to read in alphabetically based writing systems, phoneme awareness has typically been defined as a conscious awareness that spoken words are composed of speech segments that map onto alphabetic characters with a high degree of regularity. The research evaluating the relationship between deficiencies in phoneme awareness and reading difficulties further convinced me that such difficulties have a language-based origin, and I began to suspect that alphabetic mapping and visual-verbal learning problems may have a common foundation.

Visual-Auditory Verbal and Nonverbal Learning

To further evaluate the possibility that the reading difficulties experienced by some children may be caused by basic deficits in visual-verbal learning rather than basic deficits in associative or intersensory learning, we conducted yet another study that compared the performance of poor and normal readers on both intersensory and visual-verbal learning tasks (Vellutino, Steger, Harding, & Phillips, 1975). In this study, independent samples of poor and normal readers (grades 4–6) were randomly assigned to either a visual-auditory nonverbal (VANV) learning condition or a visual-verbal learning condition. The stimuli, methods, and procedures used in the VANV learning condition were identical to those used in the study conducted by Vellutino, Steger, and Pruzek (1973). Our intent was to replicate the findings of that study using independent samples of poor and normal readers. The visual-verbal learning condition was designed to simulate the process of whole-word naming in reading (often called "sight word" learning) and consisted of two subtests administered in an invariant sequence. The first subtest simulated the process of name learning and retrieval in order to assess the possibility that this rather basic aspect of language learning may be a significant source of early reading difficulty. It accordingly involved associating cartoon figures with nonsense syllables that represented the names of the figures, "wib," "pex," "mog," and "yag," respectively (see Figure 6.3-I). The second subtest was administered directly after the first and more directly simulated the process of whole-word naming in that it involved associating the nonsense syllables presented on the first task with novel nonalphabetic letter characters (see Figure 6.3-II).

Given that there were no reader group differences on the VANV learning task, the results from the VANV learning condition essentially replicated those obtained in the intersensory learning study (Vellutino, Steger, & Pruzek 1973). In contrast, there were statistically significant differences that favored the normal readers on both the name learning and whole-word naming tasks, supporting the possibility that reading difficulties in some poor readers are caused by language-based deficits that impair their ability to associate and integrate the visual and verbal counterparts of printed words as a whole. One gratuitous finding from this study is that the naming errors made by the poor readers learning to associate visual stimuli with their nonsense word counterparts were characterized by more real word substitutions (e.g., saying "fog" rather than "mog") than the naming errors of the normal readers, which were more often novel combinations of the individual phonemes in the nonsense words (e.g., saying "mag" and "yog" rather than "mog" and "yag"). This finding was taken to indicate that the normal readers were more inclined than the poor readers to code the visual stimuli phonologically and seemed to be consistent with the possibility that poor readers experience difficulties in phonological coding (Liberman & Shankweiler, 1978; Perfetti & Lesgold, 1978).

Word Identification Strategies

Although the results from the studies just discussed provided strong evidence that reading difficulties experienced by otherwise normal children are not caused by basic associative or intersensory learning deficits, they provided no direct evidence to support the hypothesis that such difficulties are caused by language-based deficits that impair the learner's ability to integrate visual and verbal stimuli. The need for such evidence motivated another study conducted in our laboratory that evaluated this hypothesis more directly (Vellutino & Scanlon, 1987a). This was a training study with an experimental design that assessed whether word identification problems in poor readers were caused by weak phonological coding or by more circumscribed difficulty in whole-word naming ("sight word" learning), perhaps caused in part by weak semantic encoding. As I indicated in a previous section, weak phonological coding could lead to difficulties in both name encoding and alphabetic mapping, which could in turn impair both whole-word naming and letter-sound decoding ability. A circumscribed difficulty in semantic encoding would be expected to impair only whole-word naming ability and leave letter-sound decoding ability intact.

A related objective of the study was to assess the relative importance of whole-word naming versus letter-sound decoding strategies in learning to read printed words. Whole-word naming is by definition a meaning-based approach to word identification that depends on ready access to a linguistic representation in the semantic network. In contrast, letter-sound decoding is a code-based approach to word identification that depends heavily on phoneme segmentation and alphabetic mapping. Our clinical experience and intuition suggested that both of these are complementary reading subskills that are necessary for learning to read successfully and conversely that deficiencies in one or the other adversely affect such learning. However, these questions had not been addressed in any of the experimental research. To fill this gap, independent samples of poor and normal readers in second and sixth grade were randomly assigned to one of five experimental conditions, three of which were experimental training conditions that simulated different approaches to reading instruction and two of which were control conditions. One of the training conditions, phonemic segmentation training (PST), simulated the code-oriented approach to word identification and involved 5 or 6 days of activities designed to foster an analytic disposition to search for letter-sound invariances in printed words. These activities included phoneme segmentation of spoken and written words and pseudowords, along with training and transfer-learning tasks that involved the decoding of pseudowords composed of novel alphabetic characters to simulate the process of learning to use letter sounds to identify printed words (see Figure 6.5). Both of these tasks involved periodic probing and feedback to encourage detection of letter-sound invariance.

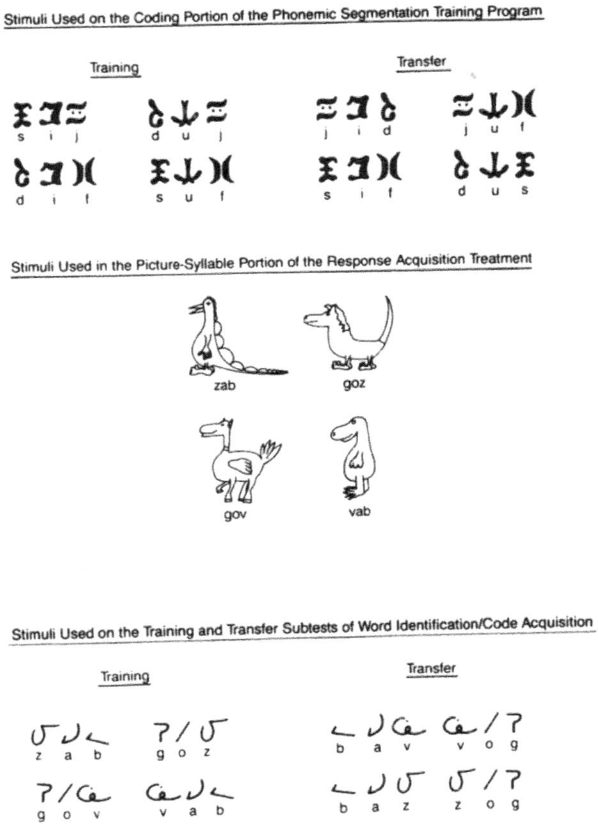

Figure 6.5. Novel alphabetic stimuli used in the phonemic segmentation training condition (top) cartoon figures used in the response acquisition condition (middle); and novel alphabetic stimuli used for the code acquisition training and transfer conditions (bottom).

A second training condition, response acquisition (RA), simulated the whole-word meaning-based approach to word identification. The children in this condition were initially presented with a phonological memory task designed to familiarize them with the nonsense words that served as the verbal response counterparts ("gov," "goz," "vab," "zab") of the visual stimuli used on the training component of the training and transfer-learning tasks (see Figure 6.5). The phonological memory task consisted of 20 free recall trials using an alternating presentation-test format, and the number of correct nonsense words recalled was recorded on each trial. After a short break, the children were presented with a paired-associate learning task on which they learned to associate the same nonsense words with cartoon-like animal figures to imbue them with meaning (see Figure 6.5). This task consisted of 15 learning trials, again using the alternating presentation-test format. The free recall task served as an operational measure of phonological coding ability, and the picture-syllable learning task served as an operational measure of name learning that was analogous to learning new vocabulary words.

Children assigned to the third experimental condition received both phonemic segmentation and response acquisition training (PSTRA), which simulated approaches to reading instruction that incorporated both code-oriented and meaning-based strategies to facilitate word identification.

After no more than a 2-day hiatus following the completion of each training program, the children were presented with new training and transfer-learning tasks (code-acquisition training and transfer) that required the decoding of written pseudowords (trigraphs) composed of novel alphabetic characters (see Figure 6.5). These were the dependent measures used to assess the effectiveness of each of the training programs, and each task involved 20 paired-associate learning trials. To assess the possibility that the failure to teach alphabetic coding skills made children more vulnerable to reversal errors (e.g., confusing "was" with "saw"), the pseudowords in the transfer task were reversed derivatives of the pseudowords in the training task ("vog," "zog," "bav," "baz"). Note also that the stimuli used as the dependent measures were completely different from the stimuli used in any of the training conditions.

As indicated, there were two control conditions. The children in the first control condition (C-1) were assigned both the training and transfer-learning tasks to assess the effects of each of the experimental conditions on both initial and transfer learning. The children in the second control condition (C-2) were assigned only the transfer-learning task to assess the effects of exposure to the training task on transfer learning, especially in terms of the tendency to make generalizations and reversal errors without the benefit of any training that could affect the tendency to make such errors.

Finally, the children in the reader groups assigned to either the treatment or control conditions were provided with (alternate form) measures of phonemic segmentation ability both before and after exposure to the conditions to which they were assigned.

Space does not permit a detailed discussion of the results obtained from this study. The data suggested that both code-oriented and meaning-based strategies for word identification were important components of both the word identification process and reading instruction insofar as the children exposed to both training conditions (PSTRA group) performed better than the children in the PST, RA, and C-1 groups on the initial learning component (code-acquisition training) of the dependent measure. The children in the PST and RA groups also performed better than the children in the C-1 group on this measure. Moreover, on the transfer-learning task (code-acquisition transfer), the children in the groups that received code-oriented training (the PST and PSTRA groups) generally performed better than the children in the groups that did not receive this training (the RA, C-1, and C-2 groups). They also made fewer generalization and intrusion errors (e.g., "was/saw" type reversals), although no fewer than the children in the C-2 control group, probably because they were not exposed to the initial learning task.

Finally, the children who received code-acquisition training (the PST and PSTRA groups) performed better than the children in any of the other groups on the posttreatment phoneme segmentation test. Note also that although the pattern of results just described was found in both the poor and normal reader groups at both grade levels, the poor readers performed worse than the normal readers on all measures. In addition, the second-grade normal readers performed as well as the sixth-grade poor readers on all measures, suggesting that a child's level of ability in both phonemic segmentation and letter-sound decoding sets upper limits on his or her reading ability.

We tentatively concluded from this pattern of results that a likely cause of reading difficulties in severely impaired readers is weak phonological coding that leads to deficiencies in name encoding, phoneme segmentation, and alphabetic mapping, which in turn lead to difficulties in acquiring both whole-word naming and letter-sound decoding skills when learning to identify printed words.

The study just described provided us with more compelling evidence than any study previously conducted in our laboratory or elsewhere that reading disability is a language-based disorder. The study was motivated by a strong, well-articulated theory that had already received considerable support in the relevant literature. Its results were generated by an experimental (randomized trials) design that incorporated theoretically well-grounded training procedures designed to assess causal relationships and minimize threats to internal validity (Shadish, Cook, & Campbell, 2002). Further, its major findings were consistent with and added to a growing body of literature that supports the phonological coding deficit theory of reading disability (see studies by Vellutino, 1979; Vellutino & Scanlon, 1982, 1987b; and Vellutino et al., 2004 for comprehensive reviews). However, not long after the article reporting the results was published, I received a letter from the late Marie Clay, the architect of "Reading Recovery," a well-known and widely used reading intervention program designed for dealing with struggling readers in the early grades. Enclosed in that letter was an article she had written entitled "Learning to be Learning Disabled" (Clay, 1987), which focused on the validity of learning disability as a psychological construct. Learning disabilities have traditionally been defined using an IQ-achievement discrepancy as the central criterion along with exclusionary criteria such as the absence of uncorrected sensory deficits, social-emotional disorder, and sociocultural and economic disadvantage. Using such exclusionary criteria, estimates of reading and other learning disabilities have typically ranged between 10% and 20% of the general population of schoolchildren.

However, in her article, Clay (1987) contended that the exclusionary criteria typically used to identify "learning disabled" children were inadequate and argued forcefully that the major impediment to the differential diagnosis of learning disabilities is the failure to control for a child's educational history. She suggested further that virtually all studies designed to evaluate process deficit theories of reading disability have been confounded by this problem and that the adverse effects of inadequate instruction, inadequate prereading experience, or a combination of both can often mask or mimic the adverse effects of constitutionally derived cognitive deficits that may lead to reading difficulties. She also suggested that what was needed to address the problem and clearly lacking in the reading disability literature was a longitudinal study that evaluated a child's prereading experience while incorporating an intervention component to help distinguish constitutionally based causes of reading difficulties from experientially and instructionally based causes. I had to agree with Clay's analysis and found her article to be quite sobering because it referred to our own research and not just the research conducted in other laboratories. In fact, it motivated a series of longitudinal/intervention studies that we ultimately conducted, two of which were specifically designed to address her question. Before describing these studies, it would be useful to comment briefly on the possibility that early reading difficulties may be caused not only by phonological coding deficits but also by deficits or dysfunctions in other language or language-based skills.

The Double Deficit Theory

Wolf and Bowers (1999) suggested that there are three subtypes of reading disability: phonological, naming, and double deficit subtypes. The phonological deficit subtype is defined using measures of phonological skills such as phoneme awareness and letter-sound decoding. The naming deficit subtype is defined using measures of naming speed such as rapid naming of letters, digits, colors, and objects. The double deficit subtype is defined using both phonological skill and naming speed measures, and both types of deficits have been said to afflict the most severely impaired readers.

Three types of evidence have been used to support Wolf and Bowers' (1999) double deficit theory. First, rapid naming and phonological tasks have been found to contribute unique variance to measures of reading ability. Second, the single and double deficit subtypes have been found to perform worse than children with no deficits on measures of reading ability. Third, the double deficit subtypes have been found to perform worse than the single deficit subtypes on measures of reading ability. However, such support is equivocal. More specifically, the results suggesting that phonological and rapid naming tasks contribute unique variance to measures of reading ability have been confounded by the failure to control for autocorrelation effects created by shared variance among phonological, rapid naming, and reading skill measures. Thus, Torgesen, Wagner, Rashotte, Burgess, and Hecht (1997) found that second-grade measures of phonological awareness accounted for unique variance on fourth-grade measures of reading ability when second-grade reading ability was controlled, whereas rapid naming of letters and digits accounted for no unique variance on the fourth-grade reading measures under the same control circumstances. These results were replicated using the same sets of measures with third- and fifth-grade children.

Similarly, the consistent finding that double deficit subtypes tend to perform below single deficit subtypes on measures of reading ability has been shown to be an artifact of the procedures used to constitute these groups such that the double deficit subtypes have tended to score lower than the single deficit subtypes on measures of phonological awareness (Schatschneider, Carlson, Francis, Foorman, & Fletcher, 2002). Third, the naming deficit subtypes have typically been found to have average reading scores, which is anomalous. Finally, slow naming speeds in severely impaired readers could be manifestations of weak phonological coding rather than a specific naming deficit of the type suggested by Wolf and Bowers (1999). Thus, although the issue remains open, the double deficit theory of reading disability is weak at best (see Vellutino et al., 2004 for a detailed review).

Semantic and Syntactic Deficits

Finally, given that reading is a language-based skill, it is important to raise the question of whether early reading difficulties may be caused by semantic or syntactic deficits in some cases. As regards the study of reading difficulties in otherwise normal children, it will suffice to point out that in several major papers that have addressed this question (Vellutino, 1979; Vellutino & Scanlon, 1982, 1987b; Vellutino et al., 2004), a large number of studies were reviewed that provided reliable and convergent evidence that semantic deficits such as deficiencies in vocabulary knowledge and semantic concept formation, along with syntactic deficits such as deficiencies in sentence comprehension, knowledge and use of inflectional morphemes and the ability to detect and repair grammatically ill-formed sentences, are consequences of prolonged reading difficulties rather than the basic causes of such difficulties. The consistent pattern of results obtained from these studies suggests that poor and normal readers tend to differ on measures of semantic and syntactic knowledge and abilities more often in contrasts made at the higher grade levels than in those made at the lower grade levels (i.e., at the beginning stages of reading development), and more often in poor readers who come from impoverished backgrounds than in those who come from relatively advantaged backgrounds. Further, reader group differences on syntactic measures have been found more often on those that tax working memory than on those that do not tax working memory (e.g., Mann, Shankweiler, & Smith, 1984; Shankweiler, Crain, Brady, & Macaruso, 1992). The latter finding is consistent with results from a large number of studies that have found strong and reliable differences between poor and normal readers on tasks evaluating working memory in these two groups, including studies we have conducted such as the training study just described among others (Vellutino et al., 2004).

Longitudinal-Intervention Studies

The Vellutino et al. (1996) Study

As indicated previously, we designed and implemented two large-scale longitudinal studies that incorporated an intervention component to distinguish constitutionally based causes of early reading difficulties from experientially and instructionally based causes of such difficulties, in accord with suggestions made by Marie Clay (1987). In the first of these studies (Vellutino et al., 1996), reading growth in children identified as struggling readers midway through first grade were tracked from the beginning of kindergarten until the end of fourth grade; that is, before and after they were identified as struggling readers. The majority of these children were provided with daily one-on-one tutoring (30-minute sessions), and the rest were provided with whichever remedial services were offered at their home schools. Intervention was initiated midway through first grade and was terminated at the end of first grade for the children who were found to be readily remediated and midway through second grade for the children who were found to be more difficult to remediate. However, after one semester of exposure to the intervention program, all of the tutored children who received project-based intervention were rank ordered on the basis of the reading growth measures administered during that semester (i.e., gain scores from December of first grade to September of second grade) and thereafter separated into four (approximately) equal groups designated as follows: very limited growth (VLG), limited growth (LG), good growth (GG), and very good growth (VGG).

For purposes of comparison, two groups of typically developing readers were also identified midway through first grade: one group consisting of children with average intelligence (AvIQNorm) and a second group consisting of children with above-average intelligence (AbAvIQNorm). Reading growth in these children was also tracked from the beginning of kindergarten through the end of fourth grade. In addition, all of the groups were compared on measures of intelligence and reading-related cognitive abilities in kindergarten, first, and third grades. Vellutino et al. (1996) found that the tutored children who were difficult to remediate differed significantly from the tutored children who were readily remediated on measures of language-based skills, especially phonological skills, which are important in learning to read, in particular, measures evaluating knowledge of letter names and sounds, phoneme awareness, letter-sound decoding, verbal memory, and name retrieval. Moreover, the children in the tutored groups performed below the children in the normal reader groups on measures of basic language processes, such as phoneme awareness, verbal memory, and name retrieval both before and after remedial intervention. In contrast, the two groups did not differ on measures of visual, semantic, and syntactic abilities, nor did they differ on measures of executive functions such as attention and concentration. But of special interest is the finding that almost 70% of the tutored children were brought to at least an average level of reading ability in one semester, and less than 5% of these children continued to perform below average on measures of word-level skills at the end of the second semester of remediation, when the intervention program was terminated. Moreover, the number of tutored children who continued to experience reading difficulties after the project ended represented only 1%–3% of the general population of schoolchildren, which is a far cry from the estimated 10%–20% who have appeared in the reading disability literature.

Finally, the intelligence measures did not distinguish among the tutored groups nor did they distinguish any of the tutored groups from a group of normal readers with average intelligence. These findings suggested that intelligence test scores do not predict reading achievement among beginning readers and that response to intervention (RTI) may be a better measure of constitutionally based reading disability than the more traditional IQ-achievement discrepancy.

The Vellutino et al. (2008) Study

The intervention study just described provided us with strong and compelling evidence that (a) most reading difficulties are caused by experiential and instructional deficits rather than constitutional deficits; (b) a small but significant percentage of impaired readers may be afflicted with language-based deficits and especially phonological deficits that impair their ability to learn to read, and (c) children who are "at risk" for early reading difficulties can be identified before being exposed to formal instruction in reading at the beginning of kindergarten if not earlier. These findings motivated us to conduct a second intervention study that adopted a "preventative approach" to early reading difficulties (Vellutino, Scanlon, Zhang, & Schatschneider, 2008). Accordingly, children in participating schools were administered a letter identification test at the beginning of kindergarten, and all of those who scored at or below the 30th percentile on the test were identified as being at risk for early reading difficulties. Half of the children in the at-risk group were randomly assigned to a project-based intervention group, wherein they received small-group supplemental instruction (three children per group) during 30-minute sessions twice weekly throughout kindergarten. The other half were assigned to a school-based comparison group, wherein they received whichever remedial services were offered by their home schools, if any. Literacy growth in all of the at-risk children was tracked through the end of kindergarten. At the beginning of first grade, the literacy skills of every available at-risk child were again evaluated, and the group was dichotomized into continued risk (CR) and no-longer-at-risk (NLAR) groups based on a composite measure derived from the test scores used to assess growth on measures of the emergent literacy skills targeted in the (project-based) kindergarten intervention program. For purposes of comparison, two groups of normal readers were also identified: one with average intelligence (AvIQNorm) and another with above-average intelligence (AbAvIQNorm). Half of the CR children received additional intervention throughout first grade, which consisted of daily one-on-one tutoring (30-minute sessions) that was comprehensive and highly individualized. The other half received school-based intervention (typically in small groups). Literacy growth among the children in all of these groups was tracked through the end of third grade, when the project ended. Measures of verbal and nonverbal intelligence from the WISC-III (Wechsler, 1991) were administered during grades 1 and 3, and measures of reading-related cognitive abilities were also administered during third grade. Finally, measures of responses to kindergarten intervention were used to classify children into the CR and NLAR groups at the beginning of first grade, and measures of response to first-grade intervention along with a measure of intelligence were used to predict reading performance at the end of second and third grade.

The results obtained from this study extend and complement the results of the Vellutino et al. (1996) study. First, approximately 84% (98/117) of the at-risk children became at least average-level readers, either through kindergarten intervention alone or through both kindergarten and first-grade intervention combined, and 73% (72/98) of the children in this group received only kindergarten intervention (Vellutino et al., 2008). All of these children continued to perform at least within the average range for the remainder of the project. Moreover, the at-risk children who received project-based supplementary intervention in kindergarten performed significantly better than the at-risk children who received no supplementary intervention in kindergarten on outcome measures of emergent literacy skills that were administered at the end of kindergarten and the beginning of first grade. In addition, the NLAR children performed much better than the CR children (and close to the levels of the normal readers) on the measures of reading-related language abilities included in the cognitive battery administered in third grade (data not shown). However, these two groups did not differ significantly on measures of nonverbal ability, in accord with results obtained in the intervention study conducted by Vellutino et al. (1996). Finally, 58% (26/45) of the CR children performed at least within the average range on all of the reading outcome measures administered at the end of first, second, and third grade and at levels that approximately matched those of the children in the NLAR and normal reader groups at all these time periods. In contrast, 42% (19/45) of the children in the CR group performed below average on the reading outcome measures at the end of second and third grade, despite performing in the low-average to average ranges on these measures at the end of first grade.

These findings were entirely consistent with the results obtained in our first intervention study (Vellutino et al., 1996) and suggested that early and long-term reading difficulties can be prevented in the large majority of at-risk children if they are identified at the beginning of kindergarten (if not sooner) and provided with the supplementary intervention needed to correct deficiencies in foundational literacy skills. The results also provided additional support for our contention that early reading difficulties in most children are caused by experiential and instructional deficits rather than biologically based cognitive deficits.

SUMMARY AND CONCLUSIONS

The study of the causes and correlates of specific reading disability (dyslexia) in otherwise normal children has been the object of considerable research throughout the 20th century, and work in this area continues to date. My colleagues and I have been conducting research in this rich area of inquiry for over four decades. We have evaluated the most prominent and influential etiological theories specifying causes of the disorder and found most of them to be invalid. Our seminal studies evaluated visual deficit theories beginning with Orton's (1925) optical reversibility theory, which suggests that reading difficulties are caused by the perception of letters and words as reversed images. When taken together, the results of these studies and those conducted elsewhere provide strong evidence that early reading difficulties are not caused by optical reversibility or any other visual deficit and that the visual abilities of poor readers are no different from those of normal readers.

We then turned our attention to several other theories that implicated dysfunction in general learning abilities, such as associative learning, intersensory learning, and attention deficits as basic causes of early reading difficulties in otherwise normal children. Despite the illogical nature of etiological theories which suggest that poor readers who have at least average intelligence may be afflicted with dysfunction in one or another of these rather basic and ubiquitous learning abilities, we conducted several studies that used experimental designs to compare the performance of poor and normal readers on associative learning tasks that placed heavy demands on these abilities. None of the studies produced any evidence to support the theories. Of special interest, however, was the finding in all of these studies that differences between poor and normal readers were obtained only on tasks that involved verbal learning and not on those that involved nonverbal learning. This finding strongly suggested that the reading difficulties experienced by children who have no other learning problems may be caused by verbal deficits, and motivated several other studies to further evaluate this possibility.

The verbal deficit studies we conducted produced strong evidence that the most severely impaired readers may be afflicted with phonological coding deficits that impair their acquisition of important reading skills such as phoneme awareness, whole-word naming, and alphabetic coding. These studies also produced strong documentation that children who are learning to read in an orthography derived from an alphabet must acquire both code- and meaning-based strategies for word identification and that failure to acquire both strategies may lead to qualitatively different types of reading difficulties. For example, the study we specifically designed to assess the differential affects of different word identification strategies produced strong experimental evidence that a child who acquires only a whole-word strategy for word identification may be more vulnerable to reversal errors such as confusing "pot" with "top" or "was" with "saw" than a child who acquires alphabetic coding skills such as phoneme awareness and knowledge of letter-sound relationships.

Finally, because none of our studies (or those conducted elsewhere) controlled for children's prereading experiences and educational histories, we conducted two major intervention studies that evaluated early reading skills and reading-related cognitive abilities, both before and after reading intervention. Each of these studies produced strong and reliable evidence that (a) early reading difficulties in the majority of beginning readers are caused by experiential and educational deficits and not by deficits in reading-related cognitive abilities, and (b) early reading difficulties in a very small percentage of such children may be caused by deficits in reading-related cognitive abilities. We will continue to conduct intervention research in the interest of developing the means to prevent early and prolonged reading difficulties. Thus, the odyssey continues.

REFERENCES

Bakker, D. J. (1972). *Temporal order in disturbed reading-developmental and neuropsychological aspects in normal and reading retarded children*. Rotterdam, The Netherlands: Rotterdam University Press.

Bannatyne, A. (1971). *Language, reading, and learning disabilities*. Springfield, IL: Charles C. Thomas.

Birch, H. (1962). Dyslexia and maturation of visual function. In J. Money (Ed.), *Reading disability: Progress and research needs in dyslexia* (pp. 161–169). Baltimore, MD: Johns Hopkins Press.

Blank, M., & Bridger, W. H. (1966). Deficiencies in verbal labeling in retarded readers. *American Journal of Orthopsychiatry, 38*, 623–834.

Brewer, W. F. (1967). *Paired associates learning of dyslexic children* (Doctoral dissertation, University of Iowa).

Clay, M. M. (1987). Learning to be learning disabled. *New Zealand Journal of Educational Studies, 22*, 155–173.

Denckla, M. B. (1972) Color naming deficits in dyslexic boys. *Cortex, 8*, 164–176.

Denckla, M. B., & Rudel, R. (1976a). Naming of pictured objects by dyslexic and other learning disabled children. *Brain and Language, 3*, 1–15.

Denckla, M. B., & Rudel, R. (1976b). Rapid automatized naming (R.A.N.): Dyslexia differentiated from other learning disabilities. *Neuropsychologia, 14*, 471–479.

Douglas, V. J. (1972). Stop, look, and listen: The problem of sustained attention and impulse control in hyperactive and normal children. *Canadian Journal of Behavioral Science, 4*, 259–281.

Downing, J. (1973). *Comparative reading: Cross national studies of behavior and processes in reading and writing*. New York, NY: Macmillan.

Eden, G. F., & Zeffiro, T. A. (1998). Neural systems affected in developmental dyslexia revealed by neuroimaging. *Neuron*, 279–282.

Elkonin, D. B. (1973). "U.S.S.R." In J. Downing (Ed.), *Comparative reading: Cross national studies of behavior and processes in reading and writing*. New York, NY: Macmillan.

Gascon, G., & Goodglass, H. (1970). Reading retardation and the information content of stimuli in paired associate learning. *Cortex, 6*, 417–429.

Herman, K. (1959). *Reading disability*. Copenhagen, Denmark: Munksgaard.

Hirsh, I. J. (1959). Auditory perception of temporal order. *Journal of the Acoustical Society of America, 31*, 759–767.

Hirsh, I. J. (1966). Audition in relation to perception of speech. In E. C. Carterette (Ed.), *Speech, language and communication, Vol. III: Brain function*. Berkeley: University of California.

Hirsh, I. J., & Sherrick, C. E. (1961). Perceived order in different sense modalities. *Journal of Experimental Psychology, 64*, 1–19.

Johnson, D., & Myklebust, H. (1967). *Learning disabilities: Educational principles and practices*. New York, NY: Grune and Stratton.

Katz, R. B., Healy, A. F., & Shankweiler, D. (1983). Phonetic coding and order memory in relation to reading proficiency: A comparison of short-term memory for temporal and spatial order information. *Applied Psycholinguistics, 4*, 229–250.

Liberman, I. Y. (1971). Basic research and speech in lateralization of language: Some implications for reading disability. *Bulletin of the Orton Society, 21*, 71–87.

Liberman, I. Y., & Shankweiler, D. (1978). Speech, the alphabet, and teaching to read. In L. Resnick & P. Weaver (Eds.), *Theory and practice of early reading*. New York, NY: Wiley.

Liberman, I. Y., Shankweiler, D., Fischer, F. W., & Carter, B. (1974). Explicit syllable and phoneme segmentation in the young child. *Journal of Experimental Child Psychology, 18*, 201–212.

Liberman, I. Y., Shankweiler, D., Orlando, C., Harris, K. S., & Berti, F. B. (1971). Letter confusion and reversals of sequence in the beginning reader: Implications for Orton's theory of developmental dyslexia. *Cortex*, 7, 127–142.

Lovegrove, W., Martin, F., & Slaghuis, W. (1986). A theoretical and experimental case for a visual deficit in specific reading disability. *Cognitive Neuropsychology, 3*, 225–267.

Mann, V. A., Shankweiler, D., & Smith, S. T. (1984). The association between comprehension of spoken sentences and early reading ability: The role of phonetic representation. *Journal of Child Language, 11*, 627–643.

Morrison, F. J, & Manis, F. R. (1982). Cognitive processes and reading disability: A critique and proposal. In C. J. Brainerd & M. Pressley (Eds.), *Verbal processes in children*. New York, NY: Springer-Verlag.

Orton, S. T. (1925). "Word-blindness" in school children. *Archives of Neurology and Psychiatry, 14*, 381–615.

Perfetti, C. A., & Lesgold, A. M. (1978). Discourse comprehension and sources of individual differences. In M. A. Just, & P. A. Carpenter (Eds.), *Cognitive processes in comprehension*. Hillsdale, NJ: Erlbaum.

Savin, H. B. (1972). What the child knows about speech when he starts to learn to read. In J. F. Kavanagh & I. G. Mattingly (Eds.), *Language by eye and by ear*. Cambridge, MA: MIT Press.

Schatschneider, C., Carlson, C. D., Francis, D. J., Foorman, B. R., & Fletcher, J. M. (2002). Relationships of rapid automatized naming and phonological awareness in early reading development: Implications for the double deficit hypothesis. *Journal of Learning Disabilities, 35*, 245–256.

Shadish, W. R., Cook, T. D., & Campbell, D. T. (2002). *Experimental and quasi-experimental designs for general causal inference*. Boston, MA: Houghton Mifflin.

Shankweiler, D., Crain, S., Brady, S., & Macaruso, P. (1992). Identifying the causes of reading disability. In P. B. Gough, L. C. Ehri, & R. Treiman (Eds.), *Reading acquisition* (pp. 275–305). Hillsdale, NJ: Erlbaum.

Steger, J. A., Vellutino, F. R., & Meshoulam, U. (1972). Visual-tactile and tactile-tactile paired associate learning in normal and poor readers. *Perceptual and Motor Skills, 35*, 263–266.

Stein, J. (2001). The sensory basis of reading problems. *Developmental Neuropsychology, 20*, 509–534.

Tallal, P. (1980). Auditory temporal perception, phonics, and reading disabilities in children. *Brain and Language, 9*, 182–198.

Torgesen, J. K., Wagner, R. K., Rashotte, C. A., Burgess, S., & Hecht, S. (1997). Contributions of phonological awareness and rapid automatized naming ability to the growth of word reading skills in second to fifth grade. *Scientific Studies of Reading, 1*, 161–185.

Vellutino, F. R. (1979). *Dyslexia: Theory and research*. Cambridge, MA: MIT Press.

Vellutino, F. R. (1987). Dyslexia. *Scientific American*, 34–41. (Reprinted in Wang, W. (1991). The emergence of language development and evolution. Readings from *Scientific American)*.

Vellutino, F. R., Fletcher, J. M., Snowling, M. J., & Scanlon, D. M. (2004). Specific reading disability (dyslexia): What have we learned in the last four decades? *Journal of Child Psychology and Psychiatry, 45*(1), 2–40.

Vellutino, F. R., Harding, C. J., Phillips, F., & Steger, J. A. (1975). Differential transfer in poor and normal readers. *Journal of Genetic Psychology, 126*, 3–18.

Vellutino, F. R., Pruzek, R., Steger, J. A., & Meshoulam, U. (1973). Immediate visual recall in poor and normal readers as a function of orthographiclinguistic familiarity. *Cortex, 9*, 370–386.

Vellutino, F. R., & Scanlon, D. M (1982). Verbal processing in poor and normal readers. In C. J. Brainerd & M. Pressley (Eds.), *Verbal processes in children* (pp. 189–264). New York, NY: Springer-Verlag.

Vellutino, F. R., & Scanlon, D. M. (1987a). Phonological coding, phonological awareness, and reading ability: Evidence from longitudinal and experimental study. *Merrill Palmer Quarterly, 33*, 321–363.

Vellutino, F. R., & Scanlon, D. M. (1987b). Linguistic coding and reading ability. In S. Rosenberg (Ed), *Advances in applied psycholinguistics* (Vol. 2 pp. 1–69). New York, NY: Cambridge University Press.

Vellutino, F. R., Scanlon, D. M., Sipay, E. R., Small, S. G., Pratt, A., Chen, R., & Denckla, M. B. (1996). Cognitive profiles of difficult to remediate and readily remediated poor readers: Toward distinguishing between constitutionally and experientially based causes of reading disability. *Journal of Educational Psychology, 88*(4), 601–638.

Vellutino, F. R., Scanlon, D. M., Zhang, H., & Schatschneider, C. (2008). Using response to kindergarten and first grade intervention to identify children at risk for long-term reading difficulties. *Reading and Writing Special Issue, 21*, 437–480.

Vellutino, F. R., Smith, H., Steger, J. A., & Kaman, M. (1975). Reading disability: Age differences and the perceptual deficit hypothesis. *Child Development, 46*, 487–493.

Vellutino, F. R., Steger, J. A., DeSetto, L., & Phillips, F. (1975). Immediate and delayed recognition of visual stimuli in poor and normal readers. *Journal of Experimental Child Psychology, 19*(2), 223–232.

Vellutino, F. R., Steger, J. A., Harding, C. J., & Phillips, F. (1975). Verbal vs. non-verbal paired associates learning in poor and normal readers. *Neuropsychologia, 13*, 75–82.

Vellutino, F. R., Steger, J. A., Kaman, M., & DeSetto, L. (1975). Visual form perception in deficient and normal readers as a function of age and orthographiclinguistic familiarity. *Cortex, 9*, 22–30.

Vellutino, F. R., Steger, J. A., & Kandel, G. (1972). Reading disability: An investigation of the perceptual deficit hypothesis. *Cortex, 8*, 106–118.

Vellutino, F. R., Steger, J. A., & Pruzek, R. (1973). Inter vs intrasensory deficit in paired associates learning in poor and normal readers. *Canadian Journal of Behavioral Science, 5*(2), 111–123.

Wechsler, D. (1991). Wechsler intelligence scale for children-III. New York, NY: Psychological Corporation.

Wolf, M., & Bowers, P. G. (1999). The double deficit hypothesis for the developmental dyslexias. *Journal of Educational Psychology, 21*, 1–24.

CHAPTER 7

SPECIFIC READING DISABILITIES

The Case for Differentiation of Assessment in Multilingual Malaysia

Lay Wah Lee

The most unifying hypothesis for dyslexia is the phonological deficit hypothesis, which suggests that children with dyslexia have specific impairments in representing, storing, and retrieving phonological information (Snowling, 2000; Wagner & Torgeson, 1987). A large-scale systematic meta-analytic review conducted recently by Melby-Lervåg, Lyster, and Hulme (2012) indicated that children with dyslexia showed a large deficit in phonological skills compared with typically developing children of the same age and reading level. Their review also showed that phonemic awareness is the strongest predictor of reading development for both English and other more consistent alphabetic orthographies. Their analyses suggested that phonological awareness is the common underlying proficiency for reading development across languages. Apart from the behavioral studies analyzed by Melby-Lervåg et al. (2012), neuroimaging studies have provided strong evidence for a common biological origin of

Understanding Developmental Disorders of Auditory Processing, Language and Literacy Across Languages: International Perspectives, pp. 147–167

dyslexia in different orthographies (Paulesu et al., 2001). Goswami et al. (2010) recently showed that despite the phonological and orthographic differences, rise-time sensitivity is a significant predictor of phonological awareness and the only consistent predictor of reading acquisition. Goswami et al. concluded that their results supported a language-universal theory of the neural basis of developmental dyslexia. The evidence from behavioral, neuroimaging, and neural studies has thus converged to indicate that the underlying cognitive deficits of dyslexia are quite universal. This universality suggests that every dyslexia assessment process shares a similar framework (Ziegler & Goswami, 2005). Consequently, it is argued in this chapter that multiple versions of a dyslexia assessment tool may not be necessary for dyslexia diagnosis even in a multilingual environment. However, although the underlying cognitive deficits of dyslexia are quite universal across languages, the differences in writing systems and instructional languages create moderate variations in phonological awareness and decoding skills across languages (Melby-Lervåg & Lervåg, 2011). These differences support the argument for the need to differentiate dyslexia assessments in a multilingual environment. It is suggested in this chapter that differentiation is the solution for dyslexia diagnosis in a multilingual environment rather than multiple versions of a single dyslexia assessment tool.

The purpose of this chapter is to propose a differentiated dyslexia assessment framework for a multilingual environment using Malaysia as a case study. To convince readers of the rationale for the proposed framework, background knowledge on the Malaysian school language systems is provided in addition to an understanding of Malay, the primary official language in Malaysia. The dyslexia assessments currently conducted in Malaysia and their prevalent problems are then discussed using a typical dyslexia assessment framework as a baseline. Solutions are subsequently offered through the proposal of a differentiated dyslexia assessment framework. This chapter argues for the differentiation of assessment at multiple levels, including the levels of assessment tasks, assessment processes, and norms. Finally, a generalized prescription for dyslexia assessment in a multilingual environment is proposed for further discussion.

MULTILINGUAL MALAYSIA

Malaysia is a multiethnic country of 27 million people, of whom 54.9% are Malay, 24.5% Chinese, 11.9% indigenous, 7.4% Indian, and 1.3% from other minorities (Department of Statistics, 2009). As a result of its multiple ethnicities and colonial history, Malaysia's community is multilingual. Standard Malay (Bahasa Malaysia), a variant of an Austronesian language (Malay) spoken in four Southeast Asian countries, is the official language of

Malaysia. English is the official second language, and Mandarin and Tamil are the third instructional languages.

This pluralism has differentiated two types of primary schools in Malaysia: the national and national-type primary schools. Malay and English are the two official languages in both types of school. However, the schools differ in their instructional languages. Malay is the primary instructional language used in national primary schools, which consist predominantly of children of Malay ethnicity. Therefore, the instructional and home languages of most of the children attending national primary schools are similar. The national-type primary schools use either Mandarin (Chinese) or Tamil as their instructional languages, apart from learning Malay and English. Most children enrolled in this stream are predominantly of Chinese or Indian ethnicity and are therefore usually trilingual. Whereas Malaysian children of Chinese ethnicity usually speak Mandarin Chinese or another Chinese dialect at home, Malaysian children of Indian ethnicity speak Tamil or other dialects. With the exception of Malay children, children encounter instructional languages at school that usually differ from their home languages.

The Malaysian school system therefore represents a microcosm of the world's writing systems, which are broadly classified into three categories, including logographic, syllabic, and alphabetic, based on the types of symbols used to represent the spoken languages. These three writing systems coexist in Malaysian schools. Mandarin Chinese, which is the instructional language in national-type Chinese primary schools, uses a logographic writing system in which a single symbol represents a whole word. Tamil, which is the instructional language in national-type Tamil primary schools, uses a syllabic writing system in which symbols represent the syllables that compose words. The symbol for a syllable usually represents a combination of consonant and vowel sounds or an individual vowel sound. However, the primary and secondary official languages in Malaysian schools have alphabetic writing systems in which a small set of basic writing symbols (the 26 letters in the English alphabet) or combinations are used to represent the phonemes of a spoken language. Phonemes are the basic sound units of spoken language (Roach, 2009).

THE MALAY WRITING SYSTEM AND ITS EFFECT ON DYSLEXIA

This section explains the Malay writing system and its possible effects on dyslexia compared with the English language. English and Malay both have alphabetic writing systems that use the same Roman alphabet and its extensions to represent phonemes in the language. The Romanized script for Malay is called Rumi. Letters or letter combinations that represent phonemes are called graphemes. The consonant phonemes represented by single-letter graphemes are very similar in both English and Malay. For example, the *k* letters used in "kite" (English) and "kita" (Malay word for "we, us") are both similarly represented by the phoneme /k/. As the basic writing blocks of both languages are similar, there are logically some similarities in the reading acquisitions of both languages. Lee (2008a) found remarkable similarities between the word-level literacy predictors in Malay compared with English. Phonological awareness is the most significant predictor, with rapid naming making independent and secondary contributions. Studies on word recognition errors in Malay have revealed phonological strategies and phonological-based errors (Lee & Wheldall, 2011). In addition, dyslexic children learning Malay have shown behavioral signs and symptoms similar to those of dyslexic children learning English (Lee, 2008b).

Beyond the similarities in the basic building blocks of both writing systems, differences appear predominantly in the orthographic transparencies and granularities of both languages. These two orthographic features are commonly used to explain the differences in reading acquisition progressions across different languages (Ziegler & Goswami, 2005).

The multiple representations in phoneme-grapheme mappings make English orthographically opaque. In English, a single phoneme can be represented by several graphemes (e.g., phoneme /k/ may be represented by graphemes *k* [as in "kite"], *c* [as in "cat"], *ck* [as in "duck"] and *ch* [as in "Christmas"]) and certain graphemes may also represent several phonemes (e.g., grapheme *ow* can be sounded as /aʊ/ [as in "cow"] and as /eʊ/ [as in "grow"]). These phoneme-grapheme mapping inconsistencies are known causes of reading difficulties among dyslexic children (Miles, 2000). In Malay, such overlaps in the phoneme-grapheme mappings only occur for the letter *e*, which represents two phonemic sounds, that is, /ə/ and /eɪ/. Despite the deviation, Malay has a consistent one-to-one phoneme-grapheme mapping compared with English and is therefore considered orthographically transparent. It has been commonly accepted that it is easier for children to learn a transparent language than an opaque language such as English (Goswami, 2008). The orthographic transparency of a language appears to promote faster reading acquisition, mainly due to its straightforward phoneme-grapheme mappings.

However, it is just as important to recognize that language transparency does not eliminate the difficulties experienced by dyslexic children. Orthographic transparency alone does not diminish the phonological deficits in these children because phonological awareness is not a language-specific mechanism. Past research on cross-linguistic transfers has shown evidence that phonological awareness is not language specific (Gomez & Reason,

2002). A strong correlation in phonological awareness across languages indicates a common underlying proficiency or a mutual processing system (Melby-Lervåg & Lervåg, 2011), suggesting that phonological awareness is not language specific. Therefore, if we accept that reading is founded in phonology, orthographic transparency alone does not decrease developmental dyslexia in any simple way (Ziegler & Goswami, 2005). Dyslexic children find it difficult to acquire even consistent orthographies due to their decreased phonological sensitivity. In other words, a child who cannot blend or segment is unable to read even if the language is transparent (Lee, 2008b). This needs to be acknowledged to avoid trivializing the problems encountered by dyslexic children when learning transparent languages. In addition, the other features of a transparent language can present reading challenges (Miles, 2000). This has also been found true for Malay. For example, research has shown that despite the transparency of the Malay language, the mere presence of digraphs and diphthongs, which are multi-letter graphemes (*ng*, *ny*, *sy*, *kh*, *gh*, *ai*, *au*, *oi*), increases word-reading errors among low-progress children (Lee & Wheldall, 2011).

Apart from orthographic transparency, Ziegler and Goswami (2005) showed that the granularity of writing systems affects reading proficiency. Granularity refers to the orthographic units of different sizes in a writing system, the largest being whole words, followed by syllables, rimes, graphemes, and letters. Most Malay words are formed by two or more distinct syllables. (Refer to a study by Lee, Low, & Abdul Rashid (2012) for a detailed description of the Malay syllabic structures.) Lee et al. (2013) showed that while about 60% of English storybook texts are monosyllabic, the majority of words in the translated Malay texts are bisyllabic (about 45%) and trisyllabic (about 35%). The most frequently occurring word structures in the Malay texts are CV+CVC, CV+CV, V+CVC and CVC+CVC bisyllabic word structures. This indicates that young Malaysian readers are most likely to encounter bisyllabic word structures. Despite the language being alphabetic, the predominance of the syllabic grain size in Malay results in a mismatch between the phonological and orthographic grain sizes. Whereas syllables are the primary phonological units, phonemes are the building blocks of orthographic print. This mismatch between grain sizes has caused confusion, as exemplified by the type of word-recognition errors made by children who are learning Malay (Lee & Wheldall, 2011). For example, children who are reading Malay have the tendency to add or delete phonemes in words to produce an erroneous CV+CV structure (e.g., "tua" [CV+V] is read as "tuya" [CV+CV]). According to Ziegler and Goswami (2005), a major cause of early reading-acquisition difficulty can be attributed to this phonological and orthographic grain-size mismatch. It would not be wrong to assume that typically developing children recover from these mismatch errors. However, these errors appear to persist among dyslexic children, as suggested by their arrested development along the continuum from the logographic to the alphabetic and finally to the orthographic phases in reading development (Frith, 1986).

Orthographies with salient syllabic features such as Malay tend to have words that are longer than English words. Despite the transparent orthography of Malay, its word-length effect poses additional challenges for dyslexic children. Word length is known to affect reading ability for both transparent and opaque languages (e.g., Davies, Cuetos, & Glez-Seijas, 2007; Ziegler, Perry, Ma-Wyatt, Ladner, & Schulte-Korne, 2003). A similar result has been found for Malay, as increasing the number of syllables in a Malay word, which concomitantly increases its length, also tends to increase its difficulty (Lee & Wheldall, 2011).

In alphabetic writing systems, written units carry both phonological and morphological information (Casalis, Colé, & Sopo, 2004). Morphology refers to an organizational level of language that deals with the smallest units of meaning, that is, the morphemes (Casalis et al., 2004). However, morphological awareness has been examined much less often than phonological awareness. As Malay is an agglutinative language, morphological awareness may exert some influence on reading acquisition. Rickard Liow and Lee (2004) found that Malay children's early spellings are based on their knowledge of syllables and morphemes despite the predictability of the phoneme-grapheme level. A more extended range of derivational morphemes has been found in Malay texts compared with English texts, as they include prefix, suffix, circumfix, reduplication, and affixed reduplication (Lee et al., 2013). At this stage, not enough local regression analysis research has been conducted to show how much additional morphological awareness can predict Malay reading acquisition compared with phonological awareness.

As has been discussed, Malay and English are both alphabetic languages with different orthographic transparencies and syllabic structures. Malay has a much more transparent phoneme-grapheme correspondence code and functions primarily at syllabic grain sizes. English has a high degree of inconsistency in phoneme-grapheme mappings for both reading and spelling, and operates at three grain sizes, including syllabic, onset/rime, and phoneme sizes. Taken together, despite the orthographic transparency of the language, Malay becomes more complex due to its salient syllabic features and rich agglutinative characteristics. Any orthographic differences found between Malay and English would naturally result in the need to differentiate the identification of dyslexic children.

A TYPICAL DYSLEXIA ASSESSMENT FRAMEWORK

Recent neuroimaging research (e.g., Paulesu et al., 2001) and behavioral studies (e.g., Ziegler et al., 2003) have pointed to a universal basis for dyslexia. This section introduces a typical dyslexia assessment framework as the baseline for a discussion of the proposed differentiated framework for Malaysia. According to Ziegler and Goswami (2005), in most languages, a dyslexia diagnosis is based on the Organization for Economic Co-operation and Development (OECD) definition of a specific problem with reading and spelling that cannot be accounted for by low intelligence, poor educational opportunities, or obvious sensory or neurological damage. A diagnosis thus requires evidence of both weaknesses in the word-recognition component and strengths in other areas of cognitive functioning. This is commonly referred to as a discrepancy profile approach. At the cognitive-linguistic level, convergent evidence has indicated that these word-level difficulties are rooted in deficits in the phonological component of language (Lyon, Shaywitz, & Shaywitz, 2003; Snowling, 2000). Whereas phonological deficits are obvious at the level of phonological recoding in opaque orthographies, extremely slow phonological recoding combined with very poor spelling exemplifies dyslexia in some transparent orthographies (e.g., German) (Ziegler & Goswami, 2005). In an operational sense, a dyslexia diagnosis can be summarized according to three main criteria and their corresponding assessment tests or tasks. These criteria and tasks are illustrated in Figure 7.1.

With reference to Figure 7.1, the first criterion (Criterion 1) characterizes dyslexia as a specific problem with reading and spelling, which can be gathered from word-reading, nonword-reading, and spelling tests. An extremely slow phonological recoding can be gathered from reading-fluency tasks using single words/nonwords and passage reading.

As specific reading problems can arise due to factors other than dyslexia (e.g., deprived educational opportunities, sensory damage, low intellect), a second exclusionary criterion (Criterion 2) is included. Poor educational opportunities and sensory damage are easier to exclude as reading disability factors. However, the decision to exclude low intellect as a factor of a specific reading problem is not as obvious. Intelligence tests have traditionally been used to exclude low intellect. However, due to the widespread criticism of the IQ-achievement discrepancy approach to identifying dyslexia (Sawyer, 2006), other alternative approaches have been proposed. One such alternative draws its inspiration from the simple view of reading (Gough & Tunmer, 1986) and includes the U.S. component model of reading (Aaron, Joshi, Gooden, & Bentum, 2008) and the U.K. two-dimensional model of language and reading impairments (Bishop & Snowling, 2004). This approach is based on the simple view that reading

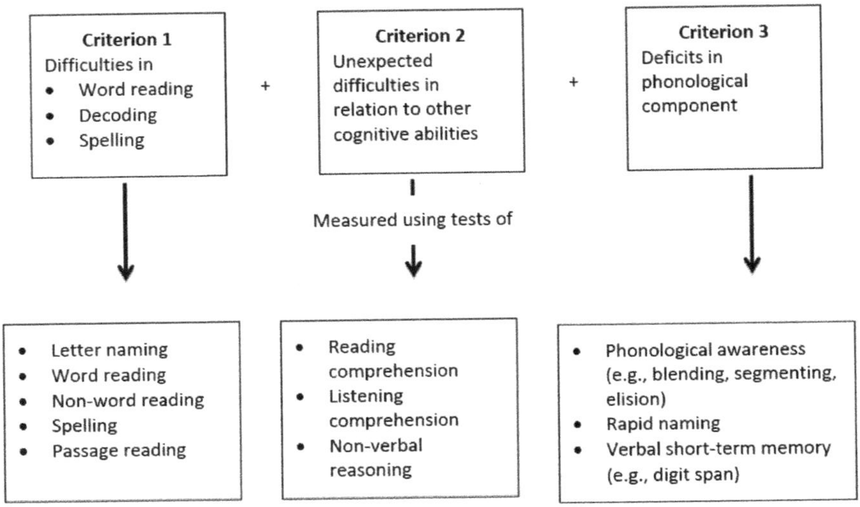

Figure 7.1. A typical dyslexia assessment framework.

involves listening and reading-comprehension assessments that contrast linguistic comprehension strengths with reading ability (Badian, 1999; Joshi, Williams, & Wood, 1998). It postulates that a child with dyslexia is able to comprehend materials that are presented orally rather than presented in print. However, this approach has not generated as much interest as the "response-to-intervention" (RTI) approach (Fletcher, Coulter, Reschly, & Vaughn, 2004; Fuchs & Fuchs, 2006). The RTI approach shifts the focus from a static assessment of a student's current skills to one that includes high quality classroom instruction and continuous progress monitoring. In the RTI approach, "a student with learning disabilities is identified as one who has *unexpected* difficulty learning and the *discrepancy* is measured relative to the expectation that most students can learn if quality instruction is provided" (Fletcher et al., 2004, p. 313).

As for the third criterion, based on research into the phonological deficits of dyslexia, we now have indicators that can positively identify dyslexia. Rather than relying on exclusionary factors (Criterion 2), specific phonological tasks may be used to positively identify dyslexia (Criterion 3). Past research has identified three major constructs in the phonological components related to dyslexia: phonological awareness, rapid naming, and verbal short-term memory tests (Snowling, 2000). Tasks such as blending, segmenting, and elision are used to identify deficits in phonological awareness; rapid naming tasks are used to identify deficits in slow phonological processing speed; and verbal short-term memory tasks measure phonological memory (Wagner, Torgesen, & Rashotte, 1999).

DYSLEXIA ASSESSMENT ISSUES IN A MULTILINGUAL ENVIRONMENT

In Malaysia, a student is considered to be dyslexic if he or she experiences significant difficulties in reading, writing, and spelling despite having a mental ability that is comparable with or above that of the average student (Haniz, 2003). While this definition is consistent with the first and second criteria in the typical dyslexia assessment framework, the third criterion is not adopted in the Malaysian definition of dyslexia, as the evidence necessary for making a causal inference has been lacking from the experimental research. In the last few years, dyslexia diagnoses in primary schools in Malaysia have followed an adapted response-to-intervention model (Fuchs & Fuchs, 2006). Students are assessed early in Year 1 and periodically after classroom instruction. Remedial teachers provide additional and more intensive remedial instruction in resource rooms for students who fail to read and write in Malay. When remedial instruction does not produce the desired outcome (usually by the end of Year 1), students are sent to medical doctors or clinical psychologists for diagnosis. In some schools, teachers administer a dyslexia checklist (Department of Special Education, 2011) to screen for students who are at risk of dyslexia before sending them for diagnosis. However, this checklist, which is used mostly in the government's national (but not national-type) primary schools, is not compulsory. The procedure encounters a grey area, as not every medical doctor and psychologist in Malaysia is familiar with dyslexia diagnosis. Those who are familiar with dyslexia diagnosis administer psychological tests in the English language. However, because such tests have not been standardized or normed in Malaysia, the data could only be interpreted subjectively. Therefore, diagnosis relies mostly on the experience of the medical practitioners and psychologists. The problem of dyslexia diagnosis is further exacerbated in no small part by the interaction of multilingualism in school and at home. The influence and interaction of a child's home language, together with the several instructional languages used at the different types of primary schools, produce multiple varieties of language background profiles. This pluralism of language profiles among children in Malaysia makes comparisons and norming processes very challenging. As dyslexia assessments are dependent on relative comparisons with peers, using a single norm as a reference base is not necessarily valid in the Malaysian context. While such situations call for differentiation at the norms level, developing a bilingual or multilingual norm is quite complex due to the different amounts of exposure to the various languages at home and in the school setting. However, in the Malaysian context, it is possible to differentiate norms by testing children based on the different school systems.

The differences in language profiles introduce other issues and have implications for dyslexia assessment. The most predominant language profile (herein called Profile 1) includes children whose first home language and primary instructional language is Malay. These children are typically of Malay ethnicity and studying in national primary schools. Although Profile 1 children are bilingual (Malay-English), they mirror a monolingual context (i.e., their home and primary school languages are similar) in terms of dyslexia assessment because English is the secondary official language in national schools. The typical assessment framework can be adopted and used to diagnose Profile 1 children. Both Malay and English are alphabetic languages, and research has shown that the predictors for reading Malay are strikingly similar to those for reading English (Lee, 2008a). Research has also shown that Profile 1 children use a phonological strategy at both the phoneme and syllable grain sizes to read and spell (Rickard Liow & Lee, 2004). However, as shown earlier in this chapter, the differences in the orthographic characteristics between the Malay and English writing systems indicate that the assessment tasks must be differentiated from those typically used for the English language. Assessment-task differentiation is explored in the subsequent section. Nevertheless, assessing dyslexia in Profile 1 children in Malaysia is essentially straightforward compared with assessing it in children whose home language is not Malay (Profile 2).

Children whose home language is not Malay (Profile 2) are typically trilingual, which adds to the complexity of their assessment. Their home language could be Mandarin, Tamil, or another ethnic language. These children attend either national or national-type primary schools. Mandarin or Tamil serve as the predominant instructional language of children who attend national-type primary schools. Profile 2 children would be much less adept at Malay than their Profile 1 counterparts.

Ziegler and Goswami (2005) pointed out that apart from a phonological deficit, an atypical reading development could arise from variations in the training environment, such as an impoverished exposure to print or an exposure to two different orthographies at once. These two factors could result in a misdiagnosis of dyslexia. In the Malaysian context, Profile 2 children would lack exposure to Malay and learn two different types of orthographic writing systems (i.e., logographic/syllabic and alphabetic) simultaneously.

No local research has highlighted the issues that may arise from diagnosing dyslexia in Profile 2 children. A search of established academic databases (such as ESCOHost) conducted in February 2013 did not uncover any Malaysian-based research that highlighted such issues. However, the search did uncover research conducted in Singapore. As Singapore and Malaysia have similar multilingual communities, the Singaporean experience may be consulted as a reference. However, it must be noted that whereas the main official language in Singaporean schools is English, that in Malaysian schools is Malay.

Dixon, Zhao, and Joshi (2010) examined the influence of first-language orthography on bilingual Mandarin-English, Malay-English, and Tamil-English children in Singapore. In their study, children whose home language was Mandarin relied on visual processing when spelling English words. The authors argued that experience with morphosyllabic Chinese characters leads to enhanced visual processing ability, which transfers to the spelling of English words. Dixon et al. cautioned that difficulties in phonological awareness and in mapping the phoneme-grapheme correspondences among bilingual Mandarin-English children should not lead to an immediate diagnosis of dyslexia. Based on such research among bilinguals with Mandarin as a first language and an alphabetic language as a second language, a similar situation could occur in the Malaysian context. Children in Malaysia whose home language is Mandarin could use visual-orthographic processes to learn Malay, especially those attending national-type Chinese schools. When children rely heavily on visual-orthographic processing, they may show weaknesses in the phonological processing tasks used to identify phonological deficits in dyslexia. Therefore, Profile 2 children could show weaknesses in the phonological component of Malay due to the influence of a logographic orthography. When diagnosing dyslexia among Profile 2 children, the first and third criteria of a typical dyslexia assessment framework could be fulfilled despite no phonological difficulties resulting from a phonological deficit at the cognitive level. Therefore, the influence of another orthography learned simultaneously, in addition to the lack of exposure to the second language, may result in atypical reading development, which could produce false positives during a dyslexia diagnosis.

We are thus led to examine the exclusionary criterion (Criterion 2) in dyslexia assessment among bilinguals. When testing bilingual children in Singapore for dyslexia using English tests, Brookes, Ng, Lim, Tan, and Lukito (2011) found that children who spoke Chinese at home tended to be at risk of dyslexia. Of those in the false positive group, 50% showed difficulties with specific language impairment or a lack of exposure to the English language. Their poor English scores were not a consequence of low intellectual ability. The administration of English tests to these bilingual children was therefore insufficient to show specificity despite English being the official language in Singaporean schools. In other words, the English tests identified weaknesses but were not specific enough to differentiate whether these weaknesses occurred due to low intellectual ability or insufficient experience with the language. Therefore, Profile 2 children in

Malaysia may not fare well on listening comprehension tests administered in Malay due to their lack of exposure to the language rather than due to a low intellect.

Taken together, a Profile 2 child may be falsely identified as dyslexic when tested in Malay due to the cross-language processing transfer from the home language and his or her lack of exposure to Malay. Such a situation of false positives would arise as long as the dyslexia assessment process is relative and dependent on comparisons with peers, especially among bilingual children. Based on the issues raised, some form of dyslexia assessment differentiation for Profile 2 children is necessary.

While there are children with other language profiles living in Malaysia, they compose the minority. For example, there are children living in urban areas whose home language is English. For such children, the use of the typical dyslexia framework, tested in English without adaptation, would be sufficient to identify dyslexia. Discussions of other minority language profiles are beyond the scope of this chapter.

THE PROPOSED DIFFERENTIATED DYSLEXIA ASSESSMENT FRAMEWORK

Based on the preceding issues, differentiating assessments at multiple levels, that is, the assessment task, assessment process, and norm levels, is proposed as a solution to the problems created by assessing dyslexia in a multilingual environment. Differentiation is broadly defined here as an adaptation of the typical dyslexia assessment framework to accommodate the different language profiles of children.

Differentiation in Terms of Assessment Tasks

The differences in orthographic characteristics invariably require a differentiation of the tasks adapted from English to Malay. Translating the tests directly from English to Malay without considering the Malay orthographic features may render the tasks less accurate or valid. Such types of differentiation include the following.

Use of Nonword Items for Blending and Segmenting Tasks

It has been found that a ceiling effect occurs in Malay for syllable blending and, to a lesser extent, syllable segmentation tasks (Lee & Wheldall, 2011). The effect occurs because syllables naturally emerge across languages (Goswami, 2008), and the predominance of syllables in Malay renders the tests easy for every student, including the weaker students (Lee & Wheldall,

2011). Therefore, to obtain variability when testing in Malay, differentiating the form of nonwords as items for syllable blending and segmentation tasks becomes necessary. The use of nonwords in blending and segmenting syllables avoids the ceiling effect and allows for a more accurate diagnosis of the phonological deficits. This idea was recently tested with 58 Profile 1 bilingual students at the primary one level. More variability was obtained when nonwords were used to test blending (M = 1.29, SD = .77) and segmenting (M = 1.59, SD = .65) than when real words were used to test blending (M = 2.82, SD = .43) and segmenting (M = 2.86, SD = .57).

Use of Multisyllabic Items Instead Of Monosyllabic Items

As previously discussed, whereas most words in Malay are bisyllabic, with CV and CVC syllables being the most prominent, early English reading materials were mostly monosyllabic (Masterson, Stuart, Dixon, & Lovejoy, 2010). This cross-language difference has influenced test construction. Whereas English tests typically use monosyllabic words, the lack of monosyllabic words and prominence of syllabic structures in Malay indicate that testing must be conducted using multisyllabic words.

Testing of Different Grain Sizes

As syllables are predominant in Malay, this grain size seems to overwhelm every other grain size (Rickard Liow & Lee, 2004) and could interfere with the tasks that test other grain sizes. The predominance of syllables in Malay interferes with phoneme blending and segmentation tasks. As students are unable to differentiate between the larger (syllable) and smaller (phoneme) grain sizes during testing, floor effects have been found to occur for phonemic blending and segmentation tasks in Malay (Lee & Wheldall, 2011). There is therefore a need to have more phoneme blending and segmentation practice items in Malay to ensure additional rehearsal before testing commences. The tasks that differentiate words via onset/rime may also be unnecessary for Malay dyslexia assessment, as the rime grain size is equivalent to phonemes in languages with CV syllable structures (Goswami et al., 2010) such as Malay. Such tasks are necessary in English, as processing onset/rime is a part of English language reading development (Goswami, 2008).

A tool involving the differentiated tasks described in this subsection was developed and validated for Malay (Lee, 2008a). Some 117 primary one students were tested using 10 subtests deemed necessary for a dyslexia assessment battery. The word-reading (α = .99), nonword-reading (α = .95), and elision (α = .94) tasks used multisyllabic items. The elision task was tested at different grain sizes (M = 6.25, SD = 5.18). However, this assessment tool must be further refined and validated with a bigger sample before it can be applied at the practical level.

Differentiation in the Assessment Procedure

Academics in Malaysia have discussed using bilingual assessment tools to assess dyslexia in the Malaysian context, that is, to administer tests in both official languages (Malay and English) or in both a child's home and school languages (e.g., Mandarin and Malay). However, it has been contended that using multilingual versions of a dyslexia assessment tool may not be the best solution. To begin with, using two versions of an assessment tool would make the final decision on dyslexia diagnoses more complicated. Further, the testing time would be considerably longer, and the child may suffer from testing fatigue.

Additional reasons for not supporting bilingual versions of a dyslexia assessment tool have been provided through linguistic analysis. For example, the use of an additional assessment tool in the second language may be redundant for Profile 1 children. If phonological deficits were identified in the more transparent Malay language, it would not be necessary to show additional phonological deficits in the opaque language. Furthermore, the use of an additional English version of the assessment tool may result in false positives due to the child's lack of exposure to the second language. We argue that it would be sufficient to use a monolingual Malay dyslexia assessment tool for Profile 1 children, even those who are Malay-English bilingual.

For Profile 2 children, the use of a Malay-English bilingual version of a dyslexia assessment tool would not solve the identified issues (false positives), as these children may lack exposure to not only Malay but also English (their third language). Further, the use of a dyslexia tool in a home language such as Chinese or Tamil would not be appropriate in the Malaysian context. We contend that such a solution would not be instructionally sound, as dyslexia is diagnosed in Profile 2 children largely to provide remediation in the nation's official languages, that is, Malay and English. It has been argued that identifying dyslexia based on the constructs of a logographic writing system (Chinese) to remediate dyslexia in Malay and English (which are alphabetic writing systems) makes no instructional sense. Chinese differs from alphabetic languages in terms of its orthographic, phonological, and morphological features. As such, different causes and risk factors may be attributed to reading problems in Chinese (Chung & Ho, 2010). Chinese research has shown that whereas both speeded naming and morphological awareness are strong correlates of developmental dyslexia (McBride-Chang et al., 2011), phonological awareness is the primary correlate in alphabetic languages. It would be more educationally sound to diagnose dyslexia in the language to be remediated. However, this returns us to the problem of false positive diagnosis. The following solutions are proposed for differentiating the assessment procedures to lessen such a problem.

Explicit Instruction in Phonological Tasks Before Testing

Rather than multilingual versions of phonological processing tests, Profile 2 children must be provided with adequate tuition or explicit instruction on phonological tasks before testing commences. Phonological task instructions given prior to testing Profile 2 children would help decrease not only the effect of poor language exposure but the effect of transferring visual-orthographic skills to the alphabetic language during the dyslexia assessment. Because practice items are currently being administered before testing, the practice item sections should be further expanded to provide adequate tuition in phonological tasks before the actual testing is conducted. This is especially important for phonological awareness tasks such as blending, segmenting, and elision. If children were able to perform phonological awareness tasks after adequate instruction, phonological processing deficits or dyslexia would naturally be excluded. If problems in the phonological awareness tasks persist after such instruction, a dyslexia diagnosis should be considered. As a precaution, it must be acknowledged that this method may not be able to specifically separate dyslexic children from children with slower learning rates. However, if a child were slow due to a global delay, he or she would exhibit delays in other processing areas, typically in terms of linguistic comprehension or nonverbal reasoning tasks (Criterion 2).

As highlighted previously, there are behavioral, neuroimaging, and neural bases for expecting phonological awareness to indicate a single ability (Goswami et al., 2010; Melby-Lervåg & Lervåg, 2011; Paulesu et al., 2001) that is not language specific (Gomez & Reason, 2002; Melby-Lervåg & Lervåg, 2011). Hence, the use of multilingual phonological tests may be redundant for bilingual children. Gomez and Reason (2002) showed the performances of Malaysian bilingual children on a phonological processing battery (PhAB) to be at least comparable with the UK norms. Their results reinforced the argument that the use of multilingual phonological tests may be redundant due to phonological deficits being language universal. If a child were to show deficits in phonological processing in the more transparent language, it may not be necessary to test for phonological processing deficits in the additional opaque language.

Listening and Reading Comprehension Tests in the Home Language/Nonverbal Reasoning Tests

Bilingual listening and reading comprehension tests administered in both a Profile 2 child's home language and primary official language may be necessary to arrive at data that rule out low intellect and improve accuracy when determining Criterion 2 in a typical dyslexia assessment. The use of listening comprehension tests in the child's home language would indicate his or her linguistic ability. However, caution would have to be exercised when making decisions, as the reading comprehension tests administered in the child's home language would not be alphabetic, and it would be harder to show a direct discrepancy between his or her linguistic skills and alphabetic reading ability. In addition, if the home language were a Chinese dialect, the spoken words would not always correspond to the written words in Mandarin. One alternative, especially for psychologists who are unable to administer tests in the home language, would be the use of nonverbal abstract reasoning tests such as the Matrix Analogies Test-Short Form (MAT-SF) (Naglieri, 1995) to gather additional information that excludes low intellect as the root cause of the child's reading problems. The MAT-SF is recommended because it is fast and easy to administer and has been used previously with Malaysian bilingual students ($\alpha = .91$) (Lee, 2008a).

Differentiation in Norming

Another consequence of multilingualism in Malaysia is the need to develop three sets of norms for the three different national primary school backgrounds when assessing dyslexia. Different sets of norms for multiple school backgrounds reflect the different sets of norms for a variety of language profiles, which may be necessary to compare peers more accurately.

A GENERAL PRESCRIPTION OF DYSLEXIA ASSESSMENT

Based on the proposed differentiation of dyslexia assessments in multilingual Malaysia, a generalized prescription for differentiation may be postulated in other multilingual environments as follows.

1. Adapting a dyslexia assessment tool from English into any other language requires understanding the orthographic features of that language in comparison with English. The assessment tasks must be differentiated in response to the orthographic features such as the depth and granularity of the language to increase the accuracy of the assessment tasks.
2. When diagnosing a child in a multilingual environment, it is important to identify the child's language profile, that is, the child's home language and the school's instructional languages. It

is subsequently important to compare the orthographic features of the child's home language and the school's instructional languages to identify the possibility of a cross-language transfer of skills that may interfere with the test results.

3. If the home and primary instructional languages are similar, dyslexia may be diagnosed solely in that language despite the child's bilingualism. In other words, it may not be necessary to consider a child's second language in testing for dyslexia.
4. If the home and primary instructional languages differ, explicit instructions of the phonological tasks must be provided in the language used for testing before the tests are administrated. Bilingual versions of the phonological tasks may not be necessary.
5. In addition, when the home and instructional languages differ, it may be necessary to administer bilingual listening and reading comprehension tests to rule out low intellect. Nonverbal reasoning tests may alternatively be used.
6. Different norms for different language profiles may be necessary, especially if the language profiles mirror different types of school systems.

The proposed prescription would require additional debate and extensive support from research evidence to test their robustness. However, at this juncture, the prescription is meant only to generate discussion. The research interest in diagnosing dyslexia in bilingual or multilingual children has been growing (Chung & Ho, 2010). Consequently, the proposed prescription should add to the debate on viable assessment solutions for bilingual and multilingual children with dyslexia.

THE WAY FORWARD

The Malay-English comparison shows that variations in orthographic transparency and in the phonological structure of alphabetic languages call for differentiating dyslexia assessments, despite the apparent similarities between the underlying cognitive and neurological bases of dyslexia. The Malaysian case study discussed in this chapter also highlights the possible problems accompanying dyslexia diagnosis in a multilingual environment. The differentiation of tasks, processes, and norms is proposed as a solution for the issues encountered during dyslexia assessments.

Empirical research must be conducted to test the robustness of the suggested prescription. First, before adapting an English dyslexia assessment tool to other languages, an orthographic analysis of the language that compares it with English should be carried out to identify the salient features that would necessitate the differentiation of tasks during the translation process.

Second, it is important to conduct research to identify the various language profiles seen in the educational environment and by extension, the cognitive profiles of children in a multilingual environment. A child's language profile influences the process and judgment involved in a dyslexia diagnosis.

Third, to identify the optimum set of tasks required for accurate dyslexia assessment when the home and school languages differ, a bilingual research design that involves correlations between similar sets of tasks in both languages must be conducted. This would help the researcher rule out redundant tasks and consolidate the tasks in a dyslexia assessment tool to an optimum number. A dyslexia tool with an optimum number of tasks that allow accurate decisions to be made on Criteria 1, 2, or 3 in the dyslexia framework is necessary in a multilingual environment.

Fourth, when the school systems are different and distinct, especially in terms of their instructional languages (such as in Malaysia), developing different norms for comparison may be necessary. This would be an extension of the recent work identifying different cognitive profiles in dyslexia diagnosis.

As previously argued, the solution for a multilingual environment is not necessarily to incorporate multiple versions of a dyslexia assessment tool. Instead, the way forward is to identify the optimum number of tests necessary to diagnose a bilingual child accurately. As the underlying cause of a reading disability is instrumental in the choice and potential effectiveness of reading interventions (Duff & Clarke, 2011), accurate assessments of bilingual children are important.

REFERENCES

Aaron, P. G., Joshi, R. M., Gooden, R., & Bentum, K. E. (2008). Diagnosis and treatment of reading disabilities based on the component model of reading: An alternative to the discrepancy model of LD. *Journal of Learning Disabilities*, *41*, 67–84.

Badian, N. A. (1999). Reading disability defined as a discrepancy between listening and reading comprehension: A longitudinal study of stability, gender differences, and prevalence. *Journal of Learning Disabilities*, *32*(2), 138–148.

Bishop, D. V. M., & Snowling, M. J. (2004). Developmental dyslexia and specific language impairment: Same or different? *Psychological Bulletin*, *130*, 858–888.

Brookes, G., Ng, V., Lim, B. H., Tan, W. P., & Lukito, N. (2011). The computerized-based Lucid Rapid Dyslexia Screening for the identification of children at risk of dyslexia: A Singapore study. *Educational & Child Psychology*, *28*(2), 33–51.

Casalis, S., Colé, P., & Sopo, P. (2004). Morphological awareness in developmental dyslexia. *Annals of Dyslexia, 54*(1), 114–138.

Chung, K. K. H., & Ho, C. S.-H. (2010). Dyslexia in Chinese language: An overview of research and practice. *Australian Journal of Learning Difficulties, 15*, 213–224.

Davies, R., Cuetos, F., & Glez-Seijas, R. M. (2007). Reading development and dyslexia in a transparent orthography: A survey of Spanish children. *Annals of Dyslexia, 57*, 179–198.

Department of Special Education. (2011). *Instrumen senarai semak disleksia*. Cetakan kedua. [Dyslexia checklist, 2nd ed.]. Retrieved February 19, 2013, from http://www.moe.gov.my/jpnperlis/v2/images/stories/download/spspk/instrumen_senarai_semak_disleksi.pdf

Department of Statistics. (2009). *Statistics handbook Malaysia*. Malaysia: Department of Statistics.

Dixon, L. Q., Zhao, J., & Joshi, R. M. (2010). Influence of L1 orthography on spelling English words by bilingual children: A natural experiment comparing syllabic, phonological and morphosyllabic first languages. *Learning Disability Quarterly, 33*, 211–221.

Duff, F. J., & Clarke, P. J. (2011). Practitioner review: Reading disorders: What are the effective interventions and how should they be implemented and evaluated? *Journal of Child Psychology and Psychiatry, 52*(1), 3–12.

Fletcher, J. M., Coulter, W. A., Reschly, D. J., & Vaughn, S. (2004). Alternative approaches to the definition and identification of learning disabilities: Some questions and answers. *Annals of Dyslexia, 54*(2), 304–331.

Frith, U. (1986). A developmental framework for developmental dyslexia. *Annals of Dyslexia, 36*, 69–81.

Fuchs, D., & Fuchs, L. (2006). Introduction to response to intervention: What, why, and how valid is it? *Reading Research Quarterly, 41*(1), 93–99.

Gomez, C., & Reason, R. (2002). Cross-linguistic transfer of phonological skills: A Malaysian perspective. *Dyslexia, 8*, 22–33.

Goswami, U. (2008). The development of reading across languages. *Annals of the New York Academy of Sciences, 1145*, 1–12.

Goswami, U., Wang, H.-L. S., Cruz, A., Fosker, T., Mead, N., & Huss, M. (2010). Language-universal sensory deficits in developmental dyslexia: English, Spanish and Chinese. *Journal of Cognitive Neuroscience, 23*(2), 325–337.

Gough, P. B., & Tunmer, W. E. (1986). Decoding, reading and reading disability. *Remedial and Special Education*, 7(2), 6–10.

Haniz, I. (2003, October). *Program bermasalah pembelajaran spesifik disleksia Kementerian Pendidikan Malaysia* [Program for dyslexia specific learning disability, Ministry of Education]. Paper presented at the 3rd National Special Education Seminar, Special Education Department, Ministry of Education, Kuala Lumpur.

Joshi, R. M., Williams, K. A., & Wood, J. R. (1998). Predicting reading comprehension from listening comprehension: Is this the answer to the IQ debate? In C. Hulme & R. M. Joshi (Eds.), *Reading and spelling: Developmental disorders* (pp. 319–327). Mahwah, NJ: Lawrence Erlbaum.

Lee, L. W. (2008a). Development and validation of a reading-related assessment battery in Malay for the purpose of dyslexia assessment. *Annals of Dyslexia, 58*, 37–57.

Lee, L. W. (2008b). Dyslexia: Different cultures, similar behavioural signs. *Dyslexia Review, 19*(3), 19–25.

Lee, L. W., Low, H. M., & Abdul Rashid, M. (2012). Word count analysis of Bahasa Malaysia textbooks for the purpose of developing a Malay reading remedial program. *Writing Systems Research, 4*(1), 103–119.

Lee, L. W., Low, H. M., & Abdul Rashid, M. (2013). A comparative analysis of word structures in Malay and English children's stories. *PERTANIKA Journal of Social Sciences & Humanities, 21*(1), 67–84.

Lee, L. W., & Wheldall, K. (2011). Acquisition of Malay language word reading skills: Lessons from low progress early readers. *Dyslexia, 17*, 19–37.

Lyon, G. R., Shaywitz, S. E., & Shaywitz, B. A. (2003). A definition of dyslexia. *Annals of Dyslexia, 53*, 1–14.

Masterson, J., Stuart, M., Dixon, M., & Lovejoy, S. (2010). Children's printed word database: Continuities and changes over time in children's early reading vocabulary. *British Journal of Psychology, 101*, 221–242.

McBride-Chang, C., Lam, F., Lam, C., Chan, B., Fong, C. Y.-C., Wong, T. T.-Y., & Wong, S. W.-L. (2011). Early predictors of dyslexia in Chinese children: Familial history of dyslexia, language delay, and cognitive profiles. *Journal of Child Psychology and Psychiatry, 52*(2), 204–211.

Melby-Lervåg, M., & Lervåg, A. (2011). Cross-linguistic transfer of oral language, decoding, phonological awareness and reading comprehension: A meta-analysis of the correlational evidence. *Journal of Research in Reading, 34*(1), 114–135.

Melby-Lervåg, M., Lyster, S.-A. H., & Hulme, C. (2012). Phonological skills and their role in learning to read: A meta-analytic review. *Psychological Bulletin, 138*(2), 322–352.

Miles, E. (2000). Dyslexia may show a different face in different languages. *Dyslexia, 6*, 193–201.

Naglieri, J. A. (1985). *Matrix Analogies Test-Short Form*. New York, NY: Psychological Corporation.

Paulesu, E., Demonet, J., Fazio, F., McCrory, E., Chanoine, V., Brunswick, N., ... Frith, U. (2001). Dyslexia: Cultural diversity and biological unity. *Science, 291*, 2165–2167.

Rickard Liow, S. J., & Lee, L. C. (2004). Metalinguistic awareness and semi-syllabic scripts: Children's spelling errors in Malaysia. *Reading and Writing, 17*(1/2), 7–26.

Roach, P. (2009). *English phonetics and phonology: A practical course* (4th ed.). Cambridge, England: Cambridge University Press.

Sawyer, D. J. (2006). Dyslexia: A generation of inquiry. *Topics in Language Disorders, 26*, 95–102.

Snowling, M. J. (2000). *Dyslexia*. Oxford, UK: Blackwell.

Wagner, R. K., & Torgesen, J. K. (1987). The nature of phonological processing and its causal role in the acquisition of reading skills. *Psychological Bulletin, 101*, 192–212.

Wagner, R. K., Torgesen, J. K., & Rashotte, C. A. (1999). *Comprehensive test of phonological processing*. Austin, TX: Pro-Ed.

Ziegler, J. C., & Goswami, U. (2005). Reading acquisition, developmental dyslexia and skilled reading across languages: A psycholinguistic grain size theory. *Psychological Bulletin, 131*(1), 3–29.

Ziegler, J. C., Perry, C., Ma-Watt, A., Ladner, D., & Schulte-Korn, G. (2003). Developmental dyslexia in different languages: Language-specific or universal? *Journal of Experimental Child Psychology, 86*, 169–193.

CHAPTER 8

VISUAL-SPATIAL ATTENTION AND ITS RELATIONSHIP WITH READING

Duo Liu

Parents and teachers frequently report that some of the errors their children make in examinations are caused by an inattention to some key words in the questions. When children are asked to copy a newly learned word, some (especially those with dyslexia) easily miss certain aspects. Likewise, people may have experienced situations such as being "blinded" to specific words (e.g., "Emergency use only" printed on a door) simply because they did not pay attention to them. These cases reveal the importance of visual-spatial attention in processing visually presented words in reading. In the research areas related to reading development and difficulties, however, little attention has been paid to the importance of attention despite an increasing number of studies that have provided positive evidence of its significance (e.g., Facoetti, Paganoni, Turatto Marzola, & Mascetti, 2000; Pammer, Lavis, Hansen, & Cornelissen, 2004; Valdois, Bosse, & Tainturier, 2004; Vidyasagar & Pammer, 2010). In this chapter, the importance of visual-spatial attention in children's reading development in alphabetic languages and Chinese is discussed and the relevant literature is reviewed.

Understanding Developmental Disorders of Auditory Processing, Language and Literacy Across Languages: International Perspectives, pp. 169–188

Visual-spatial attention, which involves the selection of stimuli based on visual-spatial location (e.g., Vecera & Rizzo, 2003), has the same elements as other types of attention, including focusing, orienting, and attentional span. Here, these elements are used to discuss the importance of visual-spatial attention in predicting reading development or identifying reading problems, following a general description of the association between visual-spatial attention and reading development. Almost all of the evidence is from studies of alphabetic languages such as English, Italian, and French. There is currently scant research on the visual-spatial attention of Chinese readers. Thus, the particular importance of visual-spatial attention in the reading development of Chinese children is subsequently discussed.

Visual-Spatial Attention and Reading Development

The first stage of reading involves the selective reception of visual information by our visual system, which corresponds with a series of saccades—short-latency ocular movements (e.g., Facoetti et al., 2000). Simply speaking, during this stage, as readers we need to disengage and shift attention from the former visual unit, focus on the current visual unit (i.e., put it in the foveal region), and sustain our focus long enough for the follow-up cognitive processing to be carried out. Meanwhile, because the current visual unit is always surrounded by "distracters" during natural reading, we also need to suppress the information coming from the periphery of the visual field, an act that is related to the inhibition aspect of attention. Moreover, a good attention span (approximately seven or eight letters at a time; e.g., Blais, Fiset, Arguin, Jolicoeur, Bub, & Gosselin, 2009) can help us cover enough information within one fixation to save our limited attentional resources from a redundant shifting of attention. Generally, the nature of reading, which is closely related to the processing of visually presented stimuli in the primary stage, determines the importance of the visual-spatial attention applied.

Researchers have debated the necessity of visual-spatial attention during reading. Some consider spatial attention necessary for visual word recognition (e.g., Stolz & McCann, 2000), while others argue that although spatial attention can facilitate word recognition, it is not a necessary condition (e.g., Brown, Gore, & Carr, 2002). For instance, using a valid/invalid cued Stroop paradigm, Brown et al. (2002) observed the Stroop effect even when a word printed in color appeared in the nontarget locations (i.e., the locations where no spatial cue had previously appeared), indicating that attention is not necessary for word processing. However, as Besner, Risko, and Sklair (2005) noted in a study conducted by Brown et al. (2002), the experimental design may not ensure that the "attended" and "unattended" stimuli are actually attended and unattended, respectively.

Besner et al. (2005) adopted a valid/invalid cued priming lexical decision paradigm to examine the necessity of visual-spatial attention in word recognition. The target was preceded by a spatial cue presented either in the target location or the opposite location. During the presentation of the spatial cue, a prime word (either identical to the target or unrelated) appeared in the opposite location. The cue validity was set as 50% (so participants had to distribute their spatial attention between two locations and then move more attention to the cued location when a cue appeared, creating a greater opportunity to pay attention to the prime word) or 100% (so participants had to focus their attention and then commit all attentional resources to the cued location when a cue appeared, making them less likely to pay attention to the prime word). An example of the presenting procedure is shown in Figure 8.1.

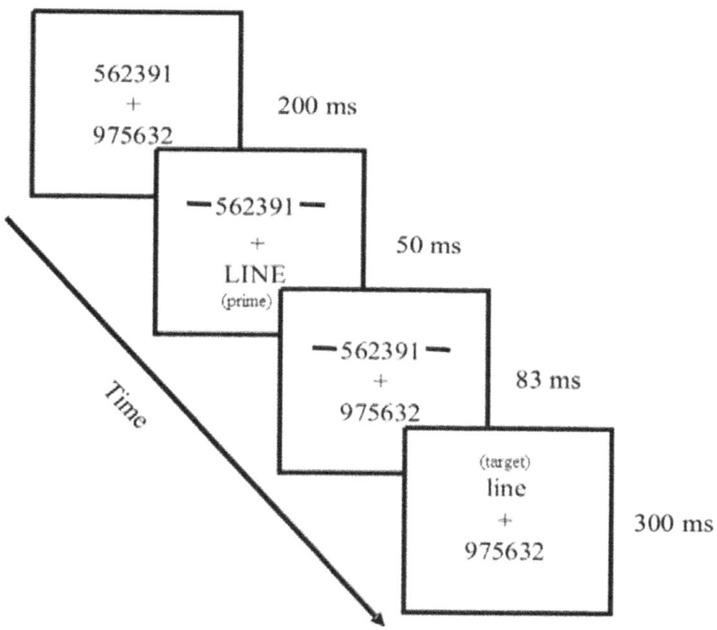

Source: Adapted from Besner et al. (2005).

Figure 8.1. An example of the sequence of events on a validly cued trial in the related condition.

Besner et al. (2005) found that when the cue was 50% valid, a repetition priming effect was observed for valid trials. However, when the cue was 100% valid, no priming effect was noted because in such situations almost all of the participants' attentional resources had been assigned to the cued location, which was opposite to the prime word location. Thus, visual-spatial attention is proven to be necessary for word recognition. The further cognitive processing (such as the mapping from orthography to semantics, which is critical for the priming effect in Besner et al., 2005) involved in reading can only happen when the attentional resources are led to the specific spatial location.

Some correlational studies have also proven the significant association between visual-spatial attention and reading performance in children. For instance, Plaza and Cohen (2007) found in their longitudinal study that the visual-spatial attention of French-speaking kindergarteners, which was measured using a serial visual search task, significantly predicted their reading and spelling performance in Grade 1, even after controlling for phonological awareness, rapid naming, and digit span (phonological memory). Similarly, in Franceschini, Gori, Ruffino, Pedrolli, and Facoetti's (2012) longitudinal study, the visual-spatial attention of Italian-speaking children, which was tested using both a serial visual search and valid/invalid cueing detection paradigm in kindergarten, was found to significantly predict their reading performance in both Grades 1 and 2, after controlling for age, IQ, speech-sound processing, cross-modal mapping skills, and rapid naming.

Orienting and Focusing of Visual-Spatial Attention and Developmental Dyslexia

Numerous studies have focused on the role of visual-spatial attention in distinguishing dyslexic children from typical readers (for reviews, see Valdois et al., 2004; Vidyasagar & Pammer, 2010). In alphabetic languages, many have argued that problems in phonological processing are the core deficit of dyslexia (e.g., Vellutino, Fletcher, Snowling, & Scanlon, 2004; Ziegler & Goswami, 2005). However, others have argued (e.g., Vidyasagar & Pammer, 2010) that reading is a process that begins with the processing of visual information and requires a series of crucial processing steps—from bottom-up, fundamental to top-down advanced steps. Every step is considered essential, and problems at any point in the process can cause difficulties in reading. It has been argued that defective visual-spatial attention might be the more fundamental reason behind reading difficulties (e.g., Bosse, Tainturier, & Valdois, 2007; Facoetti, Zorzi, & Cestnick, 2006).

There are two basic groups of studies focusing on the visual-spatial attention problems of dyslexic children: one that highlights the roles of orienting and focusing and another that concentrates on the role of visual attention span. According to the dual-route model (Coltheart, Rastle, Perry, Langdon, & Ziegler, 2001), in which visual words can be accessed through two routes—a lexical route that uses whole word direct access and a sublexical route that uses graphophonological conversion—three subtypes of developmental dyslexia are categorized: (a) surface dyslexia, which suggests a problem with the lexical route and is usually reflected in difficulty reading irregular words; (b) phonological dyslexia, which indicates a problem with the sublexical route and is reflected in difficulty decoding phonological information and reading (regular) nonwords; and (c) double-deficit dyslexia, which features problems with both routes.

It has been claimed that problems with the orienting and focusing of visual attention might be the more basic reasons for phonological dyslexia (e.g., Facoetti et al., 2006) because children with problems in these aspects find it difficult to segment and parse the detailed phonological information inside words. As Posner noted, the orienting of attention involves three basic mental operations: disengaging attention from the current location, shifting attention to the new location, and engaging attention in the new location (e.g., Posner, Walker, Friedrich et al., 1984). Dysfunction in any of these three operations causes problems in the orienting of visual-spatial attention, which correspondingly causes problems in phonological processing during reading.

The sluggish attentional shifting (SAS) theory (Hari & Renvall, 2001; Hari, Valta, & Uutela, 1999) was developed to describe the deficits of individuals with dyslexia in the orientation of attention, and a number of studies have found supporting evidence (e.g., Facoetti, Lorusso, Cattaneo, Galli, & Molteni, 2005; Facoetti, Trussardi, Ruffino et al., 2010; Lallier, Tainturier, Dering, Donnadieu, Valdois, & Thierry, 2010). According to SAS theory, individuals with dyslexia are impaired in rapid processing of stimulus sequences and have difficulty efficiently disengaging from the current item and engaging in the next item (i.e., SAS). This, in turn, is the main reason for the deficit in processing phonological information during reading.

In the study conducted by Facoetti et al. (2006), Italian-speaking dyslexic children in the nonword reading-impaired group exhibited inconsistent performances compared with dyslexic children in the intact nonword reading group and normal readers in the cued dot-detection task. The main procedure of the dot-detection paradigm is shown in Figure 8.2. Normally, a valid cue should facilitate the detection of the stimulus and an invalid cue should inhibit such detection. This pattern was observed in dyslexic children in the intact nonword reading group and normal readers. However, among the dyslexic children in the nonword reading-impaired group, the difference between valid and invalid cued conditions was not observed, especially in the right visual field. More interestingly, after controlling for age and IQ, the performance of the dyslexic children in the nonword reading-impaired group in the dot-detection paradigm significantly predicted their nonword reading performance. Given that phonological decoding is important for reading regular nonwords, the results in the study conducted by Facoetti et al. (2006) indicated that the orienting of visual-spatial attention should be critical for phonological processing. Similar results have been obtained in several other studies (e.g., Lallier et al., 2010; Facoetti et al., 2010; Hari et al., 1999).

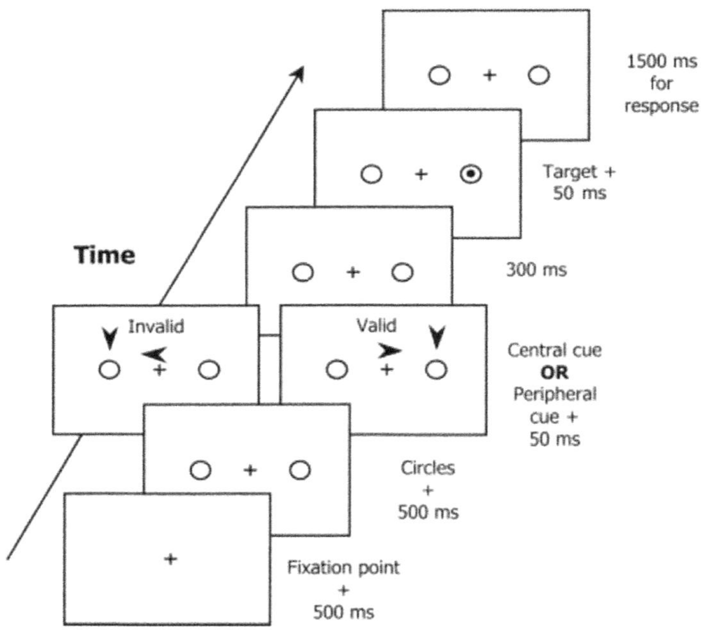

Figure 8.2. The main procedure of the dot detection paradigm used in Facoetti et al.'s (2006) study.

In addition to the deficit in the orienting of visual-spatial attention, difficulty focusing was also thought to be a reason for phonological dyslexia. The focusing of attention involves engaging, sustaining, and inhibiting. These three aspects of focusing visual-spatial attention were found to be critical during the processing of stimulus sequences and the decoding of the phonological information. Engaging can ensure that the cognitive resources are placed in the proper location. Sustaining can ensure that the stimuli at the location are processed sufficiently. Inhibiting can ensure that the processing of the current stimulus is not distracted by the surrounding stimuli.

A series of studies has provided evidence to support the perspective that children with (phonological) dyslexia exhibit an impaired focusing visual-spatial attention (e.g., Geiger, Cattaneo, & Galli et al., 2008; Ruffino, Trussardi, & Gori et al., 2010). In the study conducted by Ruffino et al. (2010), the participants were sequentially presented with two target stimuli with masks inserted before and after the presentation of each stimulus. The participants were then asked to identify the first stimulus among eight alternatives. Compared to normal readers, the processing of the first stimuli among the children with phonological dyslexia was more severely influenced by the presentation of the second stimulus, reflecting a deficit in their ability to focus their visual-spatial attention on the first (target) stimulus.

According to the "perceptual noise exclusion deficit" theory (e.g., Geiger et al., 2008; Sperling, Lu, Manis, & Seidenberg, 2005), individuals with dyslexia have a deficit in the ability to focus (particularly during the "inhibiting" process) their visual-spatial attention. According to this theory, individuals with dyslexia have difficulty suppressing the distractions generated by external noise (Sperling, Lu, Manis, & Seidenberg, 2006), possibly because they have wide and diffuse perceptual modes compared to normal readers and thus cannot efficiently focus on the targets during reading (Geiger et al., 2008). Sperling et al. (2006) found that dyslexic children exhibited much worse performance than normal readers in judging the motion of the signal dots if they were surrounded by "high external noise (i.e., signal and noise dots shared the same color and luminance). In the study conducted by Geiger et al. (2008), the participants were presented with two stimuli simultaneously: one at the center point and the other at a peripheral point, the placement of which varied from 2.5° to 12.5° from the center point, horizontally. It was found that dyslexic children had more correct responses than normal readers at the peripheral points, which indicated that the former had a wider range of visual perceptual modes and thus were less focused than the normal readers. Moreover, the crowding effect observed in letter recognition (e.g., Pelli, Farell, & Moore, 2003) when the target letter was surrounded by other letters and the recognition of the target letter was affected by the neighboring letters was found to be much worse in children with developmental dyslexia (e.g., Spinelli, De Luca, Judica, & Zocolotti, 2002). All of these findings indicate that difficulties in inhibiting distracters and focusing on the target stimuli contribute to developmental dyslexia.

Difficulty sustaining visual-spatial attention was also observed in some studies. Facoetti et al. (2000) manipulated the stimulus-onset asynchrony

(SOA) information (99 ms in the short SOA condition and 504 ms in the long SOA condition) and the size of the circle and found that in the short SOA condition, dyslexic children showed a similar pattern to normal readers (i.e., faster reaction times in the small cue trials). However, in the long SOA condition, no difference was found between small and large cue trials in dyslexic children. Because they can help participants focus, smaller cues typically facilitate processing (e.g., Eriksen & Yeh, 1985). Among dyslexic children, such an effect was only observed with short SOA, but not with long SOA, indicating that they could only exert active focus control for a relatively short period.

Together, the findings in these previous studies strongly support the importance of orienting and focusing visual-spatial attention in reading, such that difficulties in any of the steps involved in these two aspects are associated with dyslexia, particularly phonological dyslexia.

Visual-Spatial Attention Span and Reading (Difficulties)

Attention span, which is defined as "the amount of distinct visual elements that can be processed in parallel in a multi-element array" (Bosse et al., 2007), is another component of visual-spatial attention that is considered important for reading. If we only focus on one letter at a time, reading will be very inefficient. A proper size of visual attention span is necessary for reading because referring to the surrounding letters helps the reader pronounce the target letter or letter cluster correctly (e.g. the "dr" in "bedrail" should not be pronounced as /dr/) or quickly reveals whether the pronunciation can be retrieved from memory or must be spelled.

Valdois et al. (2004) developed a concept called the visual attentional window (VAW) to elaborate the importance of visual attention span in reading, following the connectionist multiple-trace memory (MTM) model of polysyllabic word reading (e.g., Ans, Carbonnel, & Valdois, 1998). The MTM model was developed by integrating and modifying the dual-route model (e.g., Coltheart et al., 2001) and the parallel distributed processing (PDP) model (e.g., Plaut, McClelland, Seidenberg, & Patterson, 1996). The basic idea was that "learning only consists of adding new separate episodic traces in memory without modifying memory structure" (Ans et al., 1998, p. 681), and thus reading is about matching the current episode (the visually presented word) with the stored multiple memory traces to select the proper reading procedure. In the MTM model, the researchers proposed two types of reading procedures: global processing, involving whole-word direct access; and analytical processing, involving the decoding of phonological information. Because readers need to directly map orthography to meaning or sound in global processing, the VAW must cover the entire sequence of the input letter string. Once global processing has failed, the VAW is narrowed so that smaller units inside the letter string can be processed analytically. Following analytical processing, letters within the VAW are activated and processed in parallel, while letters outside the VAW are activated minimally or not at all.

The MTM model suggests that global processing should facilitate familiar word reading while analytical processing should facilitate pseudoword reading. Then the different types of dyslexia can be linked with the severity of the reduction of the VAW in visual-spatial attention. A mild reduction in the VAW will influence global processing first, causing surface dyslexia, in which situation-dyslexic children exhibit particular difficulty reading irregular words because to correctly read irregular words, readers must map orthography directly with sound in a global process. Along with the reduction in the VAW, dyslexic readers will show increasing difficulties in both global and analytical reading and thus be categorized as deep dyslexics. However, deficits in phonological processing can cause phonological dyslexia, which is related to difficulty in reading pseudowords only. Therefore, researchers have proposed that both visual attention span and phonological processing deficits could be independent core deficits in dyslexic children (e.g., Valdois, Bosse et al., 2003).

In several of the empirical studies conducted by Valdois and her colleagues (e.g., Bosse et al., 2007; Bosse & Valdois, 2009; Lobier, Zoubrinetzky, & Valdois, 2012), the association between children's visual-spatial attention and reading performance was explored. In Bosse et al. (2007), French and British children were administered visual attention span tasks and other tasks, including reading tasks and tests of phonological awareness. The researchers found that phonological skills and visual attention span were unrelated to one another, and either of them could independently contribute to reading performance. In another cross-sectional study (Bosse & Valdois, 2009), similar independent contributions of visual attention span and phonological skills to word reading were observed across three grade groups of French children. Moreover, visual attention span showed a stable association with irregular word reading, but not pseudoword reading, across grades in that study, implying the importance of visual-spatial attention in global processing. The findings in these studies supported the idea that problems with visual-spatial attention span might be another core deficit of dyslexia in alphabetic languages, in addition to the problems in phonological processing. Particularly, problems with visual-spatial attention span might be more closely related to surface dyslexia caused by problems in global processing in the MTM model.

In summary, a number of studies have supported the importance of several elements of visual-spatial attention (including orienting, focusing, and attention span) in reading development and in identifying reading difficulties in alphabetic languages. Some theories have also been developed to interpret the nature of the association between visual-spatial attention and reading, specifically SAS theory (orienting), "perceptual noise exclusion deficit" theory (focusing), and VAW (attention span). More interestingly, in terms of the different types of developmental dyslexia according to the dual-route model, deficits in orienting and focusing visual-spatial attention might be more fundamental reasons for phonological dyslexia because they are critical for segmenting and parsing letter strings. Problems with attention span might thus be a core cause of surface and double-deficit dyslexia because, according to the MTM model, both global and analytical processing require some specific sizes of visual attention spans.

Evidence Against the Importance of Visual-Spatial Attention

Nevertheless, some researchers have not been fully convinced by the evidence (e.g., Vellutino et al., 2004; Ziegler, Pech-Georgel, Dufau, & Grainger, 2010). For instance, Ziegler et al. (2010) argued that because verbal materials (i.e., letters or digits) and oral report were used in the visual attention span tasks (e.g., Bosse et al., 2007), what the tasks measured might not be purely components of visual attention, but confounded by phonological processing. Therefore, in their study, Ziegler et al. (2010), used a classic two-alternative forced-choice (2AFC) *Reicher-Wheeler* paradigm to test French (both dyslexic and normal) children's visual spatial attention using both verbal (i.e., letters and digits) and nonverbal (i.e., symbols) materials.

In the 2AFC *Reicher-Wheeler* paradigm, a horizontal array of five characters was presented on the computer screen for a short time, and the participants were asked to select which of two alternatives they thought should be the character presented at that specific position, as accurately as possible (thus only accuracy was recorded). Three types of materials were involved: consonant letters presented in uppercase (B, D, F, G, K, N, L, S, and T), digits (1 to 9), and symbols (%, /, ?, @, }, <, £, §, and μ). In previous studies on adults (e.g., Mason & Katz, 1976; Tydgat & Grainger, 2009), among the letters and digits, a W-shaped serial position function was observed with the highest accuracy in the center, the lowest accuracy at positions 2 and 4, and intermediate accuracy at positions 1 and 5. In contrast, an inverted V-shaped function was observed for symbols. The crowding effect was mentioned by some researchers to explain this phenomenon (e.g., Grainger, Tydgat, & Isselé, 2010). Because letters are always displayed in a more "crowded" manner than symbols, the difference in the crowding level between positions 1 and 2 was much more significant among the letters. Thus, the decrease in the crowding of the letter in position 1 overcomes the decrease in visual acuity and prompts improved performance. However, because symbols are typically less crowded, the difference in crowding level between positions 1 and 2 was not as significant. Thus, among the symbols, the decrease in accuracy mainly reflected the influence of a decrease in visual acuity in the performance.

In Ziegler et al. (2010), differences between dyslexic and normal children were found for letters and digits, but not for symbols. Furthermore, although dyslexic children showed overall lower accuracy than normal children on the verbal materials, the patterns of their performances were quite similar. According to these results, the researchers argued that because the poor performance of dyslexic children on the visual attention task only occurred for letters and digits (both are language-related materials) and not symbols, deficits in phonological processing seem to be more significant than visual attention factors in predicting reading problems.

However, as Ziegler et al. (2010) noted, there have also been studies in which nonverbal materials were used, and the deficits in visual attention were observed in dyslexics (e.g., Facoetti et al., 2000; Pammer et al., 2004; Plaza & Cohen, 2007). Thus, the issue is far from settled. Moreover, it is still not appropriate to say that a phonological processing deficit should be "put back in the front row" (Ziegler et al., 2010) according to the current results, because the study provides no direct evidence that the phonological information in the verbal materials (i.e., digits and letters) was indeed activated during the task.

The experimental design and results of the study conducted by Ziegler et al. (2010) are questionable if we look at the details. First, in the description of the method section, the researchers should have directly borrowed the paradigm from Tydgat and Grainger (2009). However, whereas Tydgat and Grainger used 90 stimuli, Ziegler et al. (2010) only used 60 stimuli for each type of material. The Tydgat and Grainger study used a precise design to determine that 90 stimuli should be used for each type of material. As mentioned earlier, in the 2AFC *Reicher-Wheeler* paradigm, there were 5 positions and 9 optional items in each type of material. To make sure that all 9 items appeared in all 5 positions equally, there should be 45 stimuli. According to the design for each target, the correct alternative should appear twice, once below and once above the target position, to balance the button-pressing variance. Thus, 45 times 2 should be 90. For the detailed experimental design, see Tydgat and Grainger (2009). Because only 60 stimuli were involved, there may have been a problem in balancing the presentation frequency of the characters. The authors did not present any detailed information on this point, so we do not know how they addressed this issue. It is possible that some characters were not evenly presented at all 5 positions, which would cause some additional errors, particularly considering the different visual complexity of different characters.

In the results, it was noted that for symbol materials, all of the children's accuracies at positions 1, 2, 4, and 5 were close to 0.5, namely, the random level. Although the visual complexity across the three types of materials was controlled, the visual similarity of the stimuli within each type was not considered in the study, which may be why the symbol materials were more difficult to recognize or distinguish than letters or digits. Thus, it is possible that the nonsignificant difference for the symbol materials was partially caused by such a floor effect. Even with these issues not thoroughly addressed, the point indicated by Ziegler et al. (2010), that some studies only used language-related materials and thus the influence of phonological processing could not be strongly excluded, is worth considering. Therefore, more empirical studies are required to produce more reliable evidence that either supports or refutes the importance of visual spatial attention in the future. In a recent study conducted by Lobier et al. (2012), both verbal and nonverbal stimuli were involved in the visual attention span task, and the visual attention span deficit was found in both types of stimuli in dyslexic children.

The Importance of Visual Spatial Attention in Reading Chinese

The abovementioned arguments address the importance of visual-spatial attention in reading alphabetic languages, but few of the studies conducted in Chinese have directly touched on this issue, despite the fact that we believe visual-spatial attention to be particularly important for reading development in Chinese.

The role of visual processing in the reading development of Chinese children has garnered increasing attention (e.g., Ho, Chan, Tsang, & Lee, 2002; Luo, Chen, Deacon, Zhang, & Yin, 2013; McBride-Chang, Zhou, Cho, Aram, Levin, & Tolchinsky, 2011; Siok, Spinks, Jin, & Tan, 2009; Tan, Spinks, Eden, Perfetti, & Siok, 2005; Wang, Bi, Gao, & Wydell, 2010), largely due to the characteristics of the Chinese written language in terms of visual-spatial features. However, in exploring visual processing, most current studies have focused on visual perceptual skills, namely, children's ability to perceive or operate the visually presented objects. None have explicitly focused on the role of visual-spatial attention, which addresses the attention paid to the location of the visually presented stimuli, although a close relationship between visual-spatial attention and visual perception has been suggested (e.g., Luck & Ford, 1998).

The Chinese written language is a logographic system (e.g., Chen, Song, Lau, Wong, & Tang, 2003; Tan et al., 2005) with a direct visual (orthographic)-semantic link. The relatively complex two-dimensional structure and the combination of strokes and stroke patterns that create Chinese characters require fine-grained detection and identification of the visual details and their positions to identify or distinguish prints, which is closely related to visual-spatial attention. First, there are many Chinese characters that are quite similar (e.g., 大, 太, and 犬; 未 and 末; 戊, 戍, and 戌). Visual-spatial attention should be important in identifying the subtle differences in these similar characters during reading. It has been argued that during the processing of orthographic information, basic visual processing skills are necessary (e.g., McBride-Chang, Chow, Zhong, Burgess, & Hayward, 2005; Sperling et al., 2003; Stein, 2003) while visual-spatial attention should be the foundation of higher-level visual perception (Luck & Ford, 1998). Second, homographs are common in Chinese (e.g., 干 has different pronunciations and meanings in 干净 [gan1 jing4, clean] and 干活 [gan4 huo2, work]). The correct and fluent reading of these characters and words requires a proper visual attention span. For instance, covering the second character (净or 活) within one fixation will help to efficiently retrieve the correct pronunciation of the first character (gan1 and gan4, respectively, in this example).

Third, unlike the words in alphabetic languages, there is no clear boundary for multicharacter words in Chinese text. To correctly and efficiently identify a word during reading, some size of visual attention span is necessary for referring to the contextual information. Focusing and inhibiting are also needed. For example, in the sentence "其中国家名字需要单独列出", "国家 (guo2 jia1, country)" but not "中国 (zhong1 guo2, China)" should be a word. To read this sentence correctly and fluently, we need to cover at least "其中国" within one fixation so we can realize that "其中" and "国家" are two separate words in this sentence. At the same time, the word "中国" might be a distracter for processing the word "国家". Thus, we need visual-spatial attention to inhibit its processing. The importance of attention in word segmentation in Chinese has been mentioned in some previous studies (e.g., Li, Rayner, & Cave, 2009).

Given the visual complexity of Chinese characters and because they are the basic independent visual units of text, to access the meaning or sound of a Chinese character as readers we must bring enough attentional resources to the character level, including all of the important aspects of visual spatial attention such as focusing, orienting, and attention span. Chen et al. (2003) found that for older participants, the features at the character level, but not at the word level, played a crucial role in determining the pattern of eye movement, which implies that the quality of visual-spatial attention at the Chinese character level becomes increasingly important in the development of reading skills. Moreover, according to the findings in the studies conducted by Chen and his colleagues (e.g., Chen & Tang, 1998; Tang, Au Yeung, & Chen, 1997), although the attention/perceptual span is smaller than when reading alphabetic languages (e.g., English), an attention/perceptual span of 3–4 characters is required for the natural reading of Chinese.

Two recent studies (Meng, Cheng-Lai, Zeng, Stein, & Zhou, 2011; Wang et al., 2010) identified an association between the reading performance of Chinese children and the function of the visual magnocelluar pathway, which was thought to be the basic mechanism of visual-spatial attention (Vidyasagar, 1999; Vidyasagar & Pammer, 1999). Based on the features of the Chinese written languages mentioned above and the findings of these two studies, it is quite possible that visual-spatial attention is an important element of Chinese children's reading development and can be a factor in identifying Chinese children with reading difficulties. More empirical studies are required to directly examine this hypothesis.

Several studies have investigated the visual-spatial attention of Chinese readers toward different types of stimuli, although the association between visual-spatial attention and reading performance has not been mentioned. We find an exploration of the characteristics of visual-spatial attention *per se* to be important because it could provide us with a valuable reference for evaluating the visual-spatial attention of children with different reading performances. Due to the logographic feature of Chinese characters, and because they are the basic independent unit in text as symbols but are not grouped together in a crowded manner, as in letter strings, it has been proposed that the visual-spatial attention toward Chinese characters should be more like the visual-spatial attention toward symbols rather than letters in alphabetic languages (e.g., Green, Liow, Tng, & Zielinski, 1996).

Green et al. (1996) studied bilingual undergraduate students from Singapore (L1 = Chinese, L2 = English). They tested the students using the visual search paradigm and found that an M-shaped function was observed in reaction times for letters while a V-shaped function was observed for Chinese characters. The visual search paradigm is similar to the 2AFC *Reicher-Wheeler* paradigm introduced above. As some researchers have argued (e.g., Plaza & Cohen, 2007; Trick & Enns, 1998), visual search is a valid task for studying visual-spatial attention. Thus, the results obtained by Green et al. (1996) reflect the characteristics of bilingual people in terms of their visual-spatial attention toward Chinese characters, namely, it exhibited a symbol-like pattern.

In a recent study conducted by the author and colleagues, the visual-spatial attention of undergraduate students in Hong Kong was measured using the 2AFC *Reicher-Wheeler* paradigm. Five types of materials were involved: digits (0–9), letters (B, D, F, G, K, N, L, S, and T), symbols (<, ?, \, {, &, Д, §, †, and £),

Chinese characters (一, 人, 了, 十, 小, 大, 之, 七, and 上), and semantic radicals (冫, 氵, 亻, 辶, 犭, 忄, 扌, 礻, and 牜). The semantic radicals were selected because they are parts of written Chinese characters and are thus language-related stimuli. However, the semantic radicals we selected in this study were unpronounceable (with the exception of 牜, because it is derived from the Chinese character 牛), which is also a critical feature of symbols.

Generally, for digits and letters, a W-shaped position function was observed, whereas for symbols, characters, and semantic radicals, an inverted V-shaped function was observed. Thus, the symbol-like feature of Chinese characters and radicals in terms of visual-spatial attention is supported by our findings. Nevertheless, the W-shaped functions we observed for digits and letters were not as robust as those found in previous studies. It is possible that because the Chinese character is the predominant print script in Hong Kong, their frequent exposure to Chinese characters may have had some influence on these participants' visual attention span toward other types of stimuli, such as letter strings or digits. For all types of stimuli, the participants' performance (accuracy) in the center position (position 3) was much better than their performance in other positions, but this was different from the patterns found in previous studies (e.g., Tydgat & Grainger, 2009; Ziegler et al., 2010) wherein the performance in position 1 was closer to the performance in position 3. As we argued earlier, the proper processing of a specific Chinese character requires the reader to be intently focused, so the details inside can be thoroughly processed and the surrounding information can be effectively inhibited. Following the instructions of the task, the participants had to focus on the stimuli presented in position 3 and thus could only allocate limited attentional resources to the stimuli in other positions. Thus, the significantly worse performances in other positions across different types of materials indicated that the visual attention span of typical Chinese readers might be relatively smaller (Chen et al., 2003), which may be closely related to the features of the Chinese written language.

More empirical studies should be conducted to explore the developmental trajectory of visual-spatial attention toward different types of stimuli to examine whether the center-predominant visual-spatial attention to Chinese characters becomes increasingly obvious as children age and to determine when this center-predominant feature begins to be generalized to other types of stimuli. More importantly, it is necessary to explore whether the visual-spatial attention of Chinese children is correlated with their reading development, including reading accuracy and fluency, and whether deficits in visual-spatial attention could be the core reasons for developmental dyslexia in Chinese.

Interestingly, some intervention studies have been conducted in which children's visual-spatial attention was trained and an improvement in reading was observed (e.g., Facoetti, Lorusso, Paganoni, Umilta, & Mascetti, 2003; Franceschini, Gori, Ruffino, Viola, Molteni, & Facoetti, 2013, for a review see Vidyasagar & Pammer, 2010). For instance, Franceschini et al. (2013) found that playing action video games improved children's attention abilities and furthered their reading ability. Therefore, in the future, in line with establishing the importance of visual-spatial attention in Chinese children's reading development, intervention studies should also be conducted to determine the relation between these two abilities and to facilitate practical training programs that improve Chinese children's reading performance.

CONCLUSIONS

Although the main body of research in reading development still focuses on the importance of metalinguistic awareness and/or the skills directly related to the processing of language-related information, visual-spatial attention, as a relatively more fundamental cognitive ability, is drawing increased attention. There is a fair amount of empirical evidence supporting the importance of visual-spatial attention in predicting reading performance or in identifying reading difficulties. Studies have covered all of the main aspects of visual-spatial attention, including orienting, focusing, and attention span, and thus have provided a relatively comprehensive picture of the association between visual-spatial attention and reading performance. Compared to the phonological deficit hypothesis, the visual-spatial attention deficit hypothesis can explain not only phonological dyslexia, but also surface dyslexia and double-deficit dyslexia, if the different aspects of visual-spatial attention are considered.

There is still significant room for further research into the role of visual-spatial attention in reading development. For instance, some experimental paradigms should be modified to better control confounding factors (Ziegler et al., 2010). The biological mechanism of visual-spatial attention is still controversial (Vidyasagar & Pammer, 2010). The different aspects of visual-spatial attention tend to be discussed separately, and there is a lack of an integrated consideration of all aspects. Finally, only the direct effect of visual-spatial attention on reading has been investigated in almost all of the available studies. It is possible that the role of visual-spatial attention is mediated or moderated by other factors. For instance, visual perception and orthographic processing skills might be two mediators, because both are associated with visual-spatial attention and both affect reading. Vocabulary and visual memory might also be moderators because both can facilitate top-down processing and compensate for any problems caused by a visual-spatial attention deficit. All of these points deserve further research.

The Chinese written language is considered a logographic system, the processing of which should be closely related to visual-spatial attention. However, thus far, few studies have addressed this issue directly. Research in this direction would not only enrich our understanding of reading development and its related difficulties, but also provide us with more opportunities to improve the reading performance of Chinese children.

REFERENCES

Ans, B., Carbonnel, S., & Valdois, S. (1998). A connectionist multi-trace memory memory model of polysyllabic word reading. *Psychological Review, 105*, 678–723.

Besner, D., Risko, E. F., & Sklair N. (2005). Spatial attention as a necessary preliminary to early processes in reading. *Canadian Journal of Experimental Psychology, 59*, 99–108.

Blais, C., Fiset, D., Arguin, M., Jolicoeur, P., Bub, D., & Gosselin, F. (2009). Reading between eye saccades. *Plos One 4*, e6448.

Bosse, M.-L. & Valdois, S. (2009). Influence of the visual attention span on child reading performance: a cross-sectional study. *Journal of Research in Reading, 32*, 230–253.

Bosse, M.-L., Tainturier, M. J., & Valdois, S. (2007). Developmental dyslexia: The visual attention span deficit hypothesis. *Cognition, 104*, 198–230.

Brown, T. L., Gore, C. L. & Carr, T. H. (2002). Spatial attention and word recognition in Stroop color naming: Is word-recognition automatic? *Journal of Experimental Psychology: General, 131*, 220–240.

Chen, H.-C. & Tang, C. K. (1998). The effective visual field in reading Chinese. *Reading and Writing, 10*, 245–254.

Chen, H.-C., Song, H., Lau, W. Y., Wong, K. F. E., & Tang, S. L. (2003). Developmental characteristics of eye movements in reading Chinese. In C. McBride-Chang & H-C. Chen (Eds.), *Reading development in Chinese children* (pp. 157–170). London: Praeger Publisher.

Coltheart, M., Rastle, K., Perry, C., Langdon, R., & Ziegler, J. (2001). DRC: A dual route cascaded model of visual word recognition and reading aloud. *Psychological review, 108*, 204–256.

Eriksen, C. W., & Yeh, Y. (1985). Allocation of attention in the visual field. *Journal of Experimental Psychology: Human Perception and Performance, 5*, 583–595.

Facoetti, A., Lorusso, M. L., Cattaneo, C., Galli, R., & Molteni, M. (2005). Effects of visual and auditory attentional capture are both sluggish in children with developmental dyslexia. *Acta Neurobiologiae Experimentalis, 65*, 61–72.

Facoetti, A., Lorusso, M. L., Paganoni, P., Umilta, C., & Mascetti, G. G. (2003). The role of visuospatial attention in developmental dyslexia: Evidence from a rehabilitation study. *Cognitive Brain Research, 15*, 154–164.

Facoetti, A., Paganoni, P., Turatto, M., Marzola, V., & Mascetti, G. G. (2000). Visual-spatial attention in developmental dyslexia. *Dyslexia, 36,* 109–123.

Facoetti, A., Trussardi, A. N., Ruffino, M., Lorusso, M. L., Cattaneo, C., Galli, R., Molteni, M., & Zorzi, M. (2010). Multisensory spatial attention deficits are predictive of phonological decoding skills in developmental dyslexia. *Journal of Cognitive Neuroscience, 22,* 1011–1025.

Facoetti, A., Zorzi, M., Cestnick, L., Lorusso, M.L., Moltenia, M., Paganoni, P., Umilta, C., & Mascetti, G. G. (2006). The relationship between visuospatial attention and nonword reading in developmental dyslexia. *Cognitive Neuropsychology, 23,* 841–855.

Franceschini, S., Gori, S., Ruffino, M., Pedrolli, K., & Facoetti, A. (2012). A causal link between visual spatial attention and reading acquisition. *Current Biology, 22,* 1–6.

Franceschini, S., Gori, S., Ruffino, M., Viola, S., Motleni, M., & Facoetti, A. (2013). Action video games make dyslexic children read better. *Current Biology, 23,* 1–5.

Geiger, G., Cattaneo, C., Galli, R., Pozzoli, U., Lorusso, M. L., Facoetti, A., & Molteni, M. (2008). Vide and diffuse perceptual modes characterize dyslexics in vision and audition. Perception, 37, 1745–1764.

Grainger, J., Tydgat, I., & Isselé, J. (2010). Crowding affects letters and symbols differently. *Journal of Experimental Psychology: Human Perception and Performance, 36,* 673–688.

Green, D. W., Liow, S. J. R., Tng, S. K., & Zielinski, S. (1996). Are visual search procedures adapted to the nature of the script? *British Journal of Psychology, 87,* 311–326.

Hari, R., & Renvall, H. (2001). Impaired processing of rapid stimulus sequences in dyslexia. *Trends in Cognitive Science, 5,* 525–532.

Hari, R., Valta, M., & Uutela, K. (1999). Prolonged attentional dwell time in dyslexic adults. *Neuroscience Letter, 271,* 202–204.

Ho, C. S.-H., Chan, D. W.-O., Tsang, S.-M., & Lee, S.-H. (2002). The cognitive profile and multiple-deficit hypothesis in Chinese developmental dyslexia. *Developmental Psychology, 38,* 543–553.

Lallier, M., Tainturier, M. J., Dering, B., Donnadieu, S., Valdois, S., & Thierry, G. (2010). Behavioral and ERP evidence for amodal sluggish attentional shifting in developmental dyslexia. *Neuropsychologia, 48,* 4125–4135.

Li, X. S., Rayner, K., & Cave, K. (2009). On the segmentation of Chinese words during reading. *Cognitive Psychology, 58,* 525–552.

Lobier, M., Zoubrinetzky, R., & Valdois, S. (2012). The visual attention span deficit in dyslexia is visual and not verbal. *Cortex, 48,* 6, 768–773.

Luck, S. J., & Ford, M. A. (1998). On the role of selective attention in visual perception. *PNAS, 95,* 825–830.

Luo, Y., Chen, X., Deacon, H., Zhang, J., & Yin, L. (2013). The role of visual processing in learning to read Chinese characters. *Scientific Studies of Reading, 17,* 22–40.

Mason, M., & Katz, L. (1976). Visual processing of nonlinguistic strings: Redundancy effects and reading ability. *Journal of Experimental Psychology, 105,* 338–348.

Meng, X., Cheng-Lai, A., Zeng, B., Stein, J. F., & Zhou, X. (2011). Dynamic visual perception and reading development in Chinese school children. *Annals of Dyslexia, 61,* 161–176.

McBride-Chang, C., Zhou, Y., Cho, J.-R., Aram, D., Levin, I., & Tolchinsky, L. (2011). Visual spatial skill: A consequence of learning to read? *Journal of Experimental Child Psychology, 109,* 256–262.

McBride-Chang, C., Chow, B. W.-Y., Zhong, Y.-P., Burgess, S., & Hayward, W. (2005). Chinese character acquisition and visual skills in two Chinese scripts. *Reading and Writing: An Interdisciplinary Journal, 18,* 99–128.

Pammer, K., Lavis, R., Hansen, P., & Cornelissen, P. L. (2004). Symbol-string sensitivity and children's reading. *Brain and Language, 89,* 601-610.

Pelli, D. G., Farell, B., & Moore, B. (2003). The remarkable inefficiency of word recognition. *Nature, 423,* 752–756.

Plaut, D. C., McClelland, J. L., Seidenberg, M. S., & Patterson, K. (1996). Understanding normal and impaired word reading: Computational principles in quasi-regular domains. *Psychological Review, 103,* 56–115.

Plaza, M., & Cohen, H. (2007). The contribution of phonological awareness and visual attention in early reading and spelling. *Dyslexia, 13,* 67–76.

Posner, M. I., Walker, J. A., Friedrich, F. J., & Rafal, R. D. (1984). Effects of parietal injury on covert orienting of attention. *Journal of Neuroscience, 4,* 1863–1874.

Ruffino, M., Trussardi, A. N., Gori, S., Finzi, A., Giovagnoli, S., Menghini, D., Benassi, M., Bolzani, R., Vicari, S., & Facoetti, A., (2010). Attentional engagement deficits in dyslexic children. *Neuropsychologia, 48,* 3793–3801.

Siok, W. T., Spinks, J. A., Jin, Z., & Tan, L. H. (2009). Developmental dyslexia is characterized by the co-existence of visuospatial and phonological disorders in Chinese children. *Current Biology, 19,* R890–R892.

Sperling, A. J., Lu, Z.-L., Manis, F. R., & Seidenberg, M. S. (2005). Deficits in perceptual noise exclusion in developmental dyslexia. *Nature Neuroscience, 8,* 862–863.

Sperling, A. J., Lu, Z.-L., Manis, F. R., & Seidenberg, M. S. (2006). Motion-perception deficits and reading impairment: It's the noise, not the motion. *Psychological Science, 17,* 1047–1053.

Sperling, A., Lu, Z., Manis, F., & Seidenberg, M. (2003). Selective magnocellular deficits in dyslexia: A "phantom contour" study. *Neuropsychologia, 41,* 1422–1429.

Spinelli, D., De Luca, M., Judica, A., & Zoccolotti, P. (2002). Length effect in word naming in reading: Role of reading experience and reading deficit in Italian readers. *Developmental Neuropsychology, 27,* 217–235.

Stein, J. (2003). Visual motion sensitivity and reading. *Neuropsychologia, 41,* 1785–1793.

Stolz, J. A., & McCann, R. S. (2000). Visual word recognition: Re-attending to the role of spatial attention. *Journal of Experimental Psychology: Human Perception and Performance, 26,* 1320–1331.

Tan, L. H., Spinks, J. A., Eden, G. F., Perfetti, C. A., & Siok, W. T. (2005). Reading depends on writing, in Chinese. *PNAS, 102,* 8781–8785.

Tang, C. K., Au Yeung, L. H., & Chen, H.-C. (1997). The effective visual field in the reading of Chinese text. In H.-C. Chen (Ed.), *The cognitive processing of*

Chinese and related Asian languages (pp. 267–286). Hong Kong: Chinese University Press.

Trick, L. M., & Enns, J. T. (1998). Lifespan changes in attention: The visual search task. *Cognitive Development, 13,* 369–386.

Tydgat, I., & Grainger, J. (2009). Serial position effects in the identification of letters, digits, and symbols. *Journal of Experimental Psychology: Human Perception and Performance, 35,* 480–498.

Valdois, S., Bosse, M.-L., & Tainturier, M.-J. (2004). The cognitive deficits responsible for developmental dyslexia: Review of evidence for a selective visual attentional disorder. *Dyslexia, 10,* 339–363.

Valdois, S., Bosse, M.-L., Ans, B., Carbonnel, S., Zorman, M., David, D., & Pellat, J. (2003). Phonolgical and visual processing deficits can dissociate in developmental dyslexia: Evidence from two case studies. *Reading and Writing: An Interdisciplinary Journal, 16,* 541–572.

Vecera, S. P., & Rizzo, M. (2003). Spatial attention: Normal processes and their breakdown. *Neurologic Clinics of North America, 21,* 575–607.

Vellutino, F. R., Fletcher, J. M., Snowling, M. J., & Scanlon, D. M. (2004). Specific reading disability (dyslexia): What have we learned in the past four decades? *Journal of Child Psychology and Psychiatry, 45,* 2–40.

Vidyasagar, T. R. (1999). A neuronal model of attentional spotlight: Parietal guiding the temporal. *Brain Research Review, 30,* 66–76.

Vidyasagar, T. R., & Pammer, K. (1999). Impaired visual search in dyslexia relates to the role of the magnocellular pathway in attention. *Neuroreport, 10,* 1283–1287.

Vidyasagar, T. R., & Pammer, K. (2010). Dyslexia: a deficit in visuo-spatial attention, not in phonological processing. *Trends in Cognitive Sciences, 14,* 57–63.

Wang, J.-J., Bi, H.-Y., Gao, L.-Q., & Wydell, T. N. (2010). The visual magnocellular pathway in Chinese-speaking children with developmental dyslexia. *Neuropsychologia, 48,* 3627–3633.

Ziegler, J. C., & Goswami, U. C. (2005). Reading acquisition, developmental dyslexia and skilled reading across languages: A psycholinguistic grain size theory. *Psychological Bulletin, 131,* 3–29.

Ziegler, J. C., Pech-Georgel, C., Dufau, S., & Grainger, J. (2010). Rapid processing of letters, digits and symbols: what purely visual-attentional deficit in developmental dyslexia? *Developmental Science, 13,* F8–F14.

CHAPTER 9

PINYIN KNOWLEDGE AS A POTENTIALLY IMPORTANT MARKER OF EARLY LITERACY

Ying Wang, Silvia Siu-Yin Lam, Jianhong Mo, and Catherine McBride-Chang

In this chapter, we provide a selective review of the research on Pinyin knowledge and its relation to Chinese reading development. Our primary focus is elaborating the role of the Pinyin system in the Chinese reading activity of both typically developing and dyslexic children. This unique teaching and learning system provides a new perspective for understanding both Chinese reading development and disability.

We begin by introducing the characteristics of Chinese orthography, Pinyin learning and measurement, to advance a discussion of how Pinyin knowledge is related to Chinese reading skill and phonological awareness. We also discuss how phonological awareness may transfer from Pinyin to English reading as a second language. In addition, we pay special attention to the relationship between Pinyin learning and Chinese dyslexia.

Reading is a process of mapping oral language to written language. Phonological awareness has been found to be a strong predictor of young children's reading development and impairment, not only in alphabetic languages (Bradley & Bryant, 1983; Byrne & Fielding-Barnsley, 1989;

Understanding Developmental Disorders of Auditory Processing, Language and Literacy Across Languages: International Perspectives, pp. 189–206

Shankweiler, 1999; Treiman & Baron, 1983) but also in Chinese (Law, Weekes, & Wong, 2009; Share, 1995, Siok & Fletcher, 2001). In Chinese, each character corresponds to a single syllable. Moreover, there are no consonant clusters in Chinese. Thus, Chinese is relatively simple in relation to segmental phonological knowledge. Pinyin knowledge, which relies substantially on phonological coding skills, may be an ideal measure for tapping into segmental phonological awareness. Previous studies have found that Pinyin accounts for unique variances in Chinese word and character reading (Lin et al., 2010; Pan et al., 2011).

As a phonological coding system that makes use of 25 Roman letters to indicate Chinese character pronunciations, Pinyin has the potential to directly affect how the connection between Chinese spoken language and written language is formed. Pinyin consists of onsets, rimes, and lexical tones and is formally taught in mainland China in the first grade. For the purposes of our discussion, we collectively define Pinyin knowledge as invented Pinyin spelling, Pinyin letter-name knowledge, and tone representation. Pinyin knowledge has a strong relationship with Chinese word reading in initial literacy learning. For example, Lin et al. (2010) demonstrated how an invented Pinyin spelling task for kindergarten children subsequently predicted the word reading of mainland Chinese children. Wang and McBride-Chang (2012) also demonstrated kindergartners' invented Pinyin as a unique correlate of word reading in mainland Chinese children. Pinyin skills are influenced by various letter difficulties. Pan et al. (2011) not only found invented Pinyin spelling to be a sensitive predictor of a child's subsequent character recognition and dictation but also found that its predictive longitudinal effect appeared to increase over time.

What is the nature of Pinyin development? Siok and Fletcher (2001) demonstrated that Pinyin knowledge and Chinese reading share a reciprocal association from grades 2 to 5. That is, children are able to read unfamiliar Chinese characters with the aid of Pinyin, and reading success in lower grades can subsequently predict Pinyin knowledge. For children with reading disabilities, Yin and Weekes (2003) demonstrated the striking finding that Pinyin reading difficulties (e.g., confusing "b" with "p" and "n" with "l") were more common than the difficulties associated with learning to read characters in Beijing. This suggests that Pinyin reading may be a possible indicator of the phenotype for dyslexia within mainland China. McBride-Chang et al. (2011) demonstrated that mothers who highlight the phonological aspects of Pinyin tend to have children who are better at reading Pinyin. Thus, while there are likely some aspects of Pinyin learning that are innate and some that are learned via direct instruction, both are related to phonological processing in Chinese reading as they are in alphabetic languages. We highlight the unique role of Pinyin learning in mainland Chinese children's reading skills and consider whether similar findings would be found when examining Zhu-Yin-Fu-Hao in Taiwan. Such systems are important for understanding both Chinese reading development and disability.

THE MAIN CHARACTERISTICS OF CHINESE ORTHOGRAPHY

Chinese consists of not only a phonological system but also a character system. The Chinese phonological system is represented by a set of phonetic symbols called Hanyu Pinyin, which consists of a number of Roman alphabet letters similar to English and four lexical tones, with a fifth tone (i.e., the slight tone) used to differentiate the meaning denoted by a given syllable (Lin et al., 2010). In addition, the Chinese language includes a character system, and over 80% of Chinese characters are ideophonetic compounds that contain a phonological or phonetic component and a semantic radical (Kang, 1993; Zhu, 1987). The phonetic component indicates the pronunciation, and the semantic component indicates the meaning. For example, the character "清" has two radicals: the right part, which is a phonetic "青"(pronounced "*qīng*"), which signifies the sound of the character; and the left part, that is, the semantic component " 氵 " (water), which represents the meaning of the character (i.e., "clear").

Thus, unlike alphabetic languages such as English, French, and German, in which the sound is encoded in the letters, only one part of each character (the phonetic component) specifies the Chinese pronunciation (Taylor, 1995; Wu, Li, & Anderson, 1999). Most phonetic components are themselves characters with unambiguous pronunciations. For example, "木" is pronounced "*mù*" and "青" is pronounced "*qīng*." Regular compound characters are pronounced as their phonetic components, and there are irregular compound characters whose pronunciations or tones differ from the phonetic components. For example, whereas "沐" is pronounced identically to the phonetic component "木" (*mù*), "晴" is pronounced similarly to "*qíng*" (except for the tone difference) as the phonetic component "青" ("*qīng*"). This structure can make the derivation of phonological information from a given Chinese character relatively difficult if one compares the process to how phonological information is derived within words in alphabetic systems. For example, if the phonetic components themselves are characters, children must learn the pronunciation of phonetic components before they can use them as sound cues in compound characters. In addition, because phonetics do not always represent the names of compound characters phonetically but only some aspects of the holistic syllable pronunciations, children would not be able to accurately analyze the syllables if they used only the phonetic components as cues to read complex characters. For example, when faced with a new word (e.g., "sunny" or "晴"), English-speaking children pronounce or spell the word using the word's phonetic cues (e.g., "s" makes the "/s/" sound). However, Chinese children often fail to derive any explicit information within the opaque relationship between a graphic symbol and sound. For example, the compound "晴" ("*qíng*")is not pronounced identically to the phonetic component "青" ("*qīng*"). Under these circumstances, the phonological coding system known as Hanyu Pinyincan helps children learn the pronunciations of Chinese characters.

Hanyu Pinyin is a Romanized phonological transcription of Chinese characters. First introduced to the People's Republic of China following the writing reforms in 1958, it is formally used as an auxiliary alphabet in mainland China to teach first-grade children the Mandarin pronunciations of characters, with the target characters consistently presented below their Hanyu Pinyin representations. Children from Taiwan learn another alphabetic script known as Zhu-Yin-Fu-Hao before they are taught to read characters. Whenever a new character appears in Taiwan primary school textbooks, it is consistently accompanied by its Zhu-Yin-Fu-Hao representation. The teachings of Hanyu Pinyin and Zhu-Yin-Fu-Hao aim to help children achieve Chinese script recognition rather than phonological script knowledge itself. Pinyin can gradually be used as an aid for children to read new words, spell and pronounce syllables, refer to a dictionary to look up new words or characters, and read simple text during the early years of primary school (Sheridan, 1981).

Hanyu Pinyin (literally meaning "spell sound") comprises most of the 25 Roman alphabet letters used in English (there is no "v," but an additional "ü" in the Pinyin system). It also features five lexical tones, including high level, rising, falling-rising, falling, and slight tones, which are used to represent the pitch of the speech and differentiate the meaning of a given syllable. The five tones are, respectively, represented by the diacritics of macron (¯), acute accent (´), hacek (ˇ), grave accent (`), and no accent mark. The Pinyin system is commonly introduced beginning with the names of the 21 onsets, followed by 37 rimes (vowels and nasal finals) (Institute of Linguistics, 2004). The individual letter names are the same as the corresponding individual letter sounds. However, more than 30 onsets or rimes consist of two to four letters representing a single sound. For example, as in English, "*s*" and "*h*" can not only be used individually but also combined to form "*sh*" to represent a unique sound. Each of the combinations of "*ing*," "*ong*," and "*iang*" similarly represent unique phonological rimes. Thus, learning the names of the 25 letters is not enough; phoneme segmentation and combinations are also necessary for syllable reading and spelling. When children begin to learn characters, the Pinyin pronunciations are provided atop the characters in the reading text. By the end of the second year's study, Pinyin appears only atop new characters and no longer, appears with previously learned characters.

Some examples of simple characters and their Pinyin and Zhu-Yin-Fu-Hao transcriptions are provided as follows:

Pinyin	rì	yuè	shuǐ	huǒ
Character	日 (sun)	月 (moon)	水(water)	火 (fire)
Zhu-Yin-Fu-Hao	ㄖˋ	ㄩㄝˋ	ㄕㄨㄟˇ	ㄏㄨㄛˇ

Zhu-Yin-Fu-Hao (literally meaning "symbols of phonetic pronunciation") is a phonological coding script similar to Hanyu Pinyin in which a phoneme is represented by a unique character. Although it is learned during the first few weeks of first grade, children continue to use Zhu-Yin-Fu-Hao throughout their primary school years. In Zhu-Yin-Fu-Hao, the level of representation is almost always the phoneme; all of the initial consonants, simple vowels, and diphthongs are represented by their own unique characters. The only exception is a vowel followed by a nasal consonant, which is represented by one rather than two symbols. Four of the 37 Zhu-Yin-Fu-Hao symbols meet this criterion and can therefore be said to represent a rime segment rather than a phoneme. Zhu-Yin-Fu-Hao consists of 21 onsets (e.g., "ㄅ", "ㄆ", and "ㄇ") and 16 rimes (e.g., "ㄚ", "ㄛ", and "ㄜ").

Although there seems to be no direct relationship between Chinese characters and their Pinyin representations based on the appearances of alphabetic letters and ideographic characters, the regular and logical letter-sound correspondences in the Pinyin system can effectively facilitate a child's early learning of Chinese (Anderson & Li, 2006; Chung, 2002; Mingyuan, Zhu, & Ji, 1983). Children are trained extensively and explicitly to combine these onsets and rimes to form meaningful syllables. For example, they learn how to combine "*sh*" and "*a*," "*sh*" and "*an*," and "*sh*" and "*ang*" to form the syllables "*sha*," "*shan*," and "*shang*" in different tones. They are also told that syllables in different tones have different meanings. For example, when the syllable "/ma/" has a high-level tone, it means mother ("*mā*" 媽). When it has a dipping tone, it means horse ("*mǎ*" 馬). Because the letters in Hanyu Pinyin correspond to each independent phoneme, the names of characters can be learned as strings of phonemes under this approach.

Through Pinyin learning, children become aware of the onsets and rimes in Chinese syllables. Children also become more capable of pronouncing syllables written in Pinyin and reading unfamiliar characters with the aid of accompanying Pinyin transcriptions. In this way, the use of Pinyin as pronounceable alphabetic letters initially leads children to map their own visual forms (e.g., "*mā*" rather than only the graphic form "妈") to phonological entries in the spoken mental lexicon. This serves as a bridge in the earliest phases of learning. That is, with the aid of Pinyin, Chinese children find phonetic cues in the written forms when reading a word. Moreover, there may be a strong correlation between Pinyin knowledge and reading ability in the early grades. To determine the role of Pinyin in Chinese literacy acquisition, it is important to investigate the reading acquisition of mainland Chinese children.

MEASUREMENTS OF PINYIN KNOWLEDGE

Several tasks have been used in past research to measure children's Hanyu Pinyin knowledge (Lin et al., 2010; Pan et al., 2011; Wang & McBride, 2012). Pinyin letter-name knowledge and invented Pinyin spelling are two main measures that have been incorporated to test young children's Hanyu Pinyin knowledge in mainland China. In some versions of the Pinyin letter-name knowledge tasks, children are asked to name several (e.g., 12) randomly arranged Pinyin letters of the alphabet. For example, children are asked to name the letter "*k*," which is the same as the letter sound. In an invented Pinyin spelling task, children are encouraged to write out orally presented words in Pinyin, including the letters and tones within the words. All of the letters of the Pinyin alphabet (without lexical tones) are printed at the top of the answer sheet for the children's reference. This task focuses on the sounds of words rather than their meanings.

The scoring of Pinyin spelling in previous works has followed a coding scheme developed for English spelling (Tangel & Blachman, 1992). The adapted scheme has been used in Pinyin spelling codes not only to achieve the linguistic sensitivity emphasized in English but also to achieve sensitivity to lexical tones. As an example of linguistic sensitivity at the phoneme level, using "*z*" to represent "*c*" is closer linguistically according to the Pinyin system than using "*t*" to represent an "*l*" sound. This scoring method focuses on the shared and distant phonological characteristics of the phonemes of the letters. Tones 2 and 3 are identified as close tones; indeed, they are the most easily confused in Mandarin compared with the others (e.g., tones 1 and 2, tones 3 and 4). Using this method, each invented spelling item is scored on a 0–12 point scale, which includes the four dimensions of onset, rime, lexical tone and order. Onset and rime are each scored on a 5-point scale (0–4). No points are awarded when nothing is written, when Chinese characters are written, or when a picture is drawn. One point is given for writing random letters, and two points are awarded for writing a combination of closely related letters and some unrelated letters. Three points are given when only closely related letters (and no spurious letters) are written for onsets/rimes. Finally, four points are awarded for writing the correct letter(s). Lexical tones are scored on a 4-point scale (0–3) with 0, 1, 2, and 3 representing no tone, a random tone, a close tone, and a correct tone, respectively. The order of onset and rime is rated as either incorrect (0 points) or correct (1 point). Lin et al. (2010) developed this scale, which covers onset, rime, and lexical tone. In addition, the presentation order is used to better measure children's Pinyin knowledge and spelling skills. This solid measurement of Pinyin knowledge serves as a foundation for us to investigate children's Pinyin knowledge development and the relationship between Pinyin knowledge and literacy skills.

One previous study (Wang & McBride, 2012) of invented Pinyin spelling errors found that the second most frequent error made by Chinese children was their confusion of fricative consonants (e.g., "*z*" with "*zh*," "*c*" with "*s*"). Thus, to some extent, the invented Hanyu Pinyin spelling task measures phonological sensitivity. Having additional knowledge of smaller units of sound within print, such as the consonant or rime, may be helpful for children to learn Chinese characters. Indeed, awareness of the units of consonant, rime, and lexical tone plays a key role in children's Chinese reading (e.g., Siok & Fletcher, 2001). In perhaps the first study of invented Pinyin spelling in Chinese, Lin et al. (2010) found that each of these units was separately associated with Chinese preschoolers' subsequent reading skills.

THE RELATIONS BETWEEN PINYIN KNOWLEDGE AND CHINESE READING

Several studies have shown that Pinyin knowledge and Chinese reading are positively correlated (Huang & Hanley, 1997; Siok & Fletcher, 2001). Lin et al. (2010) positioned independent invented Pinyin spelling as the strongest longitudinal predictor of Chinese kindergarteners' word reading over one year. This was a stronger correlate of Chinese word reading than other phonological tasks such as syllable deletion, phoneme deletion, or letter knowledge itself. Pan et al. (2011) followed up on these children 5 years later and found that over time, with the Chinese character recognition statistically controlled, the invented Pinyin measure remained a unique predictor of subsequent Chinese reading, underscoring the measure's power for literacy acquisition in Chinese.

What are the specific ways in which Pinyin may facilitate Chinese character recognition? The Pinyin and Chinese writing systems are very different overall. First, Pinyin helps learners to derive pronunciations of Chinese characters, especially unfamiliar characters. Mapping sound onto printed forms is important when learning to read in any language. Due to the opaque orthographic nature of Chinese characters, it is difficult or almost impossible to know the pronunciations of characters merely according to their printed forms. Pinyin allows children who are encountering new characters to derive their sounds and then map the phonological representations onto the visual forms. The phonological system assists children in memorizing characters and in stabilizing phonological representations. Chinese has a complex logographic writing system that entails a great deal of visual information. Merely memorizing the visual forms when learning Chinese is daunting, but in combination with Pinyin, learners may use multiple cues to retrieve characters and store them in their memories.

Previous studies of adult learners have provided evidence in support of this idea. For example, Guan, Liu, Chan, Ye, and Perfetti (2011) tested the strategies of handwriting and Pinyin typing in learning to read Chinese. Their study demonstrated that Pinyin could help stabilize pronunciation. The adult learners who trained with Pinyin were better at pronunciation than those who trained with handwriting. Huang and Hanley (1997) further demonstrated that learning Zhu-Yin-Fu-Hao, which is similar to the Pinyin system and is used in Taiwan, helped adolescents in reading unfamiliar words.

Second, learning Pinyin could facilitate mapping between the spoken language and printed form. By the time they learn to read, children have already acquired the spoken forms of characters in their daily lives. When they begin to learn to read, they are also learning to map spoken forms onto the printed forms of characters. In alphabetic languages such as English, one of the main strategies used to promote children's early reading development is to help them resolve the transfer of grapheme-phoneme in its written form. Once a child grasps the rules, he or she is able to map the spoken language onto a written form. For example, consider a child who has already learned to say the word "cat." When the child encounters the written form of "cat," he or she is able to pronounce it if he or she knows the letter sounds connected with the string of written letters. However, this is not the case in Chinese, as characters themselves seldom give very clear clues to pronunciation.

At the same time, the introduction of Pinyin provides a connection between speech and written forms. For example, while most young Chinese children have already learned the pronunciation and meaning of the word "蘋果" ("*píng guǒ*," meaning "apple"), they do not know the written form. When they begin to learn to read with Pinyin printed atop the characters, they can retrieve the phonological representation of the characters and map the meaning onto the written forms, thereby increasing their word reading level. Without the introduction of Pinyin, it is difficult for children to read totally unfamiliar words by themselves. Therefore, Pinyin is a very useful self-learning tool when learning to read Chinese. When young children begin to read, the content mainly focuses on the things they are familiar with in their daily lives. With the help of Pinyin, they could even learn to read characters by themselves. They could also increase their fluency and speed, as they know the pronunciations of the characters that assist them in understanding the written form.

Pinyin learning is especially important for children during the early stages of learning to read Chinese. Their lack of an appropriate written vocabulary presents an obstacle to their independent reading. It is clearly difficult for young children to guess the meaning and pronunciation of a given character by using the orthographic structures of Chinese characters. Indeed, even adult foreign language learners of Chinese have not been exposed to enough written forms to make such generalizations. Children can thus make use of Pinyin to learn to recognize the characters they are familiar with in their spoken but not written forms. To a certain extent, Pinyin knowledge may assist children in overcoming early reading problems.

THE RELATIONSHIP BETWEEN PINYIN KNOWLEDGE AND SUBLEXICAL PHONOLOGY

According to the universal phonological principle suggested by Perfetti, Zhang, and Berent (1992), pronunciation is automatically activated across every writing system for skilled readers when they read printed words. For example, while reading alphabetic languages such as English, knowledge of the pronunciation of phonemes is automatically activated when reading letters. Phonological awareness and reading ability are strongly connected across alphabetic languages (e.g., Chiappe, Glaeser, & Ferko, 2007; Hulme, Snowling, Caravolas, & Carroll, 2005). Phonological awareness training can help children who experience problems when learning to read English. By improving their phonological sensitivity, children become better at spelling and word reading. Although Chinese does not involve phonemic processing because each character maps onto a syllable, Chinese characters are strongly connected with phonology in reading compared with alphabetic languages. The direct relationship between phonology and alphabetic languages is understandable in the case of English, as its printed forms are closely connected with sounds. However, how Pinyin is related to phonological awareness, and how this association affects Chinese acquisition remain in question.

Although the relationship between phonological awareness and reading in Chinese is not as obvious, as in English, an increasing number of studies have illustrated that phonological awareness is important for Chinese reading (e.g., Ho & Bryant, 1997; Tong et al., 2011). As Pinyin writing follows letter-phoneme or letter-cluster-rime conversion rules, processing

Pinyin entails both visual-orthographic and phonological components. Several studies have demonstrated that Pinyin knowledge and phonological awareness are strongly correlated. However, both syllabic and onset-rime structures, which are often included in Chinese phonological awareness tasks given how crucial these units are to Chinese speech, have been found to correlate with Chinese reading success. Phonological sensitivity coherently matches with the skills required in Pinyin knowledge.

To master the Pinyin system, one must acquire onsets, rimes, and tone representations and be able to code letters and segments and combine them into syllables. With this kind of phonology training, one may increase his or her phonological sensitivity by learning Pinyin. For example, Bertelson, Chen, and de Gelder (1997) found Hanyu Pinyin learning to significantly improve children's phonemic analysis. Ren, Xu, and Zhang (2006) conducted an intervention study of preschool children and examined the effects of learning Pinyin on phonological awareness. After a year of training, the children who trained with Pinyin were found to have enhanced their onset-rime awareness of Chinese and English. In their longitudinal study, Siok and Fletcher (2001) showed rime alliteration to be a strong predictor of Chinese reading development. Through learning Pinyin, children were able to segment a syllable into onsets and rimes and in turn combine these sounds into syllables. The children gradually become more sensitive to the phonological structure of the Chinese language via Pinyin. Huang and Hanley (1997) also trained 1st-grade students with Zhu-Yin-Fu-Hao in Taiwan, and their 10-week intervention directly increased the children's phonological awareness. Huang and Hanley found that Taiwanese children who learned Zhu-Yin-Fu-Hao performed better than Hong Kong children on the Chinese phoneme deletion test. Such studies collectively suggest that children's performances on phoneme deletion tests rely on their experience of learning an alphabetic (or other type of phonological coding) script. As suggested by Lin et al. (2010), Pinyin theoretically entails skills related to phonological sensitivity and to the integration of sound units. Pinyin may also be one type of task that taps into underlying phonological representations. Therefore, as suggested by Lin et al. (2010), Pinyin may be the clearest representation of phonological awareness in Chinese children. This suggestion bears consideration in future research.

With increasing phonological sensitivity, children may be better at learning characters that have the same components and similar pronunciations such as homophones (Ho & Bryant, 1997). For example, two characters, including "馬" ("*mǎ*," meaning "horse") and "碼"("*mǎ*," meaning "size") share the same sound but have different meanings. Children who have strong phonological representations may be better at learning to read these characters. Moreover, as mentioned previously, Chinese characters somewhat consistently contain phonetic radicals that often give clues to their pronunciations. Children with strong phonological sensitivities may also be adept at mastering this phonetic information. Hence, Pinyin knowledge and phonological sensitivity reciprocally facilitate word reading. Learning Pinyin is also clearly useful for second-language learners who are learning Chinese (Chung, 2003; Wang, Perfetti, & Liu, 2005).

The acquisition of lexical tones is also particularly important in reading Chinese because characters that share the same syllable but different tones can have completely different meanings. For example, whereas "花" ("*huā*") means "flower" when pronounced with the macron tone, and "滑" ("*huá*") means "slippery" when pronounced with the acute tone. Guan et al. (2011) found students trained with Pinyin to be better at tone accuracy. Liu et al. (in press) also demonstrated that knowledge of pitch contours via Pinyin practice could promote tone learning. It is likely that Pinyin further stabilizes the tone representations of characters and not only facilitates phonological representation but also distinguishes character meanings so that Chinese learners do not confuse characters that share the same syllable but different tones. In addition, Siok and Fletcher's (2001) study demonstrated that Hanyu Pinyin knowledge and Chinese reading have a reciprocal relationship and that this relationship may promote further phonological awareness. Hanyu Pinyin knowledge enables children to segment and process phonological segments and lexical tones. At the same time, the better children are at manipulating onsets, rimes, and lexical tones, the faster they are able to read Hanyu Pinyin and Chinese characters. In this way, both Hanyu Pinyin knowledge and Chinese reading enhance a child's phonological awareness. To some extent, learning Hanyu Pinyin promotes a child's phonological awareness as he or she becomes more sensitive to onset, rime, and lexical tone information when pronouncing Chinese characters. Thus, Hanyu Pinyin knowledge and phonological awareness may have a reciprocal relationship.

PHONOLOGICAL AWARENESS TRANSFER FROM PINYIN TO ENGLISH LEARNING

Many studies have demonstrated that because the skills acquired from one language may be transferred to other languages, children could benefit from their first language when learning a second language (Mumtaz & Humphreys, 2002; Verhoeven, 1994). For example, phonological awareness may be transferred from a first language to a second language. Chong (2005) further extended the transfer concept by examining transfers between Pinyin and English. Chong investigated a group of second-grade Hong Kong Chinese children who had received Pinyin training. In Hong Kong, Pinyin training is not typically administered in schools because

Chinese is often taught with a focus on rote memory. The Hong Kong Chinese children who had been specially trained in Pinyin were then tested to determine whether their skills in Pinyin had any association with their skills in English reading and spelling. The results showed that the Pinyin training not only facilitated their phonological awareness in general but also predicted their English pseudoword reading and nonword spelling. As suggested by Chong, orthographic Pinyin enhances a child's print-sound mapping skills, which are important for reading. The mapping of orthography onto phonology or vice versa is a key element in reading. Pinyin shares similar features with alphabetic systems such as English, and learning orthographic Pinyin (i.e., letter knowledge) could assist children in learning English reading and spelling. More importantly, to master Pinyin, children must learn to decompose phonological units, a skill quite similar to those required in English learning.

Further studies could investigate the effect of Pinyin on second-language learning. However, several points must be kept in mind when discussing the potential effects of Pinyin on reading. First, although Guan et al. (2011) found Pinyin to strengthen the linkage between phonology and character reading, Pinyin knowledge did not have a significant effect on meaning-character linkages. Such results suggested that strengthening only a phonological representation is not enough to acquire meaning. This is especially true for second-language learners, who often learn the spoken and written forms at the same time. Although they are able to acquire the sounds of the second language, these sounds do not connect directly with the meaning. Their situation is very different from that of native speakers, whose advanced knowledge of the meanings of spoken forms enables them to learn pronunciations and thereby recognize both the characters and meanings. Therefore, as suggested by Guan and colleagues, adding a meaning component to Pinyin such as an English translation may help establish the link between phonology and meaning, thereby facilitating reading as a whole.

To summarize, Pinyin knowledge facilitates a child's Chinese literacy learning in two ways. First, Pinyin represents the exact sounds of characters and can function as a self-teaching tool for children and second-language learners to recognize and read new Chinese characters. Second, Pinyin knowledge can improve a child's early phoneme awareness, syllable awareness, and tone awareness and thereby facilitate the child's early character recognition.

However, although phonological awareness is positively correlated with reading in Chinese, its causal linkage pattern is sometimes unclear. For example, Huang and Hanley (1997) investigated whether phonological awareness had any predictive power for Chinese reading among first-grade children in Taiwan. They found that the relationship between phonological awareness and reading in Chinese decreased as the children aged. What does this mean for Pinyin? It may suggest that while Pinyin is particularly useful in the initial stage of Chinese acquisition, as it becomes more automatized, additional cognitive skills (e.g., morphological awareness, vocabulary knowledge) are required to become a competent reader. Nonetheless, given the complexity of Chinese orthography, Pinyin seems to provide children with strategies in learning to read. Importantly, Pinyin is reliable and offers children a bridge to decode logographic characters with less confusion.

RELATIONSHIP BETWEEN PINYIN KNOWLEDGE AND CHINESE DYSLEXIA

Dyslexia is a specific learning disorder that occurs across orthographies. It is characterized by difficulties experienced in accurate and fluent word reading, reading comprehension, and spelling (Lyon, Shaywitz, & Shaywitz, 2003). These reading and writing impairments are shaped by the properties of the language environment involved (e.g., language characteristics, prevalent teaching methods). Whereas mainland Chinese children learn to read and write simplified Chinese characters, children from Hong Kong and Taiwan learn to read and write traditional Chinese characters. Moreover, Pinyin and Zhu-Yin-Fu-Hao are respectively used as aids to teach Chinese characters in mainland China and Taiwan. Thus, slightly different manifestations of dyslexia may be observed in different Chinese-speaking societies. One critical issue is that types of script may determine the phenotypes of dyslexia in different language environments. From a survey study of elementary school pupils from Beijing, Yin and Weekes (2003) observed that Pinyin reading difficulties (e.g., a tendency to confuse "*b*" with "*d*" and "*p*" with "*q*") are more common than the difficulties associated with learning to read characters, suggesting that the reading and writing difficulties associated with Chinese can vary according to the type of script. They also argued that the dyslexia experienced with Pinyin words is likely to have the same neurobiological origin as the dyslexia experienced with alphabetic systems such as English. According to their study, Chinese children's reading may begin with a visual/logographic phase, during which the children form arbitrary connections between visual cues and meanings in addition to character pronunciations. The second stage is the phonological phase, in which the children establish the connection from print to meaning through phonological representation. Phonological awareness is therefore particularly important during reading development. Finally, given the children's experience, their reading progresses from a phonological to an orthographic stage in which whole characters are automatically processed as a whole unit (Ho, Chan, Lee, Tsang, & Luan, 2004). Dyslexic children may therefore experience decoding difficulties that appear to be caused by phonological processing. This may be particularly clear in children who are learning to read in mainland China and Taiwan, where phonological coding systems (i.e., Pinyin and Zhu-Yin-Fu-Hao, respectively) are used to teach reading.

Yin and Weekes (2003) suggested that a phonological impairment could lead to reading problems with Pinyin words and to dyslexia with Chinese characters. Indeed, Siok and Fletcher (2001) supported the shift from the phonological to the orthographic stage. In a study by Song, Zhang, and Shu (1995), children were asked to distinguish homophones and characters with similar orthographic structures. The third-grade children tended to be less sensitive to homophones because their word reading mainly relied on a phonological pathway. For the fifth-grade children, the processing pattern tended to shift from a phonological to an orthographic-semantic pathway. The orthographic-semantic pathway is dominant in typically developing adults, perhaps because the direct pathway from an orthographic unit to a semantic representation is the most efficient due to the morphographic nature of Chinese characters. Again, as a phonological system, Pinyin plays an important role in facilitating literacy development during a child's early years via an indirect route. However, its importance decreases thereafter because readers tend to shift gradually to the more direct orthographic route.

THE IMPORTANCE OF PINYIN KNOWLEDGE FOR DYSLEXIC CHILDREN

One approach to investigating the unique role of Pinyin in reading could involve conducting comparison studies across Chinese societies (e.g., mainland China versus Hong Kong). Compared with mainland Chinese children, Hong Kong Chinese dyslexic children experience relatively low incidences of phonological deficit (Ho et al., 2004), perhaps because of the absence of a phonological coding system (i.e., Pinyin or Zhu-Yin-Fu-Hao) in Hong Kong's educational practices. In one study, Luan (2005) explored the cognitive profiles of dyslexic children in Beijing and Hong Kong. The most intriguing differences reported between the two communities surfaced in the areas of rapid naming deficits (28% of the Beijing sample versus 52% of the Hong Kong sample) and phonological awareness deficits (28% of the Beijing sample versus 12% of the Hong Kong sample). Cantonese is the dominant spoken language in Hong Kong, and no phonetic symbols are used in Cantonese to label pronunciations. Moreover, Hong Kong children are taught only by the "look and say" method, that is, they learn to read characters holistically by rote. Without the aid of a phonological coding system such as Pinyin or Zhu-Yin-Fu-Hao, they use rapid retrieval to access the names of Chinese characters. This could be a cause of the relatively important role of rapid naming in predicting dyslexia in Hong Kong. In addition, the importance of phonological sensitivity in all of its forms tends to be greater in mainland China than in Hong Kong, again due primarily to the use of Pinyin in the former but not the latter. Thus, weaknesses in Pinyin knowledge, including in letter name/sound sensitivities and awareness of onsets, rimes, and syllables, can be powerful cognitive markers for screening dyslexic children in mainland China.

Another issue of potential importance is that reading and writing difficulties may be dissociated in Chinese, perhaps more than in other orthographies (McBride-Chang & Liu, 2011). It is highly likely that a child with a word-reading problem will also experience difficulty in word writing. However, as computer usage is the international "norm," many Chinese writers type Chinese primarily using a Pinyin input method rather than character representations. In addition, given the visual complexity and the nontransparent phonology of the Chinese writing system, Chinese writing demands a complex coordination of visual-motor abilities. Because using Pinyin to write requires less effort compared with learning to write Chinese characters fluently, it is possible for Chinese children (and even some adults) to be proficient at reading Chinese and much less so at writing it. In fact, due to their widespread application of the Pinyin input method on computers and relatively little handwriting practice, typically developing individuals who rely primarily on phonological skills to retrieve characters may feel uncertain and make more errors during handwriting tasks.

CONCLUSION

The view that Pinyin knowledge plays a key role in enabling both typically developing and dyslexic children to learn to read Chinese characters is supported in two main ways. Pinyin not only directly facilitates Chinese character recognition but also improves learners' phonological sensitivity. Similar results have been found for Zhu-Yin-Fu-Hao. In addition, there are different patterns among dyslexic children with and without Pinyin knowledge in Chinese societies. However, the developmental trajectory of the effects of Pinyin and the causal relationship between Pinyin knowledge and Chinese reading require further clarification.

We anticipate that the mechanism of how Pinyin and Zhu-Yin-Fu-Hao influence Chinese and second-language learning and their relationships with phonological awareness skills will be investigated in future studies among different age groups. In addition, Pinyin and Zhu-Yin-Fu-Hao may serve as unique markers to screen and diagnose dyslexic children in mainland China and Taiwan.

REFERENCES

Anderson, R. C., & Li, W. (2006) *A cross-language perspective on learning to read.* Mahwah, NJ: Lawrence Erlbaum.

Bertelson, P., Chen, H.-C., & de Gelder, B. (1997). Explicit speech analysis and orthographic experience in Chinese readers. In H.-C. Chen (Ed.), *Cognitive processing of Chinese and related Asian languages* (pp. 27–46). Hong Kong: Chinese University Press.

Bradley, L., & Bryant, P. E. (1983). Categorizing sounds and learning to read—A causal connection. *Nature, 301*, 419–421.

Byrne, B., & Fielding-Barnsley, R. (1989). Phonemic awareness and letter knowledge in the child's acquisition of the alphabetic principle. *Journal of Educational Psychology, 81*, 313–321.

Chiappe, P., Glaeser, B., & Ferko, D. (2007). Speech perception, vocabulary and the development of reading skills in English among Korean- and English-speaking children. *Journal of Educational Psychology*, 99, 154–166.

Chong, K. Y. (2005). *The effect of Pinyin learning on the development of phonological awareness and English reading and spelling* (Unpublished master's thesis) Chinese University of Hong Kong.

Chung, K. K. H. (2002). Effective use of Hanyu Pinyin and English translations as extra stimulus prompts on learning of Chinese characters. *Educational Psychology, 22*(2), 150–164.

Chung, K. K. H. (2003). Effects of Pinyin and first language words in learning of Chinese characters as a second language. *Journal of Behavior Education, 12*(3), 207–223.

Guan, C. Q., Liu, Y., Chan, D. H. L., Ye, F., & Perfetti, C.A. (2011). Writing strengthens orthography and alphabetic-coding strengthens phonology in learning to read Chinese. *Journal of Educational Psychology, 103*(3), 509–522.

Ho, C.S.-H., & Bryant, P. (1997). Learning to read Chinese beyond the logographic phase. *Reading Research Quarterly, 32*, 279–289.

Ho, C., Chan, D., Lee, S. H., Tsang, S. M., & Luan, V. H. (2004). Cognitive profiling and preliminary subtyping in Chinese developmental dyslexia. *Cognition, 91*, 43–75.

Huang, H.-S., & Hanley, J. R. (1997). A longitudinal study of phonological awareness, visual skills and Chinese reading acquisition amongst first graders in Taiwan. *International Journal of Behavioral Development, 20*, 249–268.

Hulme, C., Snowling, M., Caravolas, M., & Carroll, J. (2005). Phonological skills are (probably) one cause of success in learning to read: A comment on Castles and Coltheart. *Scientific Studies of Reading, 9*(4), 351–365.

Institute of Linguistics, Chinese Academy of Social Sciences. (2004). *Xinhua dictionary* (10th ed.). Beijing: Commercial.

Kang, J. S. (1993). Analysis of semantics of semantic-phonetic compound characters in modern Chinese. In Y. Chen (Ed.), *Information analysis of usage of characters in modern Chinese* (pp. 68–83). Shanghai, China: Shanghai Education (in Chinese).

Law, S.-P., Weekes, B. S., & Wong, A. M.-Y. (Eds.). (2009). *Language disorders in speakers of Chinese* (pp. 138–157). Bristol, UK: Multilingual Matters.

Lin, D., McBride-Chang, C., Shu, H., Zhang, Y., Li, H., Zhang, J., ... Levin, I. (2010). Small wins big: Analytic Pinyin skills promote Chinese word reading. *Psychological Science, 21*(8), 1117–1122.

Liu, P. D., McBride-Chang, C., Wong, T. T.-Y., Shu, H., & Wong, A. M.-Y. (in press). Morphological measurement matters: Unique associations of homophone awareness and lexical compounding to word reading and vocabulary knowledge in Chinese children. *Applied Psycholinguistics*.

Luan, H. (2005). *The role of morphological awareness among Mandarin-speaking and Cantonese-speaking children.* Hong Kong, China: University of Hong Kong.

Lyon, G. R., Shaywitz, S. E., & Shaywitz, B. A. (2003). A definition of dyslexia. *Annals of Dyslexia, 53*(1), 1–14.

McBride-Chang, C., Lin, D., Liu, P. D., Aram, D., Levin, I., Cho, J.-R., ... Zhong, Y. (2011). The ABCs of Chinese: Maternal mediation of Pinyin for Chinese children's early literacy skills. *Reading and Writing, 25*(1), 283–300.

McBride-Chang, C., & Liu, D. (2011). Fundamentals of Chinese reading development and how they might affect concepts of dyslexia in Chinese. In P. McCardle, B. Miller, J. R. Lee, & O. J. L. Tzeng (Eds.), *Dyslexia across languages: Orthography and the brain-gene-behavior link* (pp. 33–43). Baltimore, MD: Brookes.

Mumtaz, S., & Humphreys, G. W. (2002). The effect of Urdu vocabulary size on the acquisition of single word reading in English. *Educational Psychology, 22*, 165–190.

Pan, J., McBride-Chang, C., Shu, H., Liu, H., Zhang, Y., & Li, H. (2011). What is in the naming? A 5-year longitudinal study of early rapid naming and phonological sensitivity in relation to subsequent reading skills in both native Chinese and English as a second language. *Journal of Educational Psychology, 103*(4), 897–908.

Perfetti, C. A., Zhang, S., & Berent, I. (1992). Reading in English and Chinese: Evidence for a "universal" phonological principle. In R. Frost (Ed.), *Orthography, phonology, morphology, and meaning* (pp. 227–248). Amsterdam, The Netherlands: North-Holland.

Ren, P., Xu, F., & Zhang, R. (2006). Effects of Pinyin learning on development of phonological awareness in kindergarten. *Acta Psychologica Sinica, 38*(1), 41–46.

Shankweiler, D. (1999). Words to meanings. *Scientific Studies of Reading, 3*, 113–127.

Share, D. L. (1995). Phonological recoding and self-teaching: Sine qua non of reading acquisition. *Cognition, 55*, 151–218.

Sheridan, E. M. (1981). Literacy and language reform in the People's Republic of China. *Reading Teacher, 20*, 804–808.

Siok, W. T., & Fletcher, P. (2001). The role of phonological awareness and visual-orthographic skills in Chinese reading. *Developmental Psychology, 37*(6), 886–899.

Song, H., Zhang, H. C., & Shu, H. (1995). The developmental shift of the role of graphic code and phonetic code in Chinese reading. *Acta Psychologica Sinica, 27*(2), 139–144 (in Chinese).

Tangel, D. M., & Blachman, B. A. (1992). Effect of phoneme awareness instruction on kindergarten children's invented spellings. *Journal of Reading Behavior, 24*, 233–258.

Taylor, I. (1995). *Writing and literacy in Chinese, Korean, and Japanese.* Philadelphia, PA: John Benjamins.

Tong, X., McBride-Chang, C., Wong, A. M.-Y., Shu, H., Reistma, P., & Rispens, J. (2011). Longitudinal predictors of very early Chinese literacy acquisition. *Journal of Research in Reading, 34*, 315–332.

Treiman, R. A., & Baron, J. (1983). Phonemic-analysis training helps children benefit from spelling-sound rules. *Memory & Cognition, 11*, 382–389.

Verhoeven, L. T. (1994). Transfer in bilingual development: The linguistic interdependence hypothesis revisited. *Language Learning, 44*, 381–415.

Wang, M., Perfetti, C. A., & Liu, Y. (2005). Chinese-English biliteracy acquisition: Cross-language and writing system transfer. *Cognition, 97*(1), 67–88.

Wang,Y., & McBride-Chang, C. (2012). *Invented Pinyin spelling and Chinese reading in kindergarten*. Poster presented at the Global Conference on Disorders in Auditory Processing, Literacy, Language and Related Sciences, 2012, Hong Kong.

Wu, X., Li, W., & Anderson, R. C. (1999). Reading instruction in China. *Journal of Curriculum Studies, 31*, 571–586.

Yin, W. G., & Weekes, B. S. (2003). Dyslexia in Chinese: Clues from cognitive neuropsychology. *Annals of Dyslexia, 53*, 255–275.

Zhu, Y. P. (1987). *Analysis of cueing functions of the phonetic in modern China.* Unpublished paper, East China Normal University, Shanghai (in Chinese).

CHAPTER 10

AN INTEGRATION OF FINDINGS ON CHINESE DYSLEXIA WITH THE APPLICATION OF JOHN MORTON'S CAUSAL MODELING FRAMEWORK

Simpson W. L. Wong

Dyslexia, a genetically based developmental disorder, has been observed in a variety of cultures. With the publication of a formal assessment tool in 2000 (HKT-SpLD; Ho, Chan, Tsang, & Lee, 2000), Chinese dyslexia can now be diagnosed, and the pace of research on the topic has accelerated, with numerous studies of various scales conducted in the last two decades. As a result, our understanding of Chinese dyslexia has been enhanced, especially in terms of cognitive (e.g., Ho, Chan, Tsang, & Lee, 2002) and neurological (e.g., Siok, Spinks, Jin, & Tan, 2009) deficits and behavioral manifestations (e.g, Chan, Ho, Tsang, Lee, & Chung, 2003). Because many of the research ideas tested in the Chinese dyslexic population are rooted in research on alphabetic languages (mostly English), the findings on Chinese dyslexics are usually compared and contrasted with other

Understanding Developmental Disorders of Auditory Processing, Language and Literacy Across Languages: International Perspectives, pp. 207–227

alphabetic readers. In the dyslexia literature, there are several competing accounts of dyslexia, and new dyslexic hypotheses emerge from time to time. Researchers studying dyslexia in nonalphabetic languages have had the inclination to replicate previous studies, resulting in projects that highlight the unique features of dyslexia in different languages. However, these research findings have been piecemeal rather than delivering a holistic picture of dyslexia in different languages. A similar situation is observed in relation to Chinese dyslexia. While there is increasing evidence of various deficits in Chinese dyslexics, the research findings have been rather scattered, and there has been no sign that efforts are being made to integrate the findings and construct comprehensive theories that might offer a better understanding of the disorder among Chinese readers. I think that it is time to review the findings on Chinese dyslexia and discuss several important issues. In this chapter, I employ John Morton's (2004) causal modeling techniques to integrate the findings on Chinese dyslexia. I hope that my effort will paint a more complete picture for researchers, practitioners, and readers who are interested in Chinese dyslexia. Specifically, I will illustrate how the level of investigation can be made clear during the research planning phrase and report finding phrase. This is an important skill because the distinction between cognitive and behavioral manifestations of dyslexia remains very vague. I aim to suggest readers with the tools link the findings reported in various scientific papers because, first, it is important to distinguish between the root causes of Chinese dyslexia and other behavioral manifestations, and second, because it is essential to possess the skills that compare and contrast different Chinese dyslexic hypotheses while identifying the connections among them. This chapter will be useful to practitioners for differentiating true dyslexia individuals from pseudodyslexic individuals whose difficulties in reading are attributed to insufficient opportunity of reading education (Gough & Tunmer, 1986).

Cognitive Demands of Reading Chinese

Cross-linguistic studies have indicated that dyslexia is a universal phenomenon. Despite its universality, the behavioral manifestations of and the cognitive deficits in dyslexia may be different across cultures. Therefore, when trying to understand Chinese dyslexia, it is necessary to identify the reading behavior of and the core mental skills needed for learning to read Chinese. This brief overview is intended to help readers differentiate between Chinese reading behavior and the cognitive skills required for Chinese word processing.

How can observing reading behavior help determine whether a Chinese child fails to read satisfactorily? Like their alphabetic counterparts, Chinese dyslexic children fail to master words at a normal pace and perform poorly in word recognition tasks (see Chan et al., 2003) for a comprehensive review of a range of reading-related behaviors in Chinese dyslexic children). They either pronounce the word wrongly or give no response. When they are asked to read a text, they show impaired reading comprehension. Another line of investigation focuses on reading fluency. The aforementioned characteristics are behavioral manifestations in terms of reading. In the following paragraphs, I will explore the causes of the disorder.

To understand the etiology of dyslexia, we need a theoretical framework. A common example is the information-processing approach, which is also known as the cognitive approach (Su, Klingebiel, & Weekes, 2010, p. 205). The diagnosis of Chinese dyslexia is based on this approach. To apply it, we first identify the linguistic features that are unique to Chinese and relate them to the cognitive skills required to process lexical information. In short, the major characteristics of Chinese orthography are as follows (Su et al., 2010, p. 203):

1. Chinese orthography is considerably complex.
2. Chinese is a tonal language.
3. The basic graphic unit of Chinese is the syllable, which maps on a meaning.

Based on these three main features, we can identify three corresponding skills needed to learn Chinese. First, good visual-orthographic skills and visual memory are required to handle the visual complexity. Second, tonal awareness is needed to differentiate between Chinese words. Third, it requires good morphological awareness to process word meanings, especially those of multisyllabic words. Logically, when researchers predict the core cognitive deficits in Chinese dyslexia, they suspect that skills that are important to Chinese acquisition are impaired in Chinese dyslexics. Indeed, research findings have shown deficits in visual-orthographic skills (Ho, Chan, Lee, Tsang, & Luan, 2004), tonal awareness (Li & Ho, 2011), and morphological awareness (Shu, McBride-Chang, Wu, & Liu, 2006) in Chinese dyslexics. Deficits in these skills are classified as metalinguistic, because they involve the skills for "thinking about the language." In this overview of cognitive demands, we have defined a scope of areas in which dyslexics would show impairment. We have also demonstrated how researchers set their hypotheses based on the cognitive demand for Chinese reading when studying Chinese dyslexia. However, the story does not end here. First, deficits in metalinguistic skills may not be an adequate explanation for dyslexia. Second, there are precursors to these metalinguistic skill deficits. Third, dyslexia is genetically based, and the links between genes and deficits should be sought. To date, researchers have independently contributed to different aspects of investigation in the field. However, the connections between multiple studies are rarely made explicit. In the following, we illustrate how findings on Chinese dyslexia can be systematically classified into behavioral, cognitive, and biological levels of investigation and linked to yield a more holistic picture.

Reading Behavior in Chinese Dyslexia

In contemporary Chinese dyslexia studies, the reading behavior that has drawn the most attention is word recognition. This skill is assessed in most Chinese dyslexia studies and is usually treated as the dependent variable when using regression analyses to evaluate the roles played by various cognitive-linguistic skills. Another reading behavior that has received researchers' attention is reading fluency and automaticity (Wong & Ho, 2010). This research direction is typically guided by the double-deficit hypothesis, which suggests that reading accuracy and fluency are two major deficit areas in dyslexia (Wolf & Bowers, 1999). Word-recognition skills and reading fluency are tested in two of the three reading subtests in the Hong Kong Test of Specific Learning Difficulties (HKT-P[II]; Ho, Chan, Chung, Tsang, Lee, & Cheng, 2007), the formal diagnostic tool developed for use in the Chinese population.

More recently, researchers have extended their area of study from the investigation of word recognition through sentence comprehension to include discourse/text comprehension (Chik et al., 2010). While this extension promotes a more holistic understanding of Chinese dyslexia, it has also hindered integration of the findings, because the cognitive skills related to word decoding differ from those linked to sentence processing. Therefore, I apply Morton's (1994) causal modeling model to link studies that report findings on the cognitive deficits that influence reading behavior.

Bridging the Phenotypes and Genotypes of Chinese Dyslexia

Dyslexia is defined and known in family and twin studies as a constitutional disorder (Olson, 2004). Therefore, its root causes should have a genetic basis, and Chinese dyslexia is no exception (Lim, Ho, Chou, & Waye, 2011). However, mapping the phenotypes and genotypes is not always easy. One reason is that many cognitive deficits are deemed unstable and can be confounded by measurement errors. Moreover, molecular genetics studies are costly and require advanced machines and techniques (Plomin, DeFries, McClearn, & McGuffin, 2008). Some of the common problems with genomic findings on dyslexia are a lack of statistical power and large discrepancies across laboratories. To yield a more stable phenotype of dyslexia, researchers have sought to identify the endophenotype (Gottesman & Gould, 2003), which is thought to be observed at lower processing levels (e.g., perceptual processing with a close link to human organs, such as the ear) or at the neurological level. Thus, once a cognitive deficit is identified, researchers conduct further studies to look for perceptual deficits and the relevant neurological markers to which they correspond. Because the phenotype-genotype relation is not simple or direct, it is important to identify the nature of dyslexia at multiple analytic levels to narrow the distance between the phenotype and genotype.

Research Directions in Chinese Dyslexia

Based on the chronological order of papers published on Chinese dyslexia, we can identify several stages in the research trend (see Wong, Xiao, & Chung, 2013 for review). First, researchers try to clarify the cognitive skills that are closely linked to Chinese reading. The second stage involves identifying subtypes and comorbid conditions. Third, Chinese dyslexia is studied among different age groups. Fourth, the nature of children at risk for dyslexia is identified. The fifth stage involves identifying the biological bases of Chinese dyslexia. In the sixth stage, researchers extend their area of study from word- to text-level processing (Xiao & Ho, 2014). The expansion of the investigation into Chinese dyslexia through these six major stages has resulted in disorganized findings.

With the identification of subtypes of Chinese dyslexia (Ho, Chan, Chung, Lee, & Tsang, 2007) and other core deficits such as dysfluency, we believe that dyslexia does not have a singular cause, and thus the cognitive profiles in the dyslexic population should be heterogeneous. Given the wide variety of accounts about what causes dyslexia, it is necessary that a tool has to be created to organize the findings.

A Brief Introduction to John Morton's (2004) Causal Modeling Framework

Morton's approach was chosen because it helps to achieve representational clarity (Morton, 2004, p. 193). Before applying the framework to Chinese dyslexia, this approach must be briefly summarized. Extending his previous work (Morton & Frith, 1995), John Morton (2004) detailed a set of ground rules enabling researchers to express and discuss the causes of developmental disorders. With the use of this causal modeling framework, competing causal theories can be expressed and compared in the form of causal relationships at behavioral, cognitive, and genetic levels of analysis. Problems or weak spots in the theories can then be isolated, and possible coherence between the theories can be discovered. The application of this causal modeling method can help to integrate the findings on Chinese dyslexia, allowing us to evaluate competing accounts. Methods of building on and modifying this causal model are outlined in Morton's book for readers who wish more details. In the following, we illustrate the application of Morton's method to integrate the findings of three major dyslexic hypotheses. When building the causal model, it is important to follow the 10 maxims outlined by Morton (2004, p. 99):

1. Start with biology.
2. Build a causal chain.
3. Give a full account.
4. Specific over general.
5. Distinguish cognitive from behavioral.
6. Be cognitively economical.
7. Correlation is not causation.
8. Avoid circularity.
9. There is no single cause of anything.
10. Nothing is determined.

Notes on the Current Experimental Paradigm of Reading Level Control

One important factor that motivates me to clarify the causes of dyslexia is that dyslexic children demonstrate not only reading problems but also other difficulties such as decreased motor (Nicolson & Fawcett, 1994) and organizational skills (Levin, 1990). Symptoms observed in dyslexic individuals could be easily mistaken for causes of reading difficulty, so when we study what causes dyslexia, we should note the distinction between symptom and syndrome (Nicolson & Fawcett, 2005). To understand how dyslexia emerges, it is essential to establish causal relationships between the factors associated with Chinese dyslexia. Interestingly, poor cognitive skills may be a result of poor reading abilities (see Stanovich, 1986). In other words, reading skills and their relevant cognitive skills could be bidirectionally linked. To tackle the confounding effect of reading experiences, reading-level design is conventionally used, in which a group of dyslexics are tested and their performance compared against a control group matched by chronological age (CA) and another matched by reading level (RL).

A discrepancy between the performances of dyslexics and CA controls is counted as a delay, whereas one between dyslexics and RL controls is considered a deficit. In most of the studies reviewed, the disorder group performed significantly worse than the CA controls, but commensurately with the RL controls (Goswami, 2003). The cognitive deficits identified in dyslexic individuals can be attributed to deficiency in reading skills that prompt the development of metalinguistic skills, and thus many of the research findings on dyslexia are confounded with reading experiences. While we have identified many of the symptoms of dyslexia, its cognitive underpinning has been limited to a few options such as phonological awareness (e.g., Snowling, 1998). That is why many researchers have argued that a deficit in phonological awareness is the core cause of dyslexia. This phonological account has also been supported by neurological and genetic findings (Klingbiel & Weekes, 2008).

Three Cognitive Deficit Hypotheses of Chinese Dyslexia (Independent Causal Models)

The aforementioned framework helps clarify the status of each piece of research evidence and integrate or disintegrate the findings to form a comprehensive picture of Chinese dyslexia. Using the "causal modeling" method (Morton, 2004), I try to distinguish the nature of observations (e.g., behavior, cognition, biology) and construct several comprehensive models that specify the causal relationships among the factors associated with Chinese dyslexia. To apply Morton's (2004) method, it is necessary to use biological findings on Chinese dyslexia. An excellent review of the neurological basis of Chinese dyslexia has been accomplished by Klingebiel and Weekes (2008), and I recommend that readers consult their findings. Studies on the genetics involved in Chinese dyslexia are still in their infancy, and my discussion is limited to a handful of recent publications.

Here, I focus on three dyslexic deficit hypotheses that have been tested in multiple studies. The main reason behind such selection is the publication of research evidence at the behavioral, cognitive, and biological levels of analysis. The models are the auditory-speech-phonological deficit hypothesis (Goswami et al., 2011), the visual-orthographic-temporal processing deficit hypothesis (Chung et al., 2008), and the morphosyntactic-lexical access deficit hypothesis (Chik et al., 2010).

In the next three paragraphs, I will describe the reading behavior and faulty computation that categorizes the cognitive skill/deficit of interest and then identify the biological markers linking the cognitive deficits.

Auditory-Speech-Phonological Deficit Hypothesis

Based on the available research findings, I first propose a causal model encapsulating the phonological, speech, and auditory accounts of Chinese dyslexia. The schematic presentation is shown in Figure 10.1. Multiple empirical studies have shown that the primary impairment in developmental dyslexia is phonological (e.g., Snowling, 1998). Chinese dyslexia is not an exception, but the deficits are usually manifested at the syllable rather than the phoneme level. More recent behavioral and neurological studies have shown that difficulties in establishing high quality phonological representations are preceded by impaired auditory processing. Several accounts of auditory deficits in Chinese dyslexia have been proposed. First, Chinese dyslexic children have difficulty processing the auditory signals with rapid changes in frequency and intensity that characterize formants (Chung et al., 2008). Using categorical perception tasks, Cheung et al. (2009) demonstrated that Chinese dyslexic children's perceptions were less categorical (as indicated by shallower identification curves) when processing tonal and aspiration contrasts. Second, Chinese dyslexic children were found to have poor rise-time discrimination, which is linked to the metrical organization of speech and to the perception of stressed and unstressed syllables (Goswami et al., 2011). Similar deficits in the discrimination of rise-time, duration, intensity, and frequency of auditory stimuli have been found in Chinese dyslexic children (Wang, Huss, Hämäläinen, & Goswami, 2012). With respect to Chinese, such deficits may affect the processing of lexical tones, which are important for discriminating between Chinese words that share the same syllable. Third, using a selective adaptation paradigm, Liu, Shu, and Yang (2009) further tested whether Chinese dyslexic children perceived speech in an allophonic mode (more sensitive to acoustic differences within a native phonetic category and less sensitive to acoustic changes across native phonetic categories). The participants were presented with a /pa/–/ta/ continuum in a nonadapted state to obtain baseline identification functions. Next, the participants were asked to join two separate adaptation sessions that were at least one day apart. In the /ta/ adaptation session, the participants heard the adaptor /ta/ repetitively before they were asked to judge whether they had heard /pa/ or /ta/. If an adaptation to /ta/ was obtained, the phoneme boundary of identification would be shifted from /pa/ to /ta/. Therefore, the participants were expected to choose /pa/ more often. As the acoustic difference between /t(a)/ and /t(e)/ belongs to a kind of allophonic mode, dyslexic children were expected to be more sensitive to the subtle acoustic differences between /t(a)/ and /t(e)/, and thus the adaptation effects of the /te/ sound on a /pa/–/ta/ continuum would be reduced. Smaller adaptation effects were found in the /te/ adaptation condition. Contrary to expectation, the dyslexic children showed fewer /ta/ adaptation effects, reflecting a difficulty in forming accurate phonological representations. Ahisssar (2007), who argued in a similar vein, found that children with phonological dyslexia failed to form perceptual anchors and thus obtained no benefit from stimulus-specific repetition. These three auditory deficit hypotheses, although describing different aspects of auditory processing, suggest that the resulting diffused and less consistent phonetic category representations affect the ability to consciously segment and manipulate phonetic categories (Wagner & Torgesen, 1987). This proposed auditory-to-phonology link has been supported by empirical evidence. In the results of hierarchical regression analyses (SEM), speech perception outcomes have predicted reading performance indirectly via phonological awareness (McBride-Chang, 1995). An interesting point to note is that more than one source of auditory impairment and neurological correlates in the "phonological" account of dyslexia have been recognized. Liu et al. (2009) argued that dyslexic children diagnosed with phonological deficits were more likely to have speech problems.

Using the abovementioned evidence, we summarize the findings on speech deficits using Morton's (2004) framework. Figure 10.1 indicates the "auditory-phonology" account of dyslexia. We also identify an important question: Can we observe all types of auditory impairments (rise-time discrimination, formant frequency and intensity detection, categorical perception of tone and aspiration, and phonemic adaptation) in children with dyslexia? If not, it is possible that some auditory problems do not cause dyslexia. Another possibility is that different auditory impairments have unique relationships with various subtypes of dyslexia; that is, auditory-phonology deficit has a biological root. In Meng et al.'s (2005) electrophysiological study, Chinese dyslexics and matched controls did not differ in mismatch negativity (MMN) to stimuli deviated in pure tone frequency (simple pure tone 1250Hz standard; 1400Hz deviant) and Chinese lexical tones. The dyslexic children, however, exhibited smaller MMN to stimuli deviated in the initial consonants, vowels, or tones of Chinese syllables (/da/-/ga/; /dan/-/dai/; /ba1/-/ba2/) and in the temporal information of composite tone patterns differing in temporal order (composite tone patterns: 2000Hz, 800Hz, 2000Hz; standard 150 and 350 ms; deviant 350 and 150 ms).

Given the multidimensional nature of speech perception, future Chinese dyslexia studies investigating a combination of auditory performances and their relations to phonological processing and representations are warranted (Zhang & McBride-Chang, 2010). It is also important to establish the developmental trajectory of auditory and phonological development in Chinese children. Moreover, the effect of phonological awareness on speech perception should not be overlooked (Eisen, Fowler, & Brady, 1995). Apart from group comparison studies, it is important to conduct experimental studies that more closely investigate the effects of impaired auditory perception on phonological awareness and word learning.

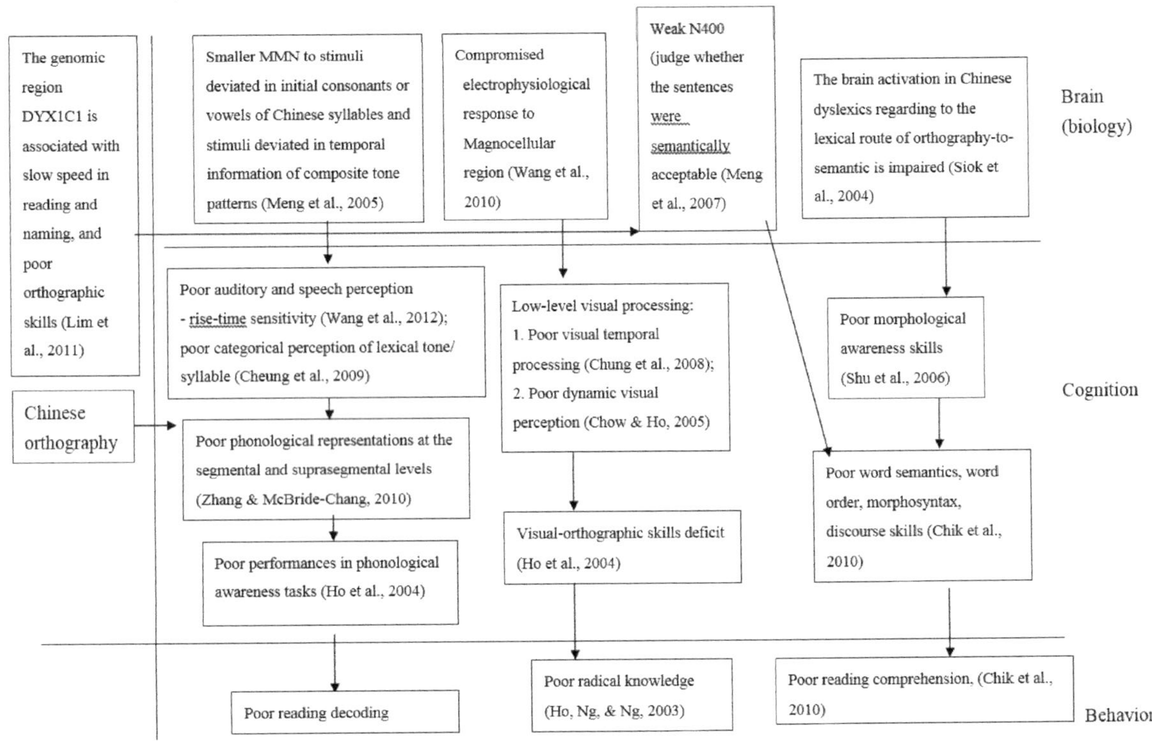

Figure 10.1. Causal analysis of Chinese dyslexia.

Visual-Orthographic-Temporal Processing Deficit Hypothesis

The visually complex Chinese script poses a heavy demand for visual skills in Chinese beginning readers. As dyslexic children do not face sight problems, we need to specify the exact visual difficulties related to their reading problems. We should also bear in mind that no physical or structural damage of eyes has been found in dyslexics. Thus, their visual impairment is reading specific. Surprisingly, recent studies have shown that dyslexic children actually have superior global visual-spatial skills (von Karolyi, Winner, Gray, & Sherman, 2003) and can discriminate between visual stimuli such as numbers and symbols, although the speed is slow (Wolf & Bowers, 1999). Using the causal modeling approach, we first define these reading-related visual problems at the behavioral level. The major problems lie in processing and organizing lexical information. For example, dyslexic children may encode the mirror image of a word or have poor memory of words (Bacon, Parmentier, & Barr, 2012).

The next step is to specify the computational algorithm that defines the cognitive skill or deficit. There are several explanations for deficits in visual-orthographic skills. Robust findings have been observed in eye-movement studies. For instance, Li and colleagues (2009) used a picture-perception task and found that dyslexic children showed significantly smaller saccade amplitude and shorter saccade distance. As a result, less textual information was extracted at each eye-fixation point. This inefficiency in informational processing concurs with the findings on dyslexics' poor visual-temporal skills. Chung et al. (2008) found that dyslexic children performed worse than the CA group but similar to the RL group in measures of the accurate processing of visual-order stimuli. Hierarchical regression analyses revealed that visual-temporal processing contributed unique variances in Chinese character recognition.

Do these visual deficits have a biological root? In a recent event-related potential (ERP) study, Wang, Bi, Gao, and Wydell (2010) employed the "cross-modal delayed response paradigm" (more specifically, the motion-onset paradigm) to examine the magnocellular pathway that processes low contrast and low spatial frequency visual stimuli in Chinese dyslexic children. They found that the mean amplitude of visual MMN in the developmental dyslexics was smaller than that detected in both the CA and RL control children. At the cognitive level, Meng, Cheng-Lai, Zeng, Stein, and Zhou (2011) reported that Chinese dyslexic children had a higher threshold than their age- and IQ-matched controls in a coherent motion detection task (Talcott, Hansen, Elikem, & Stein, 2000; Witton et al., 1998). However, no impairment was found in static pattern perception tasks, suggesting that dyslexics' visual problem lies in the magnocellular pathway.

This magnocellular deficit influenced the speed of orthographic similarity judgment even when IQ and vocabulary size were controlled for in the regression analyses. Interestingly, magnocellular deficits are confounded by the color of the visual stimuli. In Chow and Ho's (2005) study, significant mean differences were found between the blue and white conditions and between the blue and red conditions in the dyslexic group. An increase in magnocellular activity was prompted by the blue stimuli (Greer & Williams, 1995).

Another visual-orthographic deficit lies in the metalinguistic awareness of Chinese orthographic units. Past studies have shown that dyslexics exhibit poor ability to identify the phonetic and semantic radicals. The Chinese dyslexic children study also failed to acquire the orthographic skills required to make lexical decisions (Ho, Ng, & Ng, 2003). This cognitive skills deficit is consistent with the results of brain scanning studies. In an fMRI study, Siok, Spinks, Jin, and Tan (2009) showed that Chinese dyslexic children had a deficit in the left intraparietal sulcus (IPS), which is partially involved in visuospatial processing. In a study conducted by Liu et al. (2012), Chinese dyslexic children were found to have less activation in the right visual cortex, which specializes in holistic visuo-orthographic analysis. A similar abnormality was found in the bilateral occipito-temporal region, which also contributes to orthographic processing.

In a recent molecular genetics study on Chinese dyslexia, the genomic region DYX1C1 was found to be associated with Chinese dyslexia and deficits in skills such as reading and naming speed, in addition to orthographic skills (Lim et al., 2011).

The two proposed links between cognitive deficits and their related biological roots remain speculative. The cognitive-biological link needs to be tested with studies that measure cognitive skills and brain responses in the same group of children and explore the associations between eye movement and temporal deficits.

Morphosyntactic-Lexical Access Deficit Hypothesis

Morphological awareness is argued to be a crucial skill in Chinese reading acquisition. A major characteristic of Chinese characters is that a syllable maps on a morpheme. Chinese word learning involves combining morphemes to create a complex vocabulary via compounding. Moreover, due to the large number of multimorphemic words and homophones, good morphological awareness is critical for discriminating between meanings of Chinese characters across words. These morphological skills are important for reading and learning not only at the word level but also at the text level. For example, word knowledge of "書架" ("bookshelf," an object that holds books suspended in the air) can help a child predict the meaning of a new word, such as"架空" ("suspend in the air"). This skill is important in reading to learn and reading comprehension. Various studies have shown that Chinese dyslexic children have difficulty processing meaning at both the word and sentence levels (Chik et al., 2010; Meng, Tian, Jian, & Zhou, 2007).

Shu et al.'s (2006) logistic regression analyses showed that performance in morphological production tasks significantly discriminated between Chinese dyslexics and nondyslexics. Using the dual-route framework (Jackson & Coltheart, 2001), Shu, Meng, Chen, Luan, and Cao (2005) explained the nature of morphological awareness deficits based on three in-depth case studies. Two children with deep dyslexia exhibited difficulty in distinguishing between semantically related words or characters appearing in various multicharacter words. Another child, diagnosed with surface dyslexia, committed regularization (i.e., incorrect use of regularization rules to name irregular words) and homophones (inability to use a homophone of a target character to form a new word) errors. This morphological awareness impairment is thought to be closely linked to the lexical route, in which reading is achieved via orthography-to-semantic associations.

Chik and her colleagues (2010) revealed in their study that children in the dyslexic group performed significantly worse than those in the CA control group, but performed comparably with those in the RL group in Chinese word reading, sentence reading comprehension (choose a noun/verb/adjective from four choices to complete a sentence; replace an unfamiliar word), passage reading comprehension (five narratives and expository passages; multiple choice and open-ended questions), verbal working memory (listen to a sentence, answer a comprehension question, and repeat the last word), word semantics (match the target words with semantically identical or similar words), word order (arrange four to six sentence fragments to form a syntactically correct sentence), morphosyntax (locate and fill in a missing word in a sentence; detect errors in word compounds, e.g., 青年vs. 年青), and discourse skills (draw inferences between three to five sentences and then arrange them into a coherent and meaningful discourse).

The neurological marker of sentence-processing deficit has also been identified in an event-related potentials experiment. Meng et al. (2007) asked Chinese dyslexic children to judge whether certain sentences were semantically acceptable (sentences with final two-character compound words replaced by homophonic or orthographically similar characters). They found that the N400 component was weak (almost absent) when the dyslexic children judged the two types of sentences. It appeared that the Chinese dyslexics' deficits lay in using phonological and orthographic information to constrain lexical access. In another study, Siok, Perfetti,

Jin, and Tan (2004) administered lexical decision tasks in their fMRI study and showed that brain activation in Chinese dyslexics along the orthography-to-semantic lexical route is lower. This impairment is located at the left-middle-frontal gyrus, which coordinates and integrates pieces of lexical information about written characters.

Applying the causal modeling framework to integrate findings on Chinese dyslexia allows us to clarify the causal status of various cognitive deficits. It also reveals that Chinese dyslexia may be a heterogeneous disorder. Our review is corroborated by the multiple deficit hypotheses (Ho, Chan, Tsang, & Lee, 2002) and subtypes of Chinese dyslexia (Ho et al., 2004). On one hand, we look for the biology-cognition-behavior link. On the other hand, we do not limit ourselves to cause-and-effect relations when interpreting the nature of developmental disorders.

The "Developmental Neuroconstructivism" Approach

Using Morton's (2004) framework to explain Chinese dyslexia makes it clear that progress has been made in identifying the disorder's unique features and shedding light on some unresolved puzzles at the behavioral, cognitive, and biological levels. Undeniably, the causal modeling framework is useful in guiding and stimulating further research. However, it is inadequate to explain (Chinese) dyslexia through a set of unidirectional causal chains (Karmiloff-Smith, 1998) because development is not the result of predetermined epigenesis (mere triggering) but rather of probabilistic epigenesis (pushing individuals onto different developmental pathways that eventually results in reading deficits).

Thomas et al. (2009) noted the value of framing developmental disorders using the "developmental neuroconstructivism" approach. A prominent message inspired by this perspective is that deficit genes make a person more prone to developmental disorders, the outbreak of which depends on a series of dynamic man-environment interactions. Traditionally, single-point studies of dyslexia and research on disorders solely at their end state in school-aged children have dominated the field of dyslexia studies. However, according to contemporary research findings in child development, phenotypes associated with any neurodevelopmental disorders do not emerge fully blown at birth. Instead, humans develop gradually, and sometimes in transformative ways, with age. Thomas and colleagues (2009) argued that the concept of "delay," if not further elaborated, is just a redescription of behavioral data, indicating that the disorder group has produced scores and error patterns similar to those of younger typically developmental controls, with no elaboration of the causal mechanism by which this similarity may have arisen. Sooner or later, it is possible that dyslexic individuals attain a reading level comparable to typically developing individuals, as shown in reading-compensated adults (Lefly & Pennington, 1991). As Karmiloff-Smith (1998) argued, atypical development should not be considered in terms of a catalogue of impaired and intact functions in which nonaffected modules are considered to develop normally and independently of the impaired modules. It should be noted that even when normal behavioral levels are found in a developmental disorder in a given domain, they might have been achieved by different cognitive processes. Therefore, a "developmental neuroconstructivist" approach is necessary to understand the etiology of developmental disorders. Moreover, conceptualizing the ontogeny of dyslexia in a linear and unidirectional fashion—a deficit gene causes atypical neural cognitive development, constrains reading development, and results in dyslexia—is not advisable. It seems more feasible to consider dyslexia-related factors from a more dynamic perspective; that is, with multiple two-way relationships among all of the relevant factors, with genes interacting continuously with the environment and being expressed accordingly at the biological, cognitive, and behavioral levels. The so-called "developmental neuroconstructivist" approach advocates the study of developmental disorders with respect to typical development using a special kind of longitudinal design (see Thomas et al., 2009 for the details of the methodology). Conducting empirical studies based on the proposal outlined by "developmental neuroconstructivism" is a challenging endeavor. Relatively large sample sizes and testing spanning extensive age ranges over a long period, from prereading to postdiagnosis, demand significant resources and time. Despite the challenges, large-size family studies have been undertaken in different parts of the world (e.g., Choudhury & Benasich, 2003; Raskind, Hsu, Berninger, Thomson, & Wijsman, 2000). Moreover, the "developmental neuroconstructivism" approach encourages research on at-risk children and helps tackle the issue of comorbidity.

Studies of Chinese children at risk of dyslexia have revealed that such children exhibit impairment in both early phonological and nonphonological skills, which predicts the presence of dyslexia (Ho, Leung, & Cheung, 2011; Wong et al., 2012). At-risk children who later become dyslexic show a wide range of language-, phonology-, and print-related deficits. Longitudinally tracking the development of these at-risk children could have predictive power and allow for the role of each of the early skills to be studied. Early story-comprehension difficulty may hinder children's use of contextual knowledge in identifying low frequency words (Nation & Snowling, 1998). According to Liu et al. (2010), performance in sentence imitation at age 4 best discriminated between poor and adequate Chinese readers at age 7. In the same study, other factors such as grammatical knowledge at age 4, vocabulary knowledge at age 2, and articulation at age 3 predicted future dyslexia. Nonword repetition was not predictive, because Chinese syllable structure is not as complex as that of alphabetic languages. Such studies have shown that considering the periods over which difficulties unfold is important to the understanding of how Chinese dyslexia emerges.

The variations in the cognitive profiles among Chinese dyslexics can also be accounted for by the "developmental neuroconstructivist" theory. Ho and her colleagues (2004) identified seven subtypes of Chinese developmental dyslexia according to the underlying cognitive deficits: global deficit, orthographic deficit, phonological memory deficit, mild difficulty, and three other subtypes with rapid-naming-related deficits. These specific problems may be rooted in a more general deficit during the prereading period. By tracing the progression of skills through the pre- and postreading phases, we can understand how the generalist genes lead to different cognitive profiles of dyslexia (Kovas & Plomin, 2006). While the majority of Chinese dyslexic children are reported to have rapid naming and orthographic deficits, the relatively small proportion of dyslexic children whose core problems lie in phonological deficits should not be overlooked.

CONCLUSION

I have discussed two interrelated issues that deserve more attention in the study of developmental disorders, including dyslexia. First, there is still a need for greater effort in contrasting the actual causes and the contingency of dyslexia. Second, the understanding of the genetic basis of dyslexia remains incomplete. Mapping the phenotypes and genotypes of dyslexia demands a proper classification of the type of research evidence at the right level of analysis so that the phenotypes and genotypes of dyslexia can be linked at the cognitive level of analysis. Using John Morton's (2004) causal modeling method, I evaluated three Chinese dyslexic deficit hypotheses and gained a clearer picture of the etiology of Chinese dyslexia. This method helped to clarify the contributing roles of each piece of research evidence obtained from multiple Chinese dyslexia studies. Moreover, potential research gaps and new research ideas were generated from the application of the causal model (Figure 10.1). Although our discussion has centered on Chinese dyslexia, I believe that similar attempts can and should be made with other dyslexic populations, notwithstanding discrepancies in different linguistic aspects.

ACKNOWLEDGMENT

The author would like to thank Professor Dorothy Bishop for her recommendation of Professor John Morton's (2004) book. He would like to thank Professor Kevin Chung for his comments and Ms Hoyee Miao and Vina Leung for their assistance in preparing this chapter.

REFERENCES

Ahissar, M. (2007). Dyslexia and the anchoring-deficit hypothesis. *Trends in Cognitive Sciences, 11*(11), 458–465.

Bacon, A. M., Parmentier, F. B. R., & Barr, P. (2013). Visuospatial memory in dyslexia: Evidence for strategic deficits. *Memory. 21*(2),189-209.

Chan, D. W., Ho, C. S.-H., Tsang, S. M., Lee, S. H., & Chung, K. K. H. (2003). Reading-related behavioral characteristics of Chinese children with dyslexia: The use of the teachers' behavior checklist in Hong Kong. *Annals of Dyslexia, 53*, 300–323.

Cheung, H., Chung, K. K. H., Wong, S. W. L., McBride-Chang, C., Penney, T. B., & Ho, C. S.-H. (2009). Perception of tone and aspiration contrasts in Chinese children with dyslexia. *Journal of Child Psychology and Psychiatry, 50*(6), 726–733.

Chik P. P., Ho, C. S., Yeung, P. S., Wong, Y. K., Chan, D. W., Chung, K. K., & Lo, L. Y. (2010). Contribution of discourse and morphosyntax skills to reading comprehension in Chinese dyslexic and typically developing children. *Annals of Dyslexia, 62*(1), 1–18.

Choudhury, N., & Benasich, A. A. (2003). A family aggregation study: The influence of family history and other risk factors on language development. *Journal of Speech, Language and Hearing Research, 46*, 261–272.

Chow, E. M.-C., & Ho, C. S.-H. (2006). Visual motion perception in Chinese dyslexic children. *Journal of Psychology in Chinese Societies, 6*, 161–178.

Chung, K. K. H., McBride-Chang, C., Wong, S. W. L., Cheung, H., Penney, T. B., & Ho, C. S.-H. (2008). The role of visual and auditory temporal processing for Chinese children with developmental dyslexia. *Annals of Dyslexia, 58*, 15–35.

Eisen, A. W., Fowler, A. E., & Brady, S. (1995, April). *The perception and awareness of phonemes in young five-year-olds.* Paper presented at the meeting of the Society for Research in Child Development, Indianapolis, IN.

Goswami, U. (2003). Why theories about developmental dyslexia require developmental designs. *Trends in Cognitive Sciences*, 7(12), 534–540.

Goswami, U., Wang, H. L., Cruz, A., Fosker, T., Mead, N., & Huss, M. (2011). Language-universal sensory deficits in developmental dyslexia: English, Spanish, and Chinese. *Journal of Cognitive Neuroscience, 23*, 325–337.

Gottesman, I. I., & Gould, T. D. (2003). The endophenotype concept in psychiatry: Etymology and strategic intentions. *The American Journal of Psychiatry, 160*, 636–645.

Gough, P. B., & Tunmer, W. E. (1986). Decoding, reading, and reading disability. *Remedial and Special Education*, *7*, 6–10.

Greer, A., & Williams, M. (1995). *Visual timing and wavelength effects in dyslexic and normal children*. Poster presented at the meeting of the Society for Research in Child Development, Indianapolis, IN.

Ho, C. S.-H., Chan, D.W.-O., Chung, K. K., Lee, S.-H., & Tsang, S.-M. (2007). In search of subtypes of Chinese developmental dyslexia. *Journal of Experimental Child Psychology*, *97*, 61–83.

Ho, C. S.-H., Chan, D. W.-O., Chung, K., Tsang, S.-M., Lee, S.-H., & Cheng, R. W.-Y. (2007). *The Hong Kong Test of Specific Learning Difficulties in Reading and Writing for primary school students, second edition [HKT-P(II)]*. Hong Kong, China: Hong Kong Specific Learning Difficulties Research Team.

Ho, C. S.-H., Chan, D. W.-O., Lee, S.-H., Tsang, S.-M., & Luan, V. H. (2004). Cognitive profiling and preliminary subtyping in Chinese developmental dyslexia. *Cognition*, *91*, 43–75.

Ho, C. S.-H., Chan, D. W.-O., Tsang, S.-M., & Lee, S.-H. (2000). *The Hong Kong Test of Specific Learning Difficulties in Reading and Writing*. Hong Kong, China: Hong Kong Specific Learning Difficulties Research Team.

Ho, C. S.-H., Chan, D. W.-O., Tsang, S.-M., & Lee, S.-H. (2002) The cognitive profile and multiple-deficit hypothesis in Chinese developmental dyslexia. *Developmental Psychology*, *38*(4), 543–553.

Ho, C. S.-H., Leung, M.-T., & Cheung, H. (2011). Early difficulties of Chinese preschoolers at familial risk for dyslexia: Deficits in oral language, phonological processing skills, and print-related skills. *Dyslexia*, *17*(2), 143–164.

Ho, C. S.-H, Ng, T.-T., & Ng, W.-K. (2003). A "radical" approach to reading development in Chinese: The role of semantic radicals and phonetic radicals. *Journal of Literacy Research*, *35*(3), 849–878.

Jackson, N. E., & Coltheart, M. (2001). *Routes to reading success and failure: Toward an integrated cognitive psychology of atypical reading*. New York, NY: Taylor & Francis.

Karmiloff-Smith, A. (1998). Development itself is the key to understanding developmental disorders. *Trends in Cognitive Sciences*, *2*, 389–398.

Klingebiel, K., & Weekes, B. S. (2008). Developmental dyslexia in Chinese: Behavioural, genetic and neuropsychological issues. In S. P. Law, B. S. Weekes, & A. Wong (Eds.), *Disorders of speech and language in Chinese* (pp. 220–273). San Diego, CA: Plural.

Kovas, Y., & Plomin, R. (2006). Generalist genes: Implications for the cognitive sciences. *Trends in Cognitive Sciences*, *10*, 198–203.

Lefly, D. L., & Pennington, B. F. (1991). Spelling errors and reading fluency in compensated adult dyslexics. *Annals of Dyslexia*, *41*, 143–162.

Levin, B. E. (1990). Organizational deficits in dyslexia: Possible frontal lobe dysfunction. *Developmental Neuropsychology*, *6*(2), 95–110.

Li, W. S., & Ho, C. S.-H. (2011). Lexical tone awareness in Chinese children with developmental dyslexia. *Journal of Child Language*, *38*(4), 793–808.

Li, X. H., Jing, J., Zou, X. B., Huang, X., Jin, Y., Wang, Q. X., ... Yang, S. Y. (2009). Picture perception in Chinese dyslexic children: An eye-movement study. *Chinese Medical Journal*, *122*, 267–271.

Lim, C. K. P., Ho, C. S. H., Chou, C. H. N., & Waye, M. M. Y. (2011). Association of the rs3743205 variant of DYX1C1 with dyslexia in Chinese children. *Behavioral and Brain Functions, 7*, 16.

Liu, L., Wang, W.-J., You, W.-P., Li, Y., Awati, N., Zhao, X., ... Peng, D. (2012). Similar alterations in brain function for phonological and semantic processing to visual characters in Chinese dyslexia. *Neuropsychologia, 50*(9), 2224–2232.

Liu, P. H., McBride-Chang, C., Wong, A. M.-Y., Tardif, T., Stokes, S.F., Fletcher, P., & Shu, H. (2010). Early oral language markers of poor reading performance in Hong Kong Chinese children. *Journal of Learning Disabilities, 43*(4), 322–331.

Liu, W., Shu, H., & Yang, Y. (2009). Speech perception deficits by Chinese children with phonological dyslexia. *Journal of Experimental Child Psychology, 103*, 338–354.

McBride-Chang, C. (1995). Phonological processing, speech perception, and reading disability: An integrative review. *Educational Psychologist, 30*, 109–121.

Meng, X., Cheng-Lai, A., Zeng, B., Stein, J. F., & Zhou, X. (2011). Dynamic visual perception and reading development in Chinese school children. *Annals of Dyslexia, 61*, 161–176.

Meng, X., Sai, X., Wang, C., Wang, J., Sha, S., & Zhou, X. (2005). Auditory and speech processing and reading development in Chinese school children: Behavioural and ERP evidence. *Dyslexia, 11*(4), 292–310.

Meng, X., Tian, X., Jian, J., & Zhou, X., (2007). Orthographic and phonological processing in Chinese dyslexic children: An ERP study on sentence reading. *Brain Research, 1179*, 119–130.

Morton, J. (2004). *Understanding developmental disorders: A causal modeling approach*. Oxford, UK: Blackwell.

Morton, J., & Frith, U. (1995). Causal modeling: A structural approach to developmental psychopathology. In D. Cicchetti & D. J. Cohen (Eds.), *Developmental psychopathology* (Vol. 1, pp. 357–390). New York, NY: John Wiley & Sons.

Nation, K., & Snowling, M. J. (1998). Individual differences in contextual facilitation: Evidence from dyslexia and poor reading comprehension. *Child Development, 69*, 996–1011.

Nicolson, R. I., & Fawcett, A. J. (1994). Comparison of deficits in cognitive and motor-skills among children with dyslexia. *Annals of Dyslexia, 44*, 147–164.

Nicolson, R. I., & Fawcett, A. J. (2005). Developmental dyslexia, learning and the cerebellum. *Journal of Neural Transmission, 69*, 19–36.

Olson, R. K. (2004). SSSR, environment, and genes. *Scientific Studies of Reading, 8*(2), 111–124.

Plomin, R., DeFries, J. C., McClearn, G. E., & McGuffin, P. (2008). *Behavioral genetics* (5th ed.). New York, NY: Worth.

Raskind, W. H., Hsu, L., Berninger, V. W., Thomson, J. B., & Wijsman, E. M. (2000). Family aggregation of dyslexia phenotypes. *Behavior Genetics, 30*, 385–396.

Shu, H., McBride-Chang, C., Wu, S., & Liu, H. Y. (2006). Understanding Chinese developmental dyslexia: Morphological awareness as a core cognitive construct. *Journal of Educational Psychology, 98*, 122–133.

Shu, H., Meng, X., Chen, X., Luan, H., & Cao, F. (2005). The subtypes of developmental dyslexia in Chinese: Evidence from three cases. *Dyslexia, 11*, 311–329.

Siok, W. T., Perfetti, C. A., Jin, Z., & Tan, L. H. (2004). Biological abnormality of impaired reading is constrained by culture. *Nature, 431*, 71–76.

Siok, W. T., Spinks, J. A., Jin, Z., & Tan, L. H. (2009). Developmental dyslexia is characterized by the co-existence of visuospatial and phonological disorders in Chinese children. *Current Biology, 19*, 890–892.

Snowling, M. (1998). Dyslexia as a phonological deficit: Evidence and implications. *Child Psychology and Psychiatry Review, 3*, 4–11

Stanovich, K. E. (1986). Matthew effects in reading: Some consequences of individual differences in the acquisition of literacy. *Reading Research Quarterly, 21*(4), 360–407.

Su, I.-F., Klingebiel, K., & Weekes, B. S. (2010). Dyslexia in Chinese: Implications for connectionist models of reading. In N. Brunswick, S. McDougall, & P. de Mornay-Davies (Eds.), *Reading and dyslexia in different orthographies* (pp. 199–220). London, UK: Psychology.

Talcott, J. B., Hansen, P. C., Elikem, L. A., & Stein, J. F. (2000) Visual motion sensitivity in dyslexia: Evidence for temporal and motion energy integration deficits. *Neuropsychologia, 38*, 935–943.

Thomas, M. S. C., Annaz, D., Ansari, D., Scerif, G., Jarrold, C., & Karmiloff-Smith, A. (2009). Using developmental trajectories to understand genetic disorders. *Journal of Speech, Language and Hearing Research, 52*, 336–358.

Von Karolyi, C., Winner, E., Gray, W., & Sherman, G. F. (2003). Dyslexia linked to talent: Global visual-spatial ability. *Brain and Language, 85*, 427–431.

Wagner, R. K., & Torgesen, J. K. (1987). The nature of phonological processing and its causal role in the acquisition of reading skills. *Psychological Bulletin, 101*, 192–212.

Wang, H.-L. S., Huss, M., Hämäläinen, J. A., & Goswami. U. (2012). Basic auditory processing and developmental dyslexia in Chinese. *Reading and Writing: An Interdisciplinary Journal, 25*, 509–536.

Wang, J.-J., Bi, H.-Y., Gao, L.-Q., & Wydell, T. N. (2010). The visual magnocellular pathway in Chinese-speaking children with developmental dyslexia. *Neuropsychologia, 48*, 3627–3633.

Witton, C., Talcott, J. B., Hansen, P. C., Richardson, A. J., Griffiths, T. D., Rees, A., ... Green, G. G. R. (1998). Sensitivity to dynamic auditory and visual stimuli predicts nonword reading ability in both dyslexic and normal readers. *Current Biology, 8*, 791–797.

Wolf, M., & Bowers, P. G. (1999). The double deficit hypothesis for the developmental dyslexias. *Journal of Educational Psychology, 91*, 1–24.

Wong, S. W. L., & Ho, C. S.-H. (2010). The nature of the automatization deficit in Chinese children with dyslexia. *Child Neuropsychology, 16*, 405–415.

Wong, S. W. L., McBride-Chang, C., Lam, C., Chan, B., Lam, F., & Doo, S. (2012). The joint effects of risk status, gender, early literacy and cognitive skills on the presence of dyslexia among a group of high-risk Chinese children. *Dyslexia, 18*, 40–57.

Wong, S. W. L., Xiao, M. X. Y., & Chung, K. K. H. (2013). Issues of culture and language in developmental disorders: The case of dyslexia in Chinese learners. In C. R. Marshall (Ed.), *Current issues in developmental disorders* (pp. 151–170). East Sussex, UK: Psychology.

Xiao, X.-Y., & Ho, C. S.-H. (2014). Weaknesses in Semantic, Syntactic and Oral Language Expression Contribute to Reading Difficulties in Chinese Dyslexic Children. *Dyslexia, 20*(1), 74–98.

Zhang, J., & McBride-Chang, C. (2010). Auditory sensitivity, speech perception, and reading development and impairment. *Educational Psychology Review, 22*(3), 323–338.

CHAPTER 11

RELATIONSHIP BETWEEN MORPHOLOGICAL AWARENESS AND CHINESE READING DEVELOPMENT

A Treatment Study

Dustin Lau and Man Tak Leung

Reading is the process of obtaining meaning from text. Learning to read is a process through which the relations between written text and verbal language are identified for the ultimate comprehension of the written text. The process of learning to read appears to be largely uneventful in most children. However, there exists a group of children who have difficulties developing normal reading abilities, also known as children with dyslexia or reading difficulties. Understanding how and why such children have difficulty in learning to read would inform reading development theories and address how the brain organizes written and spoken forms and meanings of language, which would in turn help to explain the failure to comprehend written text. Such understanding would also direct remediation strategies for children with reading difficulties. In this chapter,

Understanding Developmental Disorders of Auditory Processing, Language and Literacy Across Languages: International Perspectives, pp. 229–247

the relationship between Chinese reading difficulties and morphological awareness is discussed.

Morphological awareness is the knowledge of and ability to reflect on and manipulate the basic meaningful linguistic units called morphemes (Kuo & Anderson, 2006). It is a cognitive ability associated with Chinese reading difficulties (e.g., Ku & Anderson, 2003; Li, Anderson, Nagy, & Zhang, 2002; McBride-Chang, Shu, Zhou, Wat, & Wagner, 2003; Wang, Cheng, & Chen, 2006). However, it is unclear why and how morphological awareness is associated with Chinese reading difficulties. We aimed to address this question in the study reported in this chapter. We begin by introducing the characteristics of Chinese and its morphology, followed by a review of studies on morphological awareness in reading Chinese, and their limitations. Finally, we report the use of a treatment study in addressing why and how morphological awareness is related to Chinese reading difficulties.

The Chinese Writing System and Its Morphology

The Chinese writing system is morphosyllabic; that is, one Chinese character usually corresponds to one syllable and one morpheme (Hoosain, 1992). For example, the character 眼 corresponds to the syllable /ngaan5/ and the morpheme [eye].

Unlike alphabetic scripts, the relationship between phonology and orthography in Chinese is very opaque. Although there is a group of Chinese characters called phonetic compound characters, consisting of phonetic radicals that give cues to their phonology, Leung and Lee (2002) reported that less than 30% of the phonetic compound characters that children learn in primary schools are regular characters with pronunciations that are identical to those of their phonetic radicals (e.g., 楓 /fung1/ [maple] and its phonetic radical 風 /fung1/ [wind]). Most phonetic compound characters learned in primary schools are irregular, and their pronunciations are different from those of their phonetic radicals (e.g., 杯 /bui1/ [cup] and its phonetic radical 不 /bat1/ [no]). Without doubt, the phonological transparency of Chinese is very low. What further jeopardizes the situation is that opacity exists in the relations between phonology and orthography on top of the relations between orthography and phonology. On average, almost three Chinese characters share each syllable in Chinese (Leung & Lee, 2002). For example, the syllable /si1/ is associated with 13 Chinese characters: 屍, 絲, 思, 師, 施, 斯, 撕, 詩, 獅, 司, 私, 廝, and 俬. The opaque relationship between orthography and phonology has been described as one of the major reasons why learning to read Chinese is so difficult (e.g., Ziegler & Goswami, 2005).

In contrast, the morphology of Chinese appears to be more reliable. In general, one character corresponds to one morpheme. For example, the Chinese word 月餅盒 /juet6 beng2 hap2/ [moon-cake box] consists of three morphemes, in which the first morpheme 月 /juet6/ means [moon], the second morpheme 餅 /beng2/ means [cake], and the third morpheme 盒 /hap2/ means [box]. Using this construct, Chinese words can be monomorphemic (e.g., 手 /sau2/ [hand] or 狗 /gau2/ [dog]) or multimorphemic (e.g., 腕錶 /wun2 biu1/ [wrist-watch] or 耳環 /ji5 waan4/ [earring]). Chinese morphemes can also be categorized into free morphemes (e.g., 頭 /tau4/ [head] or 雨 /jyu5/ [rain]) and bound morphemes (e.g., 視 /si6/ [visual], which cannot be used alone but can be combined with different morphemes to form words related to vision, such as 電視 /din6 si6/ [television] and 近視 /gan6 si6/ [short-sighted]). The three word formation rules, namely, inflection, derivation, and compounding, are also applicable to Chinese word formation. An example of Chinese inflected word is 我們 /ngo5 mun4/ [us], in which the suffix 們 /mun4/ [plural marker] is attached to the word 我 /ngo5/ [me]. An example of a Chinese derived word is 電腦化 /din6 nou5 faa3/ [computerize], in which the grammatical marker 化 /faa3/ is attached to the noun 電腦 /din6 nou5/ [computer] to change it to a verb. Finally, an example of a Chinese compound word is 金牌 /gam1 paai4/ [gold medal], in which the morpheme 金 /gam1/ [gold] is simply connected to the morpheme 牌 /paai4/ [medal] to form the whole word.[1]

Inflectional and derivational morphology are highly productive word-forming rules in English, whereas compounding is highly productive in forming new words in Chinese (Kuo & Anderson, 2006). Therefore, it is reasonable to suggest that an awareness of the contributions of constituent morphemes' meanings to the whole-word meanings of compound words is relatively more important in learning to read Chinese compared with alphabetic scripts. It is not difficult to infer that such awareness allows for the easy identification of relations between most Chinese written texts and their meanings. For example, assembling the meanings of the constituent morphemes 龜 /gwai1/ [tortoise] and 速 /cuk1/ [speed] creates the meaning of the compound word 龜速 /gwai1cuk1/ [slow]. In light of this, many studies have investigated Chinese children's awareness of the roles of constituent morphemes in compound words and how it affects their reading (e.g. Li et al., 2002; McBride-Chang et al., 2003).

Studies of Morphological Awareness and Chinese Reading

The strong relationship between morphological awareness and one's ability to read Chinese has been reported in many studies (Li et al., 2002;

McBride-Chang et al., 2003; Tong & McBride-Chang, 2010). For example, McBride-Chang et al. (2003) used an odd-man-out auditory task to assess a group of preschoolers' ability to distinguish between identical morphemes and homophones, for example, the "fung1" (風) in /daai6 fung1/ [windy] (大風) and /daa2 fung1/ [storm] (打風) corresponds to the same morpheme while that in /mat6 fung1/ [bee] (蜜蜂) does not. They reported that children's ability to distinguish between identical morphemes and homophones significantly predicted their reading ability. As mentioned above, on average, almost three Chinese characters share each syllable in Chinese. McBride-Chang et al. suggested that the homophonous nature of Chinese reinforces the importance of young Chinese children learning to distinguish among homophonic morphemes.

In the same study, McBride-Chang et al. (2003) asked their subjects to construct novel words based on morphological skills (e.g., creating the novel word /jyut6 ceot1/ [moonrise] (月出) based on the analogy of the real word /jat6 ceot1/ [sunrise] (日出)). They found that the ability to construct novel morphologically complex words significantly predicted children's reading ability. Together with the results obtained in the homophone judgment task, they concluded that young children's morphological awareness predicts their reading ability.

Subsequent studies have not only reported that good Chinese readers are better at identifying the meanings of constituent morphemes in compound words, but have also revealed that their morphological processing skills are affected by other linguistic factors. For example, Chen, Hao, Geva, Zhu, and Shu (2009) reported that children's awareness of the heads of compound nouns (e.g., /jyu5 ji1/ [raincoat] [雨衣] is a categorical item of /ji1/ [coat] (衣) but not a categorical item of /jyu5/ [rain] [雨]) was significantly related to their reading ability. In another study, Liu and McBride-Chang (2010) demonstrated that children's morphological processing of compound words is affected by the syntactic structure of the compound words. Using a priming study, Liu and McBride-Chang observed a significant semantic priming effect when both structures in prime and targets are subordinates; that is, compounds with the former morphemes modifying the latter morphemes (e.g., 白馬 /baak6 ma5/ [white horse] and 青草 / cing1 cou2/ [green grass]). This priming effect, however, was not observed when the structures were coordinates, specifically compounds with both morphemes contributing equally to the whole-word meaning (e.g., 清潔 / cing1 git3/ [clean] and 規則 /kwai1 zak1/ [rules]).

Another linguistic factor that affects the morphological processing of compound words is the boundedness of the constituent morphemes. The boundedness of morphemes refers to whether morphemes can be used independently as words. Those that can be used independently as words are free morphemes, while those that cannot are bound morphemes. Lau,

Leung, Cheung, Lui, and Tse (2011) found that children's performance in naming two-character compound words consisting of two free morphemes (FF words), for example, 醉酒/zoey3 zau2/ (*drunk*), was better than that for two-character compound words with two bound morphemes (BB words), for example, 統治 /tung2 zi6/ (*to rule*). In the subsequent experiment, they examined children's performance in naming the constituent free and bound morphemes of the FF words and BB words used in the first experiment and learned that children's naming accuracy for bound morphemes was lower than that for free morphemes. Because the frequencies of the free and bound morphemes were matched, the difference in naming accuracy suggests that children are sensitive to the boundedness of characters, such that in general, free morphemes are named better than bound morphemes. As the FF and BB words they used were matched for word and constituent morpheme frequencies, the differences in naming accuracy suggest that children are able to make use of the free morphemes in FF words to facilitate their naming performance. Lau et al. (2011) suggested that meanings carried by free morphemes can be identified when they occur freely in texts, while bound morphemes' meanings are not identifiable in isolation. The meanings of bound morphemes can only be understood by comparing the meanings of the compound words that contain the bound morphemes. In contrast, the meanings of free morphemes can be accessed directly. Consequently, free morphemes will have more concrete semantic representations in one's lexicon when compared with bound morphemes (Pastizzo & Feldman, 2004; Taft, 2003). Lau et al. (2011) suggested that the more concrete semantic representations of the free morphemes facilitate children's recognition of FF words and perform better on free morphemes in their experiments.

Apart from boundedness, the morphological processing of Chinese compound words is affected by semantic transparency. Semantic transparency refers to whether the meaning of a compound word is consistent with the meanings of its constituent morphemes. Transparent words (trans-words) are compound words whose meanings are consistent with those of their constituent morphemes, while opaque words (opaq-words) are not consistent. An example of a trans-word is 皮鞋/pei4 haai4/ [leather shoes], wherein the meanings of the constituent morphemes 皮 /pei4/ [leather] and 鞋 /haai4/ [shoes] are consistent with the meaning of the whole word. An example of an opaq-word is 馬虎 /maa1 fu1/ [careless], wherein the meanings of the constituent morphemes 馬 /maa5/ [horse] and 虎 /fu2/ [tiger] are inconsistent with the meaning of the whole word. Using a lexical decision task, Lau (2012) compared the differences in the recognition of trans- and opaq-words among a group of young children who were poor readers, a group of reading-level-matched readers, and a group of chronological-age-matched readers. Trans-words were found to be recognized faster than opaq-words in the two groups of normal readers, but the effect was absent in the poor reader group. Because the trans- and opaq-words used were matched for word frequency, constituent morpheme frequency, and boundedness, Lau suggested that good readers were aware of the transparency of the words. In contrast, because the semantic transparency effect was not significant in the poor-reader group, it indicates that poor readers were not aware of the transparency relations between compound words and their constituents.

Lau's (2012) results indicated that normal readers can manipulate free morphemes better to decode transparent words. In contrast, poor readers are less capable of doing so, possibly due to inferior morphological awareness. Lau suggested that among good readers, the overlapping between the semantic representations of the constituent morphemes and those of the trans-words facilitates the recognition and decoding of the trans-words, whereas the mismatch between the semantic representations of the constituent morphemes and those of the opaq-words inhibits the decoding of the opaq-words. Regarding poor readers, the semantic representations of the constituent morphemes of both trans- and opaq-words are not concrete enough to result in facilitation or inhibition. Therefore, their performance between trans- and opaq-words is equally poor.

To summarize, Chinese children start to demonstrate morphological processing in their use of verbal language at the preschool level (McBride-Chang et al., 2003). Later, they become aware of the linguistic properties of morphemes, which affects their processing of written compound words (Lau et al., 2011; Liu & McBride-Chang, 2010).

Relationships Between Morphological Awareness and Reading Development in Chinese

Although numerous studies have reported the strong associations between morphological awareness and reading abilities in Chinese, the nature of the relationship between morphological awareness and reading development in Chinese remains unclear. Kuo and Anderson (2006) suggested the following possible relationships between morphological awareness and reading development: (a) good morphological awareness results in good reading ability, (b) good reading ability results in good morphological awareness, and (c) the relationship is reciprocal. In other words, it is unclear whether the ill-formed semantic representations of morphemes in the poor readers' lexicons hinder their reading development, or the other way around. Alternatively, it is possible that the ill-formed semantic representations associated with morphemes hinder their reading development while simultaneously hindering the establishment of concrete semantic representations of morphemes.

The results of intervention studies conducted among typically developing children seem to support that good morphological awareness results in good reading abilities (Chow, McBride-Chang, Cheung, & Chow, 2008; Packard et al., 2006; Wu et al., 2009). For example, Packard et al. (2006) provided instructions for improving knowledge of the orthographic and morphological structures of Chinese words in an experimental group of first graders. They observed that the experimental group performed significantly better when copying Chinese characters and then writing them from memory compared to the control group. They suggested that improving children's morphological knowledge enhances their reading development.

Similar results were reported by Chow et al. (2008), who observed that training in parent-child shared book reading and metalinguistic training in morphology significantly improved preschoolers' ability to recognize Chinese characters, compared to the control group.

The results reported by Packard et al. (2006) and Chow et al. (2008) tend to support that good morphological awareness results in good reading ability.

The Current Study

If the hypothesis that "good morphological awareness will result in good reading abilities" is true, improving poor readers' morphological awareness (poor morphological awareness is removed) should improve their reading ability (poor reading is no longer observed). In contrast, if morphological awareness is improved and poor reading ability remains, then the hypothesis should be refuted. In this study, the direction of causality between morphological awareness and reading development is examined using a treatment study on a group of Chinese poor readers under the abovementioned logic.

In Hong Kong, children start to learn to read and write in kindergarten. The early Chinese reading instruction provided by teachers in kindergartens relies heavily on rote memorization, and children are required to learn Chinese characters and words as holistic units (Cheung & Ng, 2003). Without explicit morphological instruction, it is likely that poor readers will not be able to develop the morphological awareness that would allow them to demonstrate the morphological processing of compound words exhibited by their normal peers.

We aimed to improve the poor readers' morphological processing skills by explicitly and systematically introducing free morphemes and words formed by these free morphemes. In the intervention program conducted for this study, poor readers were encouraged to decode the meanings of compound words formed by the free morphemes by using the meanings of constituent free morphemes. Poor readers were also encouraged to compose real or novel compound words by combining free morphemes and to define the meanings of the newly combined compound words. Such instruction should help poor readers to establish more well-formed semantic representations of the free morphemes introduced, which should further enhance their ability to make use of free morphemes in decoding word meanings. Consequently, their reading strategies should improve. Boundedness and transparency effects should be significant in their processing of compound words after treatment (Lau, 2012; Lau et al., 2011). Finally, if better morphological processing skills help facilitate reading development, improved reading performances among the poor readers should also be observed after treatment.

To summarize, the main questions addressed here are

1. Can the morphological awareness of poor readers be enhanced through the explicit introduction of free morphemes and compound words formed by free morphemes?
2. Will enhancing the morphological awareness among poor readers consequently improve their reading ability?

METHOD

Participants

Some 20 children with reading difficulties were recruited from two mainstream schools in Hong Kong. Half of these children were allocated to the treatment group (mean age = 7.54 years, S.D. = 0.36) and the other half to the control group[2] (mean age = 7.55 years, S.D. = 0.49). Both groups were studying at the grade-2 level, and all of the children were reported by their teachers to have been diagnosed by educational psychologists with specific learning difficulties using the Hong Kong Test of Specific Learning Difficulties in Reading and Writing (Ho, Chan, Tsang, & Lee, 2000). They were assessed to have normal nonverbal intelligence (> 25 percentile in the Raven's Standard Progressive Matrices [RSPM] [Raven, 1986]) but below average Chinese reading ability (< -1.5 S.D. in the Hong Kong Graded

Character Naming Test [HKGCNT]; Leung, Lai, & Kwan, 2008). All of the children were known by the teachers to have lived and studied in Hong Kong since birth and to use Cantonese as their native language. They were all recruited in the same school area located in suburban Hong Kong, such that the social economic status of their families and parents' educational levels were relatively low across all subjects. The results of the nonverbal intelligence test and the reading tests of each group are given in Table 11.1.

Table 11.1. Age and Performance in the Nonverbal Intelligence Test and Reading Tests of the Two Groups of Participants

	Treatment Group (n = 10)		*Control Group (n = 10)*	
	Mean	*SD*	*Mean*	*SD*
Age	7.54 yrs	0.36	7.55 yrs	0.49
RSPM (standard score)	100.6	8.98	99.9	11.75
HKGCNT (raw score) (max = 150)	44.8	15.6	48.4	14.6
HKGCNT (z-score)	–2.15	0.63	–1.99	0.59

Treatment

A total of 12 group treatment sessions of 1.5 hours duration were conducted on a weekly basis by a speech therapist. At the beginning of each session, the phonological forms, orthographic forms, and meanings of 10 target free morphemes and 10 subordinate compound words formed by the target morphemes were explicitly introduced. For example, in the same session, the target morphemes 馬 /ma5/ [horse] and 車 /ce1/ [car] and the subordinate compound word 馬車 /ma5 ce1/ [carriage] were all introduced explicitly, one by one, along with the pictures representing the meanings of the corresponding words.

After the introduction section, children were engaged in language games. In different games, children were encouraged to (a) name the target morphemes and target words printed on word cards, (b) define the meanings of the target words using the meanings of the constituent morphemes, and (c) construct new/novel words using the target morphemes and define the new words' meanings, for example, the novel word 黑車 /hak1 ce1/ was constructed by one of the subjects in one session by joining the target morphemes 黑 /hak1/ [black] and 車 /ce1/ [car]. He further made use of the meanings of the constituent morphemes to define the novel word 黑車 as a "black car."

Pre- and Posttreatment Measurements

The morphological processing skills and reading abilities of both groups were measured before and after treatment.

Morphological Processing Skills

Three tests were designed to assess the participants' morphological processing skills, measured as the boundedness and semantic transparency effects, in naming the compound words and characters. Two of the tests measured the boundedness effects in naming compound words and characters, respectively, and one measured the semantic transparency effect in naming compound words.

Boundedness

One set of 18 two-character compound words that consist exclusively of free morphemes (FF words), for example, 培育 /pui4 juk6/ [nurture] and 勉勵 /min5 lai6/ [encourage], was selected. Another set of 18 two-character compound words consisting exclusively of bound morphemes (BB words), for example, 採摘 /coi2 zaak6/ [pluck] and 破爛 /po3 laan6/ [shabby], was also selected. The two sets of compound words were matched for word and constituent character frequencies. In the word-naming test, children were required to name the randomly ordered 36 compound words one by one. Naming accuracies were recorded. In the character-naming test, each child was required to name the randomly ordered 72 constituent characters one by one. Again, naming accuracies were recorded.

Semantic Transparency

One set of 24 semantically transparent two-character compound words (trans-words), for example, 商店 /soeng1 dim3/ [shop] and 疾病 /zat6 beng6/ [illness], was selected. Another set of 24 semantically opaque two-character compound words (opaq-words), for example, 拔河 /bat6 ho4/ [tug-of-war] and 和尚 /wo4 soeng2/ [monk], was also selected. The two sets of words were matched for word and constituent character frequencies, and the procedure for this task was similar to that used in the boundedness compound word naming tests.

Reading Abilities

Finally, the reading ability of the children was measured using the HKGCNT. During the test, each child was required to name 150 Chinese characters one by one. The total and the norm-referenced z-scores of each child before and after the treatment were collected.

Data Analysis

For each of the three morphological processing skills tests, a 2 (morphological conditions) X 2 (time) repeated measure ANOVA was calculated for each group of subjects. For the reading abilities test, a 2 (group) X 2 (time) repeated measure ANOVA was calculated.

RESULTS

Morphological Processing Skills

Boundedness—Character Naming

The pre- and posttreatment performances of both groups in the naming of FF and BB words are summarized in Table 11.2. The results of the repeated measures ANOVA calculated for the control group data showed that the main effects of Time and Boundedness, in addition to interaction effects, were all nonsignificant ($p > .1$). However, the results of the repeated measure ANOVA calculated for the treatment group data showed that Time had a significant main effect [$F(1, 9) = 30.819$, $p < .001$, $h_p^2 = .774$] and Boundedness had a marginally significant main effect [$F(1, 9) = 5.094$, $\eta = .05$, $h_p^2 = .361$]. The interaction effect was also significant [$F(1, 9) = 5.176$, $p < .05$, $h_p^2 = .365$]. A post-hoc analysis using Tukey's HSD test showed that the performance in naming free morphemes in the posttreatment condition was significantly higher than in the other three conditions ($p < .05$).

Table 11.2. Treatment and Control Groups' Pre- and Posttreatment Performances in Naming Bound and Free Morphemes

	Treatment Group				*Control Group*			
	Bound Morphemes		*Free Morphemes*		*Bound Morphemes*		*Free Morphemes*	
	Mean	*SD*	*Mean*	*SD*	*Mean*	*SD*	*Mean*	*SD*
Pretreatment (max =36)	3.8	1.9	4.7	2.8	4.0	1.6	4.5	2.2
Posttreatment (max =36)	8.3	4.7	13.9	6.8	4.6	1.9	4.8	2.5

Boundedness—Compound Word Naming

The pre- and posttreatment performances of both groups in the naming of free and bound morphemes are summarized in Table 3. The results of the repeated measure ANOVA calculated for the control data showed that the main effects of Time and Boundedness, along with the interaction effects, were all nonsignificant ($p > .05$). However, the results of the ANOVA calculated for the treatment group data showed a significant main effect for Time [$F(1, 9) = 22.29, p < .001, \eta_p^2 = .735$] and Boundedness [$F(1, 9) = 17.79, p < .01, \eta_p^2 = .663$]. The interaction effect was also significant [$F(1, 9) = 7.62, p < .05, \eta_p^2 = .393$]. The post-hoc analysis using Tukey's HSD test showed that the treatment group exhibited improvements in naming both BB and FF words across time ($p < .05$). Moreover, they also demonstrated better performance in naming FF words than in naming BB words in the posttreatment assessment ($p < .05$).

Table 11.3. Treatment and Control Groups' Pre- and Posttreatment Performances in Naming BB and FF Words

	Treatment Group				*Control Group*			
	BB Words		*FF Words*		*BB Words*		*FF Words*	
	Mean	*SD*	*Mean*	*SD*	*Mean*	*SD*	*Mean*	*SD*
Pretreatment (max =18)	5.1	3.4	7.5	3.0	5.0	3.5	7.2	2.9
Posttreatment (max =18)	8.9	5.0	13.0	5.4	6.5	3.9	7.6	3.4

Semantic Transparency

The pre- and posttreatment performances of both groups in the naming of trans- and opaq-words are summarized in Table 11.4. The results of the repeated measure ANOVA calculated for the control data showed that the main effect of Time was significant [$F(1, 9) = 15.00, p < .01, \eta_p^2 = .621$]. However, the main effect of Semantic Transparency and the interaction effect were both nonsignificant ($p > .05$). The results showed that the control group demonstrated general improvement in naming both trans- and opaq-words across time. However, the results of the repeated measures ANOVA calculated for the treatment group data showed a significant main effect for Time [$F(1, 9) = 15.42, p < .01, \eta_p^2 = .631$] and

Semantic Transparency, [$F(1, 9) = 19.31, p < .01, \eta_p^2 = .682$]. The interaction effect was marginally significant [$F(1, 9) = 5.04, p = .05, \eta_p^2 = .359$]. The post-hoc analysis using Tukey's HSD test showed that the treatment group demonstrated general improvement in both trans- and opaq-words across time ($p < .05$). More importantly, they demonstrated significantly better performance in naming trans-words compared to opaq-words ($p < .05$) in the posttreatment assessment.

Table 11.4. Treatment and Control Groups' Pre- and Posttreatment Performances in Naming Trans- and Opaq-Words

	Treatment Group				*Control Group*			
	Opaq-Words		*Trans-Words*		*Opaq-Words*		*Trans-Words*	
	Mean	*SD*	*Mean*	*SD*	*Mean*	*SD*	*Mean*	*SD*
Pretreatment (max =24)	8.6	3.8	11.2	5.0	8.5	3.5	10.2	4.5
Posttreatment (max =24)	14.8	5.4	20.1	6.3	9.4	3.7	11.4	4.4

Reading Ability

The pre- and posttreatment performances of both groups in the HKGCNT are summarized in Table 5. The results of the repeated measures ANOVA showed that while the main effect of Time was significant [$F(1, 9) = 35.91, p < .001, \eta_p^2 = .785$], that of Group and the interaction effects were both nonsignificant ($p > .1$). This suggests that both the treatment and control groups demonstrated similar improvements in reading ability across time.

Table 11.5. Treatment and Control Groups' Pre- and Posttreatment HKGCNT Raw Scores

	Treatment Group		*Control Group*	
	Mean	*SD*	*Mean*	*SD*
Pretreatment (max =150)	44.8	15.6	48.4	14.6
Posttreatment (max =150)	61.8	19.8	61.5	20.2

DISCUSSION

Overall, our results show that the treatment group exhibited improved morphological processing skills after treatment. Specifically, the treatment group demonstrated better performances in naming free morphemes than bound morphemes after treatment. In addition, the treatment group performed better in naming FF words than BB words after treatment. These improvements were probably due to the treatment because they were not observed in the control group.

The treatment group's better performances in naming free morphemes than bound morphemes can be attributed to the more concrete semantic representations of the free morphemes in the lexicon (Pastizzo & Feldman, 2004; Taft, 2003). The treatment group's better performance in naming FF words than BB words after treatment further supports this notion. It appears that the more concrete semantic representations of the constituent free morphemes in the lexicon facilitated the participants' recognition of the FF words.

A similar improvement was observed in the treatment group's performance in the semantic transparency test. However, it is likely that this improvement was not exclusively a result of the provided treatment because the control group also demonstrated improvements in naming both trans- and opaq-words across time. It is possible that the improvement observed in the treatment group was due to both maturation and the provided treatment.

As the treatment successfully improved the semantic representations of free morphemes in the treatment group's lexicons, we initially expected that the treatment group would also demonstrate significantly greater semantic transparency effects than the control group posttreatment. Nevertheless, this was not the case. One possible reason is that the trans-words used consisted of both free and bound morphemes. Because the treatment predominantly focused on the introduction and manipulation of free morphemes, it is reasonable to assume that the treatment only improved the semantic representations of free morphemes in the treatment group's lexicon. The semantic representations of bound morphemes remained abstract. Therefore, as the trans-words used consisted of both free and bound morphemes, it is possible that the improved semantic representations of free morphemes only facilitated some of the treatment groups' performance in naming trans-words, which was not enough to significantly demonstrate greater semantic transparency effects compared with the control group.

Finally, our results show that both groups demonstrated a similar degree of improvement in reading ability across time. This suggests that the improvement in the treatment group's reading ability was probably due to maturation instead of the provided treatment. In other words, although the treatment successfully improved some of the treatment group's morphological processing skills, the reading performances of the treatment group did not consequently improve.

Relationship Between Morphological Awareness and Reading Development

One of the major aims of the current study was to examine the direction of causality between morphological awareness and reading development. Contrary to the results reported in previous studies (Chow et al., 2008; Packard, 2006; Wu, 2009), we did not find sufficient evidence to support the notion that improved morphological awareness results in improved reading ability. Although we successfully improved some of the morphological processing skills in the treatment group, the improvement did not significantly improve reading ability.

Although we did not find sufficient evidence to support the causal role of morphological awareness in reading development, the results of this study should not be considered counterevidence against the notion. Previous studies have suggested that a number of cognitive skills, such as phonological processing skills, orthographic knowledge, verbal language, and rapid processing, are related to reading development (Bishop & Snowling, 2004; Ho, Chan, Lee, Tsang, & Luan, 2004; Nagy, Berninger, Abbott, Vaughan, & Vermeulen, 2003). It is possible that the treatment group in our study was not only deficient in morphological processing skills, but also in other cognitive skills related to reading development. If this is true, improving their morphological processing skills without improving other cognitive skills might not successfully lead to improved reading performance. One major limitation of this study is that we did not obtain the overall cognitive profiles of the participants. As a result, we cannot be sure whether our participants were also deficient in other cognitive skills. It is suggested that participants' complete cognitive profiles should be obtained in future studies. Those with multiple deficits could then be excluded from the treatment and control groups so that testing the relations between morphological awareness and reading development would be possible.

Another explanation for the failure to improve the treatment group's reading ability is that we did not successfully enhance the treatment group's performance in the semantic transparency test. As discussed, the improvement that the treatment group exhibited in the semantic transparency test posttreatment could be due to both maturation and the provided treatment. Furthermore, because the treatment successfully improved the treatment group's semantic representations only of free morphemes but not the bound morphemes in their lexicons, it is possible that the treatment group's improvement in morphological processing skills was not large enough to result in a significant improvement in reading ability. It is recommended that future studies involve more treatment sessions and focus on the consolidations of semantic representations of both free and bound morphemes. With improvements in both free and bound morphemes, the treatment group would be expected to demonstrate a greater improvement in reading ability.

Pedagogical Implications

The results of this study imply the importance of intervention. The successful improvement of children's morphological processing skills suggests that it is possible to improve poor readers' cognitive deficits and thus alter their reading strategies through the explicit introduction of free morphemes and compound words formed by free morphemes. As described, future training in morphological processing skills should focus more on the consolidation of semantic representations of both free and bound morphemes. Children are expected to adopt the new analytic reading strategies to help them to decode compound words.

Given that the treatment and control groups differed in morphological processing skills but not in reading abilities in the posttreatment measurements, it is unclear whether treatment intended to improve morphological processing skills should be recommended to poor readers. Nevertheless, it still suggests that poor readers would benefit from training in morphological processing skills. As described, one possible explanation of why the treatment group failed to outperform the control group in the posttreatment measurements of reading ability is that they might have deficits in other cognitive skills related to reading development apart from morphological processing skills (Ho et al., 2004). Because training in morphological skills will not improve poor readers' other cognitive deficits, it is unreasonable to expect that the treatment group would exhibit dramatic improvement in overall reading ability. This, however, does not necessarily mean that training poor readers to improve their morphological skills is a useless endeavor. Morphological training is necessary. If it is true that poor readers have multiple cognitive deficits (Ho et al., 2004), training in other cognitive skills would likewise not improve their morphological processing skills. Therefore, it is suggested that interventions for children with poor reading ability focus on their cognitive deficits. It appears that training in every individual cognitive deficit will be necessary, because training just one skill does not seem to improve any others. Future intervention studies are necessary to support this suggestion.

Limitations of the Current Study

The limitation of not obtaining complete cognitive profiles of the subjects was discussed above. Another major limitation of the current study concerns the small sample size. Given that there were only 10 children each in the treatment and control groups, it is highly likely that the results obtained were affected. Although we successfully recruited 20 poor readers with similar backgrounds, the fact that they had to be randomly assigned to two groups considerably reduced the possible effect size that could be obtained. It is suggested that in future studies, a larger number of students should be recruited to avoid this issue. Another solution is to explore the possibility of using other research designs such as obtaining multiple baselines in a single group of poor readers instead of using the group comparison design.

CONCLUSION

To conclude, we demonstrated that it is possible to improve poor readers' morphological processing skills by introducing free morphemes and teaching morphological parsing skills. Although improved morphological processing skills did not significantly improve the poor readers' reading ability, we hypothesize that the involvement of other deficient cognitive skills among poor readers hinders their improvement in reading ability. The insignificant improvements in the treatment group's ability to decode semantically transparent words may also suggest that their morphological processing skills did not improve sufficiently, given that their semantic representations of the bound morphemes remained abstract, to result in significant improvement in reading ability. Further studies are needed to confirm the hypotheses.

NOTES

1. There are two exceptions. First, when one character corresponds to two or more morphemes that correspond to different syllables. For example, the character 少 is pronounced as /siu3/ when it refers to the meaning of [young] and is pronounced as /siu2/ when it refers to the meaning of [little in quantity]. Second, binding words and loan words, which consist of two or more characters but correspond exclusively to single morphemes. A binding word consists of two characters in which the individual characters carry no morphemic status but must combine with one another to create a single morpheme, and the two characters can only occur in that one word (Taft, Liu, & Zhu, 1999). An example of a binding word is 忐忑 /taan2 tik1/

[uneasy], in which the single characters 忐 and 忑 do not carry any meanings in isolation and do not occur in other words other than the meaningful word 忐忑. Loan words are words "copied from another language in which the individual characters have been chosen purely so that the sound of the resulting Chinese word will approximate its pronunciation in the original language" (Taft et al., 1999). An example of a loan word is 巴士 /baa1 si2/ [bus], which approximates the pronunciation of the word "bus" in English.

2. The same treatment program used in this study was applied to the control group children 3 months after the posttreatment data collection.

REFERENCES

Bishop, D. V. M., & Snowling, M. J. (2004). Developmental dyslexia and specific language impairment: Same or different? *Psychological Bulletin, 130*(6), 858–886.

Chen, X., Hao, M., Geva, E., Zhu, J., & Shu, H. (2009). The role of compound awareness in Chinese children's vocabulary acquisition and character reading. *Reading and Writing, 22*, 615–631.

Cheung, H., & Ng, L. (2003). Chinese reading development in some major Chinese societies: An introduction. In C. McBride-Chang & H.-C. Chen (Eds.), *Reading development in Chinese children* (pp. 3–17). Westport, CT: Praeger.

Chow, B. W. Y., McBride-Chang, C., Cheung, H., & Chow, C. S. L. (2008). Dialogic reading and morphology training in Chinese children: Effects on language and literacy. *Developmental Psychology, 44*(1), 233–244.

Ho, C. S.-H., Chan, D. W.-O., Lee, S.-H., Tsang, S.-M., & Luan, V. H. (2004). Cognitive profiling and preliminary subtyping in Chinese developmental dyslexia. *Cognition, 91*, 43–75.

Ho, C. S.-H., Chan, D. W.-O., Tsang, S.-M., & Lee, S.-H. (2000). *The Hong Kong Test of Specific Learning Difficulties in Reading and Writing*. Hong Kong, China: Hong Kong Specific Learning Difficulties Research Team.

Hoosain, R. (1992). Psychological reality of the word in chinese. In H. Chen & O. J. L. Tzeng (Eds.), *Language processing in chinese* (pp. 111–130). Amsterdam: North-Holland.

Ku, Y.-M., & Anderson, R. C. (2003). Development of morphological awareness in Chinese and English. *Reading and Writing: An Interdisciplinary Journal, 16*, 399–422.

Kuo, L.-J., & Anderson, R. C. (2006). Morphological awareness and learning to read: A cross-language perspective. *Educational Psychologist, 41*(3), 161–180.

Lau, D. K. Y. (2012). Compound word processing: Development and disorder (Unpublished PhD thesis). University of Hong Kong, Hong Kong.

Lau, D. K. Y., Leung, M.-T., Cheung, H., Lui, M., & Tse, A. W.-C. (2011). The development of morphemic processing in reading Chinese compound words. *Asia-Pacific Journal of Speech, Language and Hearing, 14*(1), 13–22.

Leung, M.-T., Lai, A., & Kwan, E. S. M. (2008). *The Hong Kong Graded Character Naming Test*. Hong Kong, China: Centre of Communication Disorders.

Leung, M.-T., & Lee, A. (2002). *The Hong Kong corpus of primary school Chinese*. Paper presented at the ninth meeting of the International Clinical Phonetics and Linguistics Association.

Li, W., Anderson, R. C., Nagy, W., & Zhang, H. (2002). Facets on metalinguistic awareness that contribute to Chinese literacy. In W. Li, J. S. Gaffney, & J. L. Packard (Eds.), *Chinese children's reading acquisition: Theoretical and pedagogical issues* (pp. 87–106). Boston, MA: Kluwer.

Liu, P. D., & McBride-Chang, C. (2010). Morphological processing of Chinese compounds from a grammatical view. *Applied Psycholinguistics, 31,* 605–617.

McBride-Chang, C., Shu, H., Zhou, A., Wat, C. P., & Wagner, R. K. (2003). Morphological awareness uniquely predicts young children's Chinese character recognition. *Journal of Educational Psychology, 95*(4), 743–751.

Nagy, W., Berninger, V. W., Abbott, R. D., Vaughan, K., & Vermeulen, K. (2003). Relationship of morphology and other language skills to literacy skills in at-risk second-grade readers and at-risk fourth-grade writers. *Journal of Educational Psychology, 95*(4), 730–742.

Packard, J. L., Chen, X., Li, W., Wu, X., Gaffney, J. S., Li, H., & Anderson, R. C. (2006). Explicit instruction in orthographic structure and word morphology helps Chinese children learn to write characters. *Reading and Writing, 19,* 457–487.

Pastizzo, M. J., & Feldman, L. B. (2004). Morphological processing: A comparison between free and bound stem facilitation. *Brain and Language, 90*(1), 31–39.

Raven, J. C. (1986). *Hong Kong supplement to guide to the standard progressive matrices.* Hong Kong, China: HKSAR Government, Education Department.

Taft, M. (2003). Morphological representation as a correlation between form and meaning. In E. Assink & D. Santa (Eds.), *Reading complex words* (pp. 113–137). New York, NY: Kluwer Academic/Plenum.

Taft, M., Liu, Y., & Zhu, X. (1999). Morphemic processing in reading chinese. In J. Wang, A. Inhoff & H. Chen (Eds.), *Reading chinese scripts: A cognitive analysis* (pp. 91–114). Hillsdale, NJ: Lawrence Erlbaum Associates.

Tong, X., & McBride-Chang, C. (2010). Longitudinal predictors of very early Chinese literacy acquisition. *Journal of Research in Reading, 33,* 1–18.

Wang, M., Cheng, C., & Chen, S.-W. (2006). Contribution of morphological awareness to Chinese-English biliteracy acquisition. *Journal of Educational Psychology, 98*(3), 542–553.

Wu, X., Anderson, R. C., Li, W., Wu, X., Li, H., Zhang, J., ... Gaffney, J. S. (2009). Morphological awareness and Chinese children's literacy development: An intervention study. *Scientific Studies of Reading, 13*(1), 26–52.

Ziegler, J. C., & Goswami, U. (2005). Reading acquisition, developmental dyslexia, and skilled reading across languages: A psycholinguistic grain size theory. *Psychological Bulletin, 131*(1), 3–29.

ABOUT THE EDITORS/AUTHORS

ABOUT THE EDITORS

Kevin K. H. Chung is the head and professor in the Department of Special Education and Counselling of the Hong Kong Institute of Education. He was the Associate Dean (Research) 07/2008–08/2010, the Faculty of Education Studies, Coordinator, KRA: Learning and Assessment. Prior to joining the Institute, he was assistant professor and program director of MED and PCAES (special and inclusive education) at the University of Hong Kong. He was also a high school teacher in Sydney for more than 4 years before embarking on an academic career. He completed his undergraduate and postgraduate studies at the University of New South Wales in Sydney. He has won research grants from General Research Fund, Quality Education Fund, and Hong Kong Jockey Club Charities Trust. His research interests are developmental dyslexia and learning disabilities, literacy acquisition, assessment and instruction, cognitive development, and cognitive neuroscience of language. E-mail: kevin@ied.edu.hk

Kevin C. P. Yuen is assistant professor and associate head at the Department of Special Education and Counselling at the Hong Kong Institute of Education. Dr. Yuen is a qualified audiologist and a speech-language therapist. He received his undergraduate degree in speech and hearing sciences and master's degree in audiology from the Faculty of Education,

The University of Hong Kong. He received his doctor of philosophy degree from the Faculty of Medicine, the Chinese University of Hong Kong. Dr. Yuen has a strong research interest in sound perception and speech recognition of normal hearing and hearing-impaired children in both quiet and noise environments. He investigated the contribution of frequency-specific temporal envelope and periodicity components (without any fine structure components) for lexical tone recognition in normal hearing and hearing-impaired listeners. Dr. Yuen has developed the Cantonese Lexical Neighborhood Test, the Computerized Cantonese Disyllabic-Word Lexical Tone Identification Test in Noise, and the Computerized Mandarin Pediatric Lexical Tone & Disyllabic-Word Picture Identification Test in Noise to serve the Cantonese- and Mandarin-speaking populations in Hong Kong and Mainland China. One of his key future research areas is to identify and remediate young individuals in the Chinese communities with Auditory Processing Disorder (APD) and to investigate the impact of APD on speech and language development, learning, and academic performance. E-mail: cpyuen@ied.edu.hk

Dennis McInerney is Chair Professor of Educational Psychology at the Hong Kong Institute of Education having served for a period of time as Associate Vice-President (Research and Development). Prior to this he was Research Professor and Associate Dean (Education Research) at the National Institute of Education, Nanyang Technological University, Singapore having also served as Vice-Dean (Research and Methodology) within the Centre for Research in Pedagogy and Practice. Previous to this Professor McInerney was Research Professor and Associate Director of the Self Research Centre at the University of Western Sydney. Professor McInerney has published over 300 research articles in refereed journals and book chapters, edits two international research monographs and has written a number of textbooks including *Educational Psychology: Constructing Learning* (Pearson 6th Edition, 2014) which is a bestselling educational psychology text in Australia; *Developmental Psychology for Teachers* (Allen & Unwin, 2006); *Helping Kids Achieve Their Best: Understanding and Using Motivation in the Classroom* (Information Age Publishing, 2005), and *Publishing Your Psychology Research* (Sage and Allen & Unwin, 2001). Professor McInerney's major areas of research interest are cross-cultural studies of learning and motivation, self-processes and adaptive psychological determinants of school behavior (such as self-regulation, self-concept, metacognition, learning styles etc), and instrument design and validation. E-mail: dennismm@ied.edu.hk

ABOUT THE AUTHORS

Piers Dawes is a research fellow with the Audiology and Deafness Research Group in the School of Psychological Sciences at the University of Manchester, UK. His background is in experimental psychology and speech and language therapy. He is interested in the cognitive aspects of hearing, and his research interests include hearing loss, auditory processing, and developmental psychology from childhood to old age, hearing genetics, auditory plasticity, and developmental disorders. E-mail: piers.dawes@manchester.ac.uk

Kenneth Hugdahl is professor of biological psychology at the Department of Biological and medical psychology, University of Bergen, Norway since 1984, and adj. professor at the Division of Psychiatry, Haukeland University Hospital, Bergen, Norway since 2006. He is also the head of the Bergen fMRI Group since 1994. Previous to this he was at the University of Uppsala in Sweden and has been guest professor at the Neuropsychiatric Institute, UCLA, 1991. He has published extensively in the areas of hemispheric asymmetry, auditory and speech perception, and dyslexia, in particular, the sue of dichotic listening procedures, and including three edited volumes on hemispheric asymmetry and brain laterality, published by MIT Press between 1995 and 2010. Kenneth Hugdahl has been chief editor of the *Scandinavian Journal of Psychology*, and associate editor and on the editorial board for numerous journals, including *Laterality, Brain and Cognition, Psychophysiology, Child Neuropsychology*, and *Frontiers in Human Neuroscience*. E-mail: Hugdahl@psybp.uib.no

Silvia Siu-Yin Lam is currently studying in an Mphil program in psychology at the Chinese University of Hong Kong. Her central research interest is about language and literacy development, both in normal and atypical development. She is interested in studying the relationship between motor skills and children's literacy abilities. E-mail: sylam@psy.cuhk.edu.hk

Dr. Dustin Lau has worked as a speech therapist and clinical instructor in a variety of settings that equipped him with frontline experience working with clients with different communication disorders. His research interests lie mainly in clinical psycholinguistics and neurolinguistics. While most of his work has focused on reading development in Chinese developmental dyslexia in Chinese, and its assessment and treatment, he is also interested in conducting research on language development and disorders. E-mail: Dustin.lau@polyu.edu.hk

Lay Wah Lee is currently associate professor at the School of Educational Studies, Universiti Sains Malaysia. Previous to this, she was the chairperson of the special education program. She is the curriculum developer of both the BEd (Special Education) and the forthcoming MEd (special education) program. Her research is primarily focused on dyslexia, learning disabilities, special educational technology, and visual impairment. She has published quite extensively in journal papers, book chapters, and produced a number of teaching and learning products, including award-winning open educational web portals for special education, notably *ePKhas* and *eKodBraille*. E-mail: lwah@usm.my

Man Tak Leung is associate professor of the Department of Chinese and Bilingual Studies, Faculty of Humanities, Hong Kong Polytechnic University. He received his speech pathologist qualification from Lincoln Institute of Health Sciences, Australia, and his PhD degree from the University of Hong Kong. Dr. Leung specializes in research and teaching on language processing, acquired language disorders, and children reading development. He has developed several treatment approaches for dyslexic students and has gained substantial experience in conducting school-based treatment in Hong Kong. He has published articles, books, and book chapters on corpus linguistics, reading and its relationship with cognitive, psychological and linguistic development, standardized assessment, and treatment for dyslexia. E-mail: mantak.leung@polyu.edu.hk

Duo Liu is now assistant professor in the Department of Special Education and Counseling of the Hong Kong Institute of Education. He got his PhD from the Department of Psychology of the Chinese University of Hong Kong. His current research interests focus on cognitive development, especially on language and literacy development and difficulties, and metalinguistic processing and developmental models. E-mail: duoliu@ied.edu.hk

Jenny H. Y. Loo is currently the principal audiologist at the Center for Hearing Intervention and Language Development, Department of Otolaryngology, Head & Neck Surgery, National University Hospital in Singapore. She also holds a joint appointment at the National University of Singapore as a senior lecturer for the postgraduate audiology program. Jenny has many years of clinical experience working with hearing impaired children and adults, as well as in assessing children with auditory processing disorder. Her research interest mainly focused on the assessment and management of auditory processing disorder, where she has published a few peer-reviewed papers in this area. Her most recent work involves research on the hearing and auditory processing of elderly with dementia. E-mail: Jenny_LOO@nuhs.edu.sg

Catherine McBride-Chang is professor in developmental psychology at the Chinese University of Hong Kong. Her main research interests are in the development and impairment of reading across languages and cultures. She wrote a book in 2004 on this topic, entitled *Children's Literacy Development*. Catherine McBride-Chang currently serves as an editor for two journals and one encyclopedia. She is the incoming president of the Society for the Scientific Studies of Reading. E-mail: cmcbride@psy.cuhk.edu.hk

Carol Miller is associate professor of communication sciences and disorders and linguistics at Penn State University and a member of Penn State's Center for Language Science. She was previously a research associate at Purdue University. Carol's research focuses on typical and atypical language development, with an emphasis on specific language impairment (SLI). She studies people with SLI from preschool to adulthood. An overall theme of her work is trying to understand how cognitive and perceptual abilities interact with language in development. Her research on auditory processing in SLI has been funded by the National Institutes of Health. Carol has served as an associate editor for language for the *Journal of Speech, Language, and Hearing Research*. E-mail: cam47@psu.edu

Jianhong Mo is currently working on her PhD under the supervision of Professor McBride at the Chinese University of Hong Kong, Hong Kong. Jianhong has a strong interest in children's reading and writing difficulties. Her research is primarily focused on the area of cognitive correlates of reading and writing disorders. She participated in a project (supported by the Innovation Funds of the National Ministry of Science and Technology, China) focused on designing a computer-based version of a cognitive assessment system (CAS) for learning disabled children as a master's student. She has co-written book chapters in the area of Chinese dyslexia and Chinese-English bilingual transfer, as well as a conference paper in the area handwriting and writing composition. E-mail: lanny.mjh@gmail.com

David Moore is professor of otolaryngology and associate director of the Communication Sciences Research Center at Cincinnati Children's Hospital, Cincinnati, Ohio. Educated (PhD, Monash University) in Australia, he spent 22 years at Oxford University on projects including auditory spatial hearing, biology of deafness, and the consequences of otitis media. He became professor of auditory neuroscience in 2000. As Director of the Medical Research Council Institute of Hearing Research, Nottingham (2002–2012), he focussed on auditory development and learning in humans. In 2008, he also co-founded the National Biomedical Research Unit in Hearing (NBRUH), re-funded in 2011. He has been a visiting scientist at the University of California, Irvine; the University of Washington, Seattle; New York University; and Northwestern University, Chicago. He was the founder of MindWeavers PLC, creating digital learning experiences based on world-leading brain science. In 2010, he was awarded the George Davey Howells prize for editing the *Oxford Handbook of Auditory Science*. E-mail: david.r.moore@cchmc.org

Frank R. Vellutino holds the rank of distinguished professor at the University at Albany, the State University of New York. He currently holds joint appointments in the Department of Psychology (Cognitive Psychology Program) and the Department of Educational and Counseling Psychology. He is also the director of the University's Child Research and Study Center, a research and student training center. Dr. Vellutino currently teaches graduate courses in knowledge acquisition, which emphasize cognitive, perceptual, memory, and language development. Most of his research has been concerned with reading development, the cognitive underpinnings of reading, and the relationship between reading difficulties and various aspects of language and other cognitive abilities. His research has generated numerous articles in refereed journals, in addition to a seminal book summarizing work in the study of dyslexia (*Dyslexia: Theory and Research*, MIT Press, 1982) and numerous book chapters addressing the causes and correlates of developmental reading difficulties. E-mail: fvellutino@albany.edu

Ying Wang is currently working on her PhD under the supervision of Professor McBride in the Chinese University of Hong Kong. Ying has a strong interest in early literacy development and education. Her research is primarily focused on correlates of Chinese children's early reading and writing skills, with particular interest in early literacy interventions for young children. She has published some papers in the core periodicals of Chinese psychology and written some conference papers. E-mail: yingwang@psy.cuhk.edu.hk

Simpson W. L. Wong is assistant professor in the Department of Psychological Studies, the Hong Kong Institute of Education. He received his doctorate in experimental psychology at the University of Oxford. Besides his recent interest in behavioral genetics, Wong has focused on developmental dyslexia and second-language acquisition. He also has research interests in acoustic phonetics and health psychology. E-mail: wlswong@gmail.com

Printed and bound by CPI Group (UK) Ltd, Croydon, CR0 4YY
15/09/2026
14962370-0005